AIRWAY MANAGEMENT IN EMERGENCIES

AIRWAY MANAGEMENT IN EMERGENCIES

GEORGE KOVACS, MD

Professor
Department of Emergency Medicine
Dalhousie University
Nova Scotia, Halifax, Canada

and

J. ADAM LAW, MD

Professor
Departments of Anesthesiology and Surgery
Dalhousie University
Nova Scotia, Halifax, Canada

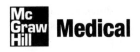

New York   Chicago   San Francisco   Lisbon   London   Madrid   Mexico City
Milan   New Delhi   San Juan   Seoul   Singapore   Sydney   Toronto

The McGraw·Hill Companies

Airway Management in Emergencies

1234567890   DOC/DOC   0987

ISBN: 978-0-07-147005-6
MHID: 0-07-147005-0

This book was set in Garamond Light by International Typesetting and
Composition.
The editors were Anne Sydor and Karen G. Edmonson.
The production supervisor was Catherine H. Saggese.
The cover designer was Mary McKeon.
The indexer was Susan Hunter.
RR Donnelley was printer and binder.

This book is printed on acid-free paper.

Library of Congress Cataloging-in-Publication Data
Kovacs, George, MD.
    Emergency airway management / George Kovacs, J. Adam Law.
        p. ; cm.
    ISBN 978-0-07-147005-6
    1. Respiratory emergencies.   2. Respiratory intensive care.
3. Airway (Medicine)   4. Respiratory organs—Obstructions.   I. Law,
J. Adam.   II. Title. [DNLM: 1. Airway Obstruction—therapy.
2. Emergencies.   3. Intubation, Intratracheal—methods.
WF 145 K88e   2008]
RC735.R48K68   2008
616.2′00425—dc22

                                                    2007015952

From GK. To my partner in life, Sandra Kovacs, and my four children, Hannah, Maya, Ben, and Aaron: thank you for your love, tolerance, and support.

From JAL. For Trevor, Simon, and Julia—may your love of life and learning always be with you—and my wife Kate, for her support and loyalty. Thanks must also go to my parents, for laying the foundation, and to fellow AIME contributors and instructors, for making a difference.

Contents

Editors and Lead Authors

GEORGE KOVACS, MD, MHPE, FRCPC
Professor, Department of Emergency Medicine
Dalhousie University
Halifax, Nova Scotia, Canada

J. ADAM LAW, MD, FRCPC
Professor, Departments of Anesthesiology and Surgery
Dalhousie University
Halifax, Nova Scotia, Canada

Contributing Authors

GRAHAM BULLOCK, MD, FRCPC
Associate Professor, Department of Emergency Medicine
Dalhousie University
Halifax, Nova Scotia, Canada

SAM CAMPBELL, MB BCH, CCFP(EM)
Associate Professor, Department of Emergency Medicine
Dalhousie University
Halifax, Nova Scotia, Canada

T.J. COONAN, MD, FRCPC
Professor, Departments of Anesthesiology and Surgery
Dalhousie University
Halifax, NS Canada

PAT CROSKERRY, PHD, MD, CCFP(EM)
Professor, Department of Emergency Medicine
Dalhousie University
Halifax, Nova Scotia, Canada

KIRK MACQUARRIE, MD, FRCPC
Assistant Professor, Departments of Anesthesiology
    and Surgery
Dalhousie University
Halifax, Nova Scotia, Canada

WILLIAM A MCCAULEY, MD, MHPE, FRCPC
Associate Professor, Division of Emergency Medicine
University of Western Ontario
London, Ontario, Canada

DAVID A PETRIE, MD, FRCPC
Associate Professor, Department of Emergency Medicine
Dalhousie University
Director, Division of Emergency Medical Services
Halifax, Nova Scotia, Canada

JOHN A ROSS, MD, FRCPC
Professor, Departments of Emergency Medicine and
    Anesthesiology
Head, Department of Emergency Medicine
Dalhousie University
Chief, Department of Emergency Medicine, Queen
    Elizabeth II Health Sciences Centre
Halifax, Nova Scotia, Canada

CHRISTIAN M. SODER, MD, FRCPC
Associate Professor, Departments of Anesthesiology
    and Pediatrics
Dalhousie University
Chief, Department of Pediatric Critical Care, IWK Health
    Centre
Halifax, Nova Scotia, Canada

JOHN M TALLON, MD, FRCPC
Associate Professor, Departments of Emergency Medicine
    and Surgery
Dalhousie University
Medical Director, Nova Scotia Trauma Program and
    Queen Elizabeth II Health Sciences Centre Trauma
    Program
Halifax, Nova Scotia, Canada

Illustrations

TIM FEDAK, BSc, PhD
Halifax, Nova Scotia, Canada

JIRI J. DUBEC, MD, CCFP (EM)
Surrey, British Columbia, Canada

JANET DAVISON, BFA
Chamonix, France

Photography

JOSEPH O'LEARY
Halifax, Nova Scotia, Canada

Foreword

George Kovacs and Adam Law have created a text that covers the physiology, anatomy, techniques, and devices of emergency airway management in a readable, concise, and practical manner. The well thought out outlines, interesting clinical cases, and recommended approaches have evolved from real world practice. This teaching method is clearly a result of the authors' extensive clinical expertise, but also comes from their vast experience running training courses and supervising physicians in training. The rare combination of both an emergency medicine and anesthesia perspective is also apparent. The imaging and line art assembled within these pages comes from years of academic focus and a real passion for the topic. I especially appreciate the juxtaposition of beautifully prepared drawings with fluoroscopy images and direct laryngoscopy imaging. Overall, this text is a great addition to the educational resources available to emergency airway providers.

Richard M. Levitan, MD

Preface

Acute-care clinicians are well aware of the alphabetical "ABC" (airway, breathing, circulation) directive of resuscitation. This term has been widely disseminated through programs such as Advanced Trauma Life Support (ATLS) and Advanced Cardiac Life Support (ACLS). In fact, both courses have contributed significantly to improving awareness of resuscitation priorities required in managing patients rendered critically ill from trauma or cardiac events. Indeed, many hospital administrators require active certification in these programs (and others) for clinicians working in environments such as the emergency department (ED). However, from a real-world perspective, it is the "A" of the ABCs that often poses the greatest challenge, or produces significant anxiety in the clinician.

As a relatively new specialty, Emergency Medicine has appropriately taken on responsibility for airway management in the ED. The first described use of pharmacologic aids, including neuromuscular blockers, to facilitate intubation outside the operating room precipitated turf battles, out of concerns for safety. However, the need for nonanesthesiologists to gain expertise in acute airway management could not be disputed for long. Over time, appeased by observed good clinical practice, and supported by the literature, the opposition has appropriately waned.

Clearly the term "acute-care clinician" is not defined by emergency medicine alone. Be it a general practitioner in a small community hospital, a general surgeon, internist, intensivist, paramedic, nurse, physician assistant, or respiratory therapist, the airway belongs to the most skilled clinician available at the bedside when time and urgency mandate immediate action. Declaring "ownership" of the airway should not be based on departmental borders, but rather, on whether the clinician has the required knowledge and skills to safely manage the patient.

It has become apparent that the "A" needs to come out of the "ABCs" to stand alone as an educational focus. The perceived deficit in clinician confidence in acute airway management has led to the development of several focused educational programs to address these needs. This text is based in part on the manual used in one such program (AIME—Airway Interventions and Management in Emergencies). In delivering this course and similar educational content to thousands of clinicians over the years, the lead authors of this text have gained significant insight into the issues surrounding improving airway management knowledge and skills.

A team of emergency physicians and anesthesiologists has written this text. The goal is to support the educational needs of all medical and allied health clinicians involved in the care of acutely ill patients requiring airway management in an emergency setting.

George Kovacs, MD
J. Adam Law, MD

Acknowledgments

This book has roots as the informal manual to accompany a one-day airway course (AIME—Airway Interventions and Management in Emergencies) for delivery to Canadian emergency physicians. The Canadian Association of Emergency Physicians (CAEP), and in particular Ms. Vera Klein and Dr. Tim Allen were instrumental in supporting the development of this educational program, for delivery in communities in need. The entire founding course faculty has contributed to this book: all continue to teach the course across Canada and must be acknowledged for their enthusiasm and dedication.

We also wish to thank the Department of Emergency Medicine at Dalhousie University, and in particular Ms. Corrine Burke for administrative assistance. For peer review, we are indebted to Drs. T.J. Coonan, Ian Morris, Michael Murphy, Hugh Devitt, Orlando Hung and Ron Stewart, as well as Mr. Paul Brousseau. Finally, many thanks to Mr. Derek Leblanc, the Atlantic Health Training and Simulation Centre, and Emergency Health Services (EHS) Nova Scotia for the opportunity to test and develop our educational material.—GK and JAL.

CHAPTER 1

Introduction

▶ INTRODUCTION TO AIRWAY MANAGEMENT IN EMERGENCIES

▶ Case 1.1

You are in the emergency department (ED) at 3 a.m. when you get a "heads up" from the nurse that paramedics are 3 minutes out with a 20-year-old posthanging victim. The paramedics were unable to intubate the patient at the scene. On arrival in the ED, the patient, a large (100 kg), bearded male, is immobilized on a backboard and is posturing. He has noisy upper airway sounds and is producing pink, frothy pulmonary edema. His oxygen saturation (SaO_2) is 82% with assisted bag-mask ventilation.

The emergency care of this patient illustrates several layers of complexity in airway management decision making. Acute-care clinicians must consider two often competing issues—prevalence and acuity—in their diagnosis and management of a patient.[1] More simply, they must be prepared to manage "what is common and what can kill." Even in high volume clinical settings, high-acuity scenarios involving airway management and resuscitations make up only a small fraction of presenting cases. However, in spite of the small numbers, clinicians must be

prepared with the cognitive, psychomotor, and affective skills required to competently manage patients such as the one presented above. These core competencies in airway management are summarized in Table 1–1.

Clinical competence is best viewed as a continuum, varying from being considered simply safe, to being an expert. Ideally, clinicians with acute-care responsibilities should strive to attain an expert skill level in airway management. It may not be realistic to expect expertise "out of the gate" from any training program; however, with appropriate learning experiences, clinicians *can* acquire and maintain the knowledge and skills needed to safely manage the vast majority of airway emergencies. A novice making the statement that he has "never intubated the esophagus" may be viewed as skilled by a second novice. However, to the veteran clinician, the statement is simply a sign of inexperience. In other words, if you haven't experienced difficulty, you will remain inexperienced!

Procedural skill competence is dependent on sound decision making, but is also predicated upon practice in an observed setting, with timely feedback.[2] This practice should ideally begin with simulation (e.g., using airway training mannequins) and then move to a controlled setting such as the operating room. How much experience is required to learn and maintain competency in various airway skills? Investigators examining the learning curve for direct

▶ **TABLE 1–1** AIRWAY MANAGEMENT CORE COMPETENCIES

Cognitive	Psychomotor	Affective

• Indications for advanced airway management
• Relevant airway anatomy and physiology
• Predictors of the difficult airway
• Approach to the difficult airway—whether predicted or not
• Indications and contraindications for rapid sequence intubation and awake intubation
• Airway pharmacology
	• Bag mask ventilation (including response to difficulty)
	• Direct laryngoscopy and intubation (including response to difficulty)
	• Alternative intubation techniques
	• Rescue oxygenation techniques, including extraglottic devices and cricothyrotomy
		• Crisis Resource Management skills:
		  • Anticipation and planning
		  • Leadership and communications
		  • Situation awareness
		  • Team dynamics

laryngoscopy and intubation have estimated that up to 50 intubations are required before a predetermined level of proficiency is reached.[3–6] Although a prerequisite minimum number of intubations alone will never guarantee competence or ensure safety, the message that volume matters and practice improves skills cannot be disputed.

Skills transfer from simulation to the live setting is not perfect, and depends in part on the degree of similarity between the two settings.[7,8] Although the airway equipment used in both simulation and "live" airway management is identical, the physical tissue interface used in most simulators is still relatively immature compared to the human patient. Imperfect as the simulation setting may be, it does provide the opportunity to attain the psychomotor skills needed for many tools and techniques. In addition, instructors can manipulate the clinical context to provide the learner with an opportunity to address various cognitive and human factors issues related to airway management.

Prior to this patient's arrival (and during the resuscitation) it is likely that the clinician will have to acknowledge and deal with immediate psychological (affective) issues. The ability to effectively manage the patient *in extremis* requires more

than cognitive and psychomotor skill.[9] Excitement, fear, and/or anxiety are all very real "gut" emotions that even experienced clinicians will feel on hearing the heads-up about this patient. Professional athletes and actors acknowledge a certain performance-enhancing effect associated with the stress of high-stakes events in their respective areas of expertise. Unprepared, however, in times of extreme stress or near disaster, it has been said that 10% of individuals will naturally lead, 10% will be incapacitated, and the remainder will neither lead nor flounder, but *are* able to follow.[10] Successful resuscitative airway management requires effective anticipation, communication, and leadership skills in a team setting.

The major challenge in teaching and learning airway management for emergencies is to create an integrated cognitive, psychomotor, and affective network that promotes easy retrieval and a rapid appropriate response to change. Medical administrators, educators, and learners all seem to have a natural affinity for line diagrams and algorithms. Rare is the medical text that does not include such figures, and this book is no exception (e.g., Fig. 11–3, and Fig. 12–1). These algorithms support the three major questions that must be addressed to manage the airway, reinforced by experience, knowledge, and skill:

A. Is the procedure indicated?
B. What is the safest and most efficacious way to proceed when difficulty is anticipated (see Fig. 11–3)?
C. How will you respond to difficulty once encountered (see Fig. 12–1)?

Efforts to simplify airway management decision making have become somewhat clouded in recent years by attempts to produce the "Holy Grail" of airway tools. Such tools are often marketed as requiring minimal skills and possessing the potential to render the term "difficult airway" obsolete. To this exploding equipment industry can be added a growing body of literature on managing the difficult airway. Is this devotion appropriate, or overkill? In actual fact, we have not arrived at the point where airway management decisions are black and white, or our tools foolproof. Claims that standard skills such as direct laryngoscopy are soon to become procedures of the past are likely premature. In addition, this direction carries a significant risk of compromising the acquisition and maintenance of competence in needed core skills.

Successful airway management of the previously described case should not be defined simply by the correct placement of an endotracheal tube. At the end of the day, success must be measured by positive patient outcomes. To improve these outcomes, the clinician must work at enhancing the knowledge and skills needed for successful airway management in emergencies.

REFERENCES

1. Kovacs G, Croskerry P. Clinical decision making: an emergency medicine perspective. *Acad Emerg Med.* 1999;6(9):947–952.
2. Kovacs G, Bullock G, Ackroyd-Stolarz S, et al. A randomized controlled trial on the effect of educational interventions in promoting airway management skill maintenance. *Ann Emerg Med.* 2000;36(4):301.
3. Charuluxananan S, Kyokong O, Somboonviboon W, et al. Learning manual skills in spinal anesthesia and orotracheal intubation: is there any recommended number of cases for anesthesia residency training program? *J Med Assoc Thai.* 2001;84 Suppl 1:S251–S5.
4. de Oliveira Filho GR. The construction of learning curves for basic skills in anesthetic procedures: an application for the cumulative sum method. *Anesth Analg.* 2002;95(2):411–416.
5. Konrad C, Schupfer G, Wietlisbach M, et al. Learning manual skills in anesthesiology: Is there a recommended number of cases for anesthetic procedures? *Anesth Analg.* 1998;86(3):635–639.
6. Mulcaster JT, Mills J, Hung OR, et al. Laryngoscopic intubation: learning and performance. *Anesthesiology.* 2003;98(1):23–27.
7. Issenberg SB, McGaghie WC, Hart IR, et al. Simulation technology for health care professional skills training and assessment. *JAMA.* 1999;282(9):861–866.
8. Hall RE, Plant JR, Bands CJ, et al. Human patient simulation is effective for teaching paramedic students endotracheal intubation. *Acad Emerg Med.* 2005;12(9):850–855.
9. Schull MJ, Ferris LE, Tu JV, et al. Problems for clinical judgement: 3. Thinking clearly in an emergency. *CMAJ.* 2001;164(8):1170–1175.
10. Leach J. Why people 'freeze' in an emergency: temporal and cognitive constraints on survival responses. *Aviat Space Environ Med.* 2004;75(6):539–542.

CHAPTER 2

Definitive Airway Management: When Is It Time?

▶ KEY POINTS

- The basic goals of airway management are oxygenation and ventilation. Initially, this may require simple airway opening maneuvers and bag-mask ventilation (BMV) support.
- The indications for intubation are to (a) **obtain and maintain** the airway, (b) **correct** abnormalities of gas exchange (c) **protect** the airway, and (d) secure the airway early in the face of **predicted clinical deterioration**.

▶ INTRODUCTION

Successful airway management requires competent decision-making and good procedural skills. The decision of whether a patient requires definitive airway management must be made early in the clinical assessment. In the spontaneously breathing patient, there is often a significant delay in making this decision. This chapter reviews the presentation of patients requiring basic airway support, as well as the indications for endotracheal intubation.

▶ CASE PRESENTATIONS

Consider the following patient presentations:

▶ Case 2.1

A 20-year-old male with a fracture/dislocation of his ankle has had it reduced under "procedural sedation". Some time later, the spouse of the patient in the adjoining bay comes to get help. She reports that the 20-year old is blue and does not appear to be breathing. *The blood pressure (BP) is 170/90, heart rate (HR) is 100, respiratory rate (RR) 4, and the oxygen saturation (SaO$_2$) is 65% on room air.*

▶ Case 2.2

A 45-year-old female presents to the emergency department (ED). Shortly before, while at home, she had complained of a sudden-onset severe headache, then collapsed. She was transported by ambulance. On arrival, she is receiving oxygen, but is unresponsive and has snoring respirations. *The BP is 180/100, HR 55, RR 25, SaO$_2$ 92% with nonrebreathing face mask (NRFM), and the Glasgow Coma Scale (GCS) is 7.*

▶ **Case 2.3**

A 35-year-old female, 8 months pregnant, was involved in a motor vehicle collision (MVC). At the scene she was complaining of right-sided chest discomfort and pain in what appeared to be a broken right arm. She was transported by ambulance to the ED "backboarded and collared." She is now unconscious, and has snoring respirations. *Only her systolic BP is obtainable at 50/, HR 140, RR 35; SaO$_2$ is unobtainable on a 40% simple facemask, and her GCS is 7.*

▶ **Case 2.4**

A 55-year-old male was in a house fire. Although his burns seemed limited, 6 hours after the injury he started complaining of shortness of breath, and subsequently developed stridor on inspiration. *His BP is 160/90, HR 90, RR 30, SaO2 92% with NRFM, and his GCS is 15.*

▶ **Case 2.5**

A 35-year-old female, well known in the intensive care unit, has been receiving maximal medical therapy for an acute exacerbation of asthma. She remains "tight" and is moving very little air. Although her SaO$_2$ is 91% with oxygen, she is visibly tired and getting drowsy. *Her BP is 170/100, HR 120, RR 30, SaO$_2$ 91% with NRFM, and her GCS is 14.*

The patients described in the above cases all require urgent airway management. The ultimate goal of resuscitation efforts and airway management is gas exchange, with oxygen delivery the priority. Although many clinicians view endotracheal intubation as the definitive intervention of airway management, other maneuvers, often perceived as basic, are all potentially life saving. Recognition of the obstructed airway, airway opening maneuvers, the administration of high flow oxygen, and bag-mask ventilation (BMV) are all crucial airway management skills. In most cases it would be inappropriate to proceed with intubation before any of these basic life support (BLS) interventions had first been attempted.

Despite the importance of BLS maneuvers as initial steps in correcting or maintaining oxygenation, many patients will go on to require endotracheal intubation. A cuffed endotracheal tube (ETT) placed below the cords provides both airway protection and an efficient means of providing gas exchange. Although extraglottic devices such as the Laryngeal Mask Airway (LMA) or Esophageal-Tracheal Combitube (ETC) are also very effective at providing gas exchange, placement of an ETT remains a gold standard for airway management in emergencies.

▶ **INDICATIONS FOR ENDOTRACHEAL INTUBATION**

There are four broad categories of indication for endotracheal intubation in emergencies:

A. To **obtain and maintain** a patent airway (e.g., in the face of an obstructed airway from any cause).
B. To **correct** deficient gas exchange (i.e., hypoxia and/or hypercarbia).
C. To **protect** the airway (e.g., against aspiration of gastric contents or blood).
D. To preempt **predicted clinical deterioration** (to one of the above three situations).

Obtain and Maintain

Airway obstruction can occur from functional, pathologic, or mechanical causes. Functional obstruction can occur in the patient with a depressed level of consciousness, as loss of muscular tone results in posterior relaxation of the soft palate, tongue, and epiglottis toward the posterior pharyngeal wall. Functional obstruction will most often be alleviated by BLS maneuvers such as head tilt or chin lift (unless contraindicated by C-spine precautions in the trauma patient), or, more effectively, a **jaw thrust**. If respiratory effort is still present, adequate gas exchange can then resume, although intubation may still be indicated to **maintain** ongoing airway patency. In the apneic patient, initial BLS maneuvers are still indicated to assess and establish airway patency, but positive pressure ventilation with BMV will be the next step to reoxygenate the patient. Here again, unless the cause of the apnea can be rapidly corrected, intubation will be indicated to maintain a patent airway.

Pathologic airway obstruction may result from an intrinsic process such as edema, hematoma, infection, or tumor, while mechanical obstruction can occur from extrinsic processes such as excessive application of cricoid pressure or foreign body. Pathologic airway obstruction is rarely quickly corrected and often requires intubation to obtain and maintain a patent airway while the underlying cause of obstruction is addressed.

Regardless of the nature of obstruction, it is crucial that the signs and symptoms of obstruction (discussed in more detail in Chap. 4) be recognized early and addressed promptly to safely secure the airway.

Correction of Gas Exchange

Cellular metabolism and function depends on the delivery and uptake of oxygen. Oxygen delivery in turn depends on adequate lung function, sufficient hemoglobin levels, and an effective cardiac output. In return, carbon dioxide (CO_2) produced as a byproduct of cellular metabolism must be delivered to the lungs for removal by ventilation.

Respiratory failure is a clinical term describing inadequate pulmonary gas exchange. Inadequate oxygenation (hypoxemia) can be quantified through the measurement of arterial blood gases (ABGs) or estimated noninvasively using pulse oximetry. Early clinical effects of hypoxemia are not always readily apparent. Cyanosis is a late clinical sign of hypoxemia and may be absent in profoundly anemic patients or in those with dark skin. Ventilation refers to the mechanics of effective gas exchange, and is commonly quantified using arterial P_{CO_2}. An acutely elevated P_{CO_2} is often clinically apparent as CO_2 narcosis with a diminished level of consciousness, frequently combined with an inadequate respiratory effort.

Despite the fact that respiratory failure can be determined by ABGs (i.e., P_{O_2} less than 60 mm Hg/P_{CO_2} greater than 60 mm Hg), **the decision to intervene with airway and ventilatory support should be a clinical one, and in most situations, precede ABG testing.**

Although failure of oxygenation and ventilation usually occur together, this is not always the case. Critically ill asthmatics may be able to maintain an SaO_2 above 90% with supplemental oxygen, but still require ventilatory support as they fatigue. Furthermore, a patient in circulatory shock may have no ventilatory abnormalities but may still require intubation to optimize oxygen delivery.

Included in this category is the need for "pulmonary toilet," that is, the suctioning of secretions from the lower airway of patients who cannot adequately cough.

Protection

The awake patient with intact airway reflexes is able to respond to secretions or other material threatening the airway by swallowing and/or coughing. Although the gag reflex is commonly assessed as a measure of airway protection, its utility has been questioned following findings that up to a third of the general population has an attenuated or absent gag reflex.[1,2] Furthermore, testing for the gag reflex can itself be hazardous, with the risk of provoking vomiting.

As with any reflex, intact and coordinated sensory and motor pathways must exist through a central connection.[3] Protective airway reflexes become diminished as the patient's level of consciousness decreases. Rigid suction should always be available during airway interventions and the clinician should be prepared to rapidly suction and safely reposition the patient.

The patient's ability to swallow and cough may be thought of as confirming intact protective reflexes. However, the effectiveness of these reflexes in managing significant vomitus or blood in a patient with a depressed level of consciousness is always uncertain. The presence of pooled secretions or fluid in the posterior pharynx is strongly suggestive of impaired airway protective reflexes, as is the ability to tolerate an oropharyngeal airway.

The Glasgow Coma Scale (GCS) is often used as a gross marker of a patient's ability to protect the airway.[4] The Advanced Trauma Life Support (ATLS) program recommends that patients with a GCS below 8 should be intubated, unless a rapid improvement in level of consciousness occurs or is anticipated.[5] Unfortunately, clinical application of the GCS is fraught with difficulties as a prospective decision tool.[6–8] Rather than rigidly using a certain GCS cutoff, the patient's clinical ability to handle secretions should be assessed in conjunction with level of consciousness (as measured by GCS or otherwise).

▶ Predicted Clinical Deterioration

The foregoing discussion refers to assessing the patient's immediate need for intubation. However, the clinician should always be thinking of the patient's expected clinical course. This includes consideration of the patient's presenting condition, potential for deterioration, and other factors such as the need to facilitate emergent investigations (e.g., computed tomography [CT] scan) or transportation to another institution. In this population, intubation may be desirable in anticipation of the patient's risk of deteriorating, which would require intubation in a less favorable environment (where adequately trained personnel or appropriate equipment may be lacking), or at a time when intubating may be significantly more difficult, for example, due to progressive airway edema.

It must be appreciated that active airway interventions such as intubation are not without complications. Intubation for the indications of obtaining and maintaining a patent airway and correction of gas exchange may be mandated urgently as part of the "ABCs" (airway, breathing, circulation) of resuscitation. On the other hand, intubation for the sole indication of airway protection or predicted clinical deterioration is somewhat different, especially in a patient who is currently maintaining a patent airway with adequate gas exchange. In this latter situation, risk/benefit analysis may point to deferring the procedure until better conditions and expert personnel are available.

▶ CASE REVIEW

The five cases presented earlier will be reviewed here, with reference to the four categories of indication for intubation discussed above.

▶ Case 2.1

A 20-year-old male with a fracture/dislocation of his ankle has had it reduced under "procedural sedation". Some time later, the spouse of the patient in the adjoining bay comes to get help. She reports that the 20-year old is blue and doesn't appear to be breathing. *The blood pressure (BP) is 170/90, heart rate (HR) is 100, respiratory rate (RR) 4, and the oxygen saturation (SaO$_2$) is 65% on room air.*

With the relief of pain following reduction of his fracture, the patient became bradypneic, as he had lost much of the stimulus that was competing with the respiratory depressive effect of the sedative/analgesic combination. Visible cyanosis is a late sign of oxygen desaturation. The patient should be briefly assessed for airway patency and respiratory effort. His airway should be opened with head tilt/chin lift/jaw thrust, and if spontaneous respirations do not resume, positive pressure BMV with oxygen should be rapidly instituted. Naloxone administration (with or without the benzodiazepine antagonist Flumazenil) will probably result in a rapid return of spontaneous respirations and consciousness, and intubation will most likely not be needed. Other clinical states which may be reversible before intubation is required, include the following:

- Ventricular arrhythmias—may respond to defibrillation.
- Hypoglycemia—may respond to glucose.
- Anaphylaxis—may respond to epinephrine.

Concomitant basic airway management may well still be indicated in these scenarios, and depending on the response to treatment, intubation may also be required.

► Case 2.2

A 45-year-old female presents to the emergency department (ED). Shortly before, while at home, she had complained of a sudden-onset severe headache, then collapsed. She was transported by ambulance. On arrival, she is receiving oxygen, but is unresponsive and has snoring respirations. *The BP is 180/100, HR 55, RR 25, SaO$_2$ 92% with non-rebreathing face mask (NRFM), and the Glasgow Coma Scale (GCS) is 7.*

In assessing the ABCs in this patient, snoring is likely to be indicative of functional airway obstruction, due to the patient's obtunded state. Other signs of functional obstruction may be present, such as supra- and intercostal indrawing, and a "rocking" pattern of respiration, whereby the chest falls and the abdomen rises with attempted inspiration. The airway should be opened with head tilt/jaw thrust. An oral airway can be inserted. If the airway is now patent, oxygen by nonrebreathing face mask should be administered. The patient will require intubation for a number of reasons: airway maintenance, airway protection, and predicted clinical course. The condition of this patient is too tenuous for her to be sent to the diagnostic imaging department without having an airway secured by intubation.

► Case 2.3

A 35-year-old female, 8 months pregnant, was involved in a motor vehicle collision (MVC). At the scene she was complaining of right-sided chest discomfort and pain in what appeared to be a broken right arm. She was transported by ambulance to the ED "backboarded and collared." She is now unconscious, and has snoring respirations. *Only her systolic BP is obtainable at 50/, HR 140, RR 35; SaO$_2$ is unobtainable on a 40% simple facemask, and her GCS is 7.*

This patient also has an airway which is functionally obstructed at initial presentation. As a trauma victim with a depressed level of consciousness, C-spine precautions are in effect. However, the front of the cervical collar should be removed and replaced with manual in-line stabilization. A jaw thrust may be performed to open the airway, but head tilt and chin lift should be omitted. 100% oxygen should be administered. Concomitantly, the patient must be removed from the supine position, as a supine hypotension syndrome due to the gravid uterus causing aorto-caval compression may be causing or contributing to the hypotension. A wedge should be placed under the right side of the spine board. Fluid resuscitation should be initiated, and vital signs reevaluated. In this case, relief of caval compression helped restore preload, and BP rapidly reached 100/70. The patient regained consciousness, and now maintaining her own airway, did not acutely require intubation.

▶ Case 2.4

A 55-year-old male was in a house fire. Although his burns seemed limited, 6 hours after the injury he started complaining of shortness of breath, and subsequently developed stridor on inspiration. *His BP is 160/90, HR 90, RR 30, SaO$_2$ 92% with NRFM, and his GCS is 15.*

The patient with an inhalational thermal injury can develop progressive airway edema which may eventually threaten airway patency. Critical narrowing at the laryngeal inlet is often heralded by inspiratory stridor. Stridor should generally be regarded as a sign of impending complete airway obstruction. Intubation is indicated in this patient to obtain and maintain a patent airway and for predicted clinical deterioration. While making preparations for intubation, elevation of the head of the bed and the administration of a helium-oxygen mixture (if immediately available) may help temporize the situation.[9]

The patient described in Case 2.5 is maintaining her airway at present, and requires no basic airway intervention other than oxygen administration. However, intubation is indicated for impaired gas exchange (her Pco$_2$ is steadily climbing), and predicted clinical deterioration. The patient has received maximal medical

▶ Case 2.5

A 35-year-old female, well known in the intensive care unit, has been receiving maximal medical therapy for an acute exacerbation of asthma. She remains "tight" and is moving very little air. Although her SaO$_2$ is 91% with oxygen, she is visibly tiring and getting drowsy. *Her BP is 170/100, HR 120, RR 30, SaO$_2$ 91% with NRFM, and her GCS is 14.*

---

therapy and her condition will worsen as she tires. Hypoxia will ensue and as her CO$_2$ narcosis progresses, she may also be unable to protect her airway.

▶ SUMMARY

In the foregoing cases, some patients required immediate attention with basic airway opening maneuvers and only temporary airway support, while others went on to require intubation. Either way, an initial assessment of airway patency and effectiveness of gas exchange should always be made. **Noninvasive maneuvers to maintain oxygenation and ventilation should be undertaken as needed, while a determination is made about the subsequent need for intubation.** Intubation may be needed to obtain and maintain an airway, correct gas exchange, protect the airway, or for an anticipated adverse predicted clinical course.

REFERENCES

1. Bleach NR. The gag reflex and aspiration: a retrospective analysis of 120 patients assessed by videofluoroscopy. *Clin Otolaryngol Allied Sci.* 1993;18(4):303–307.
2. Davies AE, Kidd D, Stone SP, et al. Pharyngeal sensation and gag reflex in healthy subjects. *Lancet.* 25, 1995;345(8948):487–488.
3. Altschuler SM. Laryngeal and respiratory protective reflexes. *Am J Med.* 3, 2001;111 (Suppl 8A):90S–94S.

4. Mackay LE, Morgan AS, Bernstein BA. Swallowing disorders in severe brain injury: risk factors affecting return to oral intake. *Arch Phys Med Rehabil.* 1999;80(4):365–371.

5. *Advanced Trauma Life Support for Doctors.* American College of Surgeons; 2004; No. 46.

6. Gill M, Windemuth R, Steele R, et al. A comparison of the Glasgow Coma Scale score to simplified alternative scores for the prediction of traumatic brain injury outcomes. *Ann Emerg Med.* 2005;45(1): 37–42.

7. Gill MR, Reiley DG, Green SM. Interrater reliability of Glasgow Coma Scale scores in the emergency department. *Ann Emerg Med.* 2004;43(2):215–223.

8. Al-Salamah MA, McDowell I, Stiell IG, et al. Initial emergency department trauma scores from the OPALS study: the case for the motor score in blunt trauma. *Acad Emerg Med.* 2004;11(8):834–842.

9. Ho AM, Dion PW, Karmakar MK, et al. Use of heliox in critical upper airway obstruction. Physical and physiologic considerations in choosing the optimal helium:oxygen mix. *Resuscitation.* 2002;52(3): 297–300.

CHAPTER 3

Airway Physiology and Anatomy

▶ KEY POINTS

- Oxygen delivery depends on having an adequate pump (cardiac output), carrier (hemoglobin), and oxygen saturation.
- Time to desaturation is extended by meticulous attention to preoxygenation, and shortened by factors that adversely affect oxygen storage (the functional residual capacity, FRC) and consumption (VO_2).
- Pulse oximetry may be inaccurate in low-flow clinical conditions.
- The epiglottis is an important landmark in airway management, and should be a source of reassurance, not anxiety.
- Attempts to lift the tongue prematurely during direct laryngoscopy, before the hyoepiglottic ligament is engaged at the base of the vallecula, will often result in an inadequate view of the glottic inlet.
- The maximal outer diameter of a tube or cannula placed through the cricothyroid membrane should be no greater than 8.5 mm.
- The Cormack-Lehane (C-L) classification and percentage of glottic opening (POGO) score both provide a means of describing glottic visualization. A modified version of the C-L classification may help the clinician decide how best to proceed with endotracheal intubation.

- When managing a child's airway, it is important to appreciate that there are more anatomical and physiologic similarities to adults than differences. The Broselow tape can significantly assist the practitioner in assembling equipment for the critically ill child.

▶ AIRWAY PHYSIOLOGY: INTRODUCTION

Hypoxia is a common terminal event in the critically ill patient. Human cells require oxygen for vital metabolic processes. Although cells in some organs can survive without oxygen for short periods of time via less efficient anaerobic metabolism, cells in vital organs such as heart and brain function only by aerobic metabolism. As oxygen stores are limited in the human body, these organs require a continual supply of oxygen molecules to function and survive: death follows quickly in the absence of oxygen delivery.

▶ THE OXYGEN ECONOMY

As in most economies, cells operate on a supply and demand system. The currency is oxygen. Cellular survival depends on an appropriate match between oxygen delivery (DO_2) and consumption (VO_2).

Alveolar Ventilation

Oxygen in the atmosphere* moves along a pressure gradient, through the respiratory tract and alveoli, via arterial blood and capillaries to tissues and cells. In the alveoli, the partial pressure of oxygen (PAO_2) drops from 150 mm Hg to around 100 mm Hg, due to the balance of oxygen uptake by the pulmonary capillaries and its supply by ventilation. The partial pressure of deoxygenated blood in the pulmonary capillaries, returned to the lungs via the pulmonary arteries, is about 40 mm Hg. Oxygen thus diffuses from the alveoli to the pulmonary capillaries along a pressure gradient.

In a perfect lung, blood leaving the pulmonary capillaries via the pulmonary veins would be fully oxygenated, that is, with no alveolar/arterial PO_2 difference. In practice, this does not happen because of a number of factors:

- **Ventilation-perfusion mismatch:** Ideally all alveoli would receive an equal share of alveolar ventilation and all pulmonary capillaries would receive an equal share of cardiac output. In reality, some alveoli are relatively overventilated, while some are relatively overperfused.
- **Shunt** occurs when alveoli are perfused but receive no ventilation (an extreme form of ventilation-perfusion [VQ] mismatch). Deoxygenated blood has no chance to become oxygenated and returns to the pulmonary veins still in a deoxygenated state. While physiologic drainage of intrinsic cardiac (thebesian) and bronchial veins

into the pulmonary venous blood will always create a small degree of shunt, other causes include atelectasis, lung consolidation with fluid-filled alveoli, or small airway closure.

- **Diffusion abnormalities:** Generally, diffusion of oxygen from alveolus to capillary along the pressure gradient is complete by the time blood has traveled only one-third of the way along the capillary. Diffusion is generally completed even if cardiac output is increased (e.g., in exercise). Thus, the contribution of any impairment in diffusion to an alveolar/arterial PO_2 difference will be minimal in the absence of significant pulmonary disease.

Oxygen Transport in the Blood

Following its entry by diffusion into blood, oxygen is carried in two ways:

- **In combination with hemoglobin:** Each gram of hemoglobin can chemically combine with a maximum of 1.31 mL of oxygen: this is termed the *oxygen capacity*. Thus, with a blood hemoglobin concentration of 15 g/dL (150 g/L), each liter of blood can carry (150 g/L × 1.31 mL/g) = 197 mL of oxygen. The term *oxygen saturation* (SaO_2) describes the percentage of hemoglobin which is combined with oxygen.
- **Dissolved in plasma and intracellular fluid:** At atmospheric pressure, 0.3 mL/dL (or 3 mL/L) of oxygen are carried in physical solution. Although a very small proportion, this amount increases to 20 mL/L by breathing 100% oxygen, and can be raised even further under hyperbaric conditions.

The **arterial oxygen content** thus reflects the hemoglobin concentration, its percent saturation with oxygen, and the amount of dissolved

---

*Air is composed of 21% oxygen, 78% nitrogen, and 1% other gases, at a pressure of 760 mm Hg at sea level. The partial pressure of oxygen when first inspired is therefore (760) (.21) = 159 mm Hg. Inspired air is humidified in the upper airway, and as the total pressure exerted by a mixture of gases is equal to the partial pressure of each of the component gases, the partial pressure of water vapor (47 mm Hg) drops the partial pressure of inspired oxygen, thus: (760–47) (.21) = 150 mm Hg.

oxygen. In a patient with a hemoglobin of 15 g/dL and an SaO_2 of 95%, the arterial oxygen content will be (.95 × 150 g/L × 1.31 mL/g) + 3 mL/L dissolved O_2 = 190 mL/L.

The relationship between the arterial partial pressure of oxygen (PaO_2) and SaO_2 is described by the oxyhemoglobin dissociation curve (Fig. 3–1). The flat upper portion of the curve indicates that with an initial fall in PaO_2, the SaO_2 falls little, and the arterial oxygen content is little changed. However, as the PaO_2 continues to fall below 60 mm Hg, the slope of the curve becomes steeper. While this steeper part of the slope reflects easier offloading of oxygen to the tissues, it also implies that once oxygen desaturation begins, its progression is quick. The linear portion of this curve can be estimated by the 90–60, 60–30 rule of thumb, whereby an SaO_2 of 90% corresponds roughly to a PaO_2 of 60 and an SaO_2 of 60% corresponds to a PaO_2 of 30.

The total quantity of oxygen available to the tissues in one minute is termed **oxygen delivery** (DO_2), and equals the cardiac output × arterial oxygen content. With a typical cardiac output of 5 L/min, DO_2 is 5 L/min × 190 mL/L = approximately 1000 mL O_2/min. In the healthy, resting patient, **VO_2** is 250 mL/min, that is, 25% of available oxygen is consumed. Thus, the hemoglobin in mixed venous blood is 95% − 25% = 70% saturated. This 70% oxygen saturation of venous blood represents an important reserve from which tissues can extract extra oxygen when compensating for decreased DO_2. Below a critical value of DO_2, however, compensation no longer occurs and evidence of tissue hypoxia occurs.

The foregoing discussion on DO_2 is clinically relevant, as it points to areas which can result in inadequate tissue oxygenation (i.e., tissue **hypoxia**):

A. **Low cardiac output** (*stagnant or circulatory hypoxia*). Even with a normal arterial oxygen content, circulatory failure can result

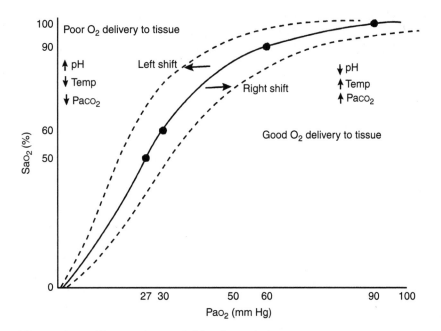

Figure 3–1. The oxyhemoglobin dissociation curve.

in failure of tissue oxygenation, due to lack of delivery of oxygen to the tissues. This can happen globally, or regionally, with inadequate blood flow to a particular organ. Initially, tissues will compensate by increasing oxygen extraction, but as perfusion worsens, this becomes insufficient and tissue hypoxia develops.

B. **Low arterial oxygen saturation** (*hypoxic hypoxia*). This is defined as an inadequate arterial PO_2. This may result from many causes, including decreased inspired partial pressure of oxygen (e.g., at altitude); hypoventilation from central (e.g., due to sedative medications) or peripheral (e.g., functional airway obstruction) causes; or from inadequate alveolar-capillary transfer (e.g., from V-Q mismatch, shunt, or diffusion abnormalities).

C. **Low hemoglobin concentration** (*anemic hypoxia*). With profound anemia, oxygen content will fall in proportion to the hemoglobin concentration, even with a normal PaO_2. A compensatory increase in cardiac output may occur, but if or when this can no longer be sustained, tissue hypoxia occurs. Alternatively, if hemoglobin is rendered incapable of carrying oxygen, for example, by carbon monoxide poisoning, a similar reduction in DO_2 can occur.

D. **Histotoxic hypoxia**. In spite of normal delivery of oxygen to the tissues, cellular metabolic processes utilizing oxygen can be impaired, an example of which is cyanide poisoning.

In the critically ill patient, VO_2 is often increased, a factor over which we have little control in the short term. Thus, in the early phase of resuscitation, attention must be directed to maximizing DO_2, by avoiding oxygen desaturation, *as well as* by maintaining or restoring cardiac output and hemoglobin concentration. If tissue oxygenation demands are not met, anaerobic metabolism occurs, leading to lactic acid production and metabolic acidosis.

This in turn can affect the efficacy of pharmacologic and other therapy.

Oxygen Stores

Oxygen stores in the body are sufficiently limited that life cannot be sustained for more than a few minutes once breathing stops. Oxygen is stored mainly in the blood and lungs, with small amounts bound or dissolved in tissues. Blood stores depend on the blood volume and hemoglobin concentration. Lung stores of oxygen depend on the alveolar PO_2 and the lung volume at end expiration (the **functional residual capacity [FRC]**, about 35 cc/kg or 2.5 L). This volume of 2.5 L contains a reservoir of 2500 mL x .21 (the FiO_2) = 500 mL of oxygen. With threatened hypoxemia, only part of the oxygen stored in the blood (mainly bound to hemoglobin), is released before a critical decrease in blood PaO_2 has occurred (Fig. 3–1). The better reservoir for oxygen is the FRC of the lungs, particularly if **preoxygenation** has been undertaken prior to apnea: this can increase the FRC oxygen stores from 500 mL to 2500 mL (the FRC of 2500 mL x 1.0 [the FiO_2]), 80% of which can be used before the PaO_2 falls below normal. Preoxygenation of a patient using 100% oxygen, applied via a tightly fitting face mask, prolongs the time to desaturation after onset of apnea by many minutes, compared to a patient breathing room air.[1] This is shown in Fig. 3–2, using data derived from healthy elective surgical patients. Shown in the same graph is the markedly shortened apnea time available in the patient with an FRC decreased by obesity. Other conditions that may lessen the effectiveness of preoxygenation by limiting FRC include advanced pregnancy and any process that limits the patient's ability to take a deep breath (e.g., rib fractures, pneumothorax, pulmonary contusion). The critically ill patient has also been shown to benefit less from preoxygenation,[2] as fever, trauma, and other physiological stressors increase metabolic demands and the rate of VO_2.

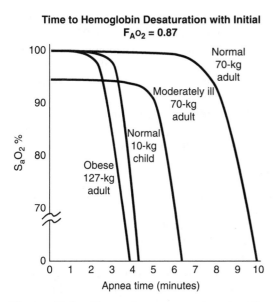

Figure 3–2. Times to oxygen desaturation following onset of apnea in preoxygenated elective surgical patients (From Benumof J,[1] with permission).

▶ MONITORING OXYGENATION

Signs and symptoms of hypoxemia include tachycardia, dysrhythmias, tachypnea, dyspnea, cyanosis, and mental status changes. All are non-specific and of little value in reliably detecting hypoxemia. The clinician should be well-versed in the advantages and limitations of methods available for monitoring the oxygenation status of the critically ill patient.

Cyanosis

Cyanosis is a bluish discoloration of skin and mucus membranes which occurs with oxygen desaturation. The presence of cyanosis should be used as an indication to more objectively monitor and manage who is most likely a hypoxemic patient. Cyanosis will appear at an SaO_2 of 85%–90%, although variation exists. It will be less apparent in the anemic patient, and more readily visible in the polycythemic patient.

The clinician should recognize that other factors may contribute to the appearance of cyanosis. Decreased tissue blood flow can cause so-called peripheral cyanosis, whereby apparent cyanosis occurs even with a normal arterial oxygen content. This can be observed in patients with hypothermia, decreased cardiac output, or in some, simply when placed in the supine or Trendelenburg position. Ambient lighting differences can affect how easily cyanosis is detected, and certain drugs (e.g., benzocaine) can cause the appearance of cyanosis, also with a normal arterial oxygen content.

Arterial Blood Gases

Arterial blood gas monitoring is the gold standard for monitoring blood oxygen tension. Although invasive, it has the advantage of also giving information about carbon dioxide and acid-base status: many contemporary point-of-care blood-gas analyzers can also deliver other blood chemistry results. However, it is important to recognize that even with a normal PaO_2 (and SaO_2), tissue hypoxia can occur from low cardiac-output states, anemia, or failure of the tissues to utilize oxygen. In addition, regional hypoxia in a vital organ (e.g., brain or heart) can cause morbidity or death in a normally oxygenated patient.[3]

Pulse Oximetry

Pulse oximeters noninvasively measure the percentage of hemoglobin that is saturated with oxygen. A transcutaneous probe (usually applied to a digit) emits light at two different wavelengths. One wavelength is absorbed by oxyhemoglobin in the tissues, and one by deoxyhemoglobin. The relative absorption of each wavelength enables the processor to calculate the proportion of hemoglobin which is saturated. The technique is enhanced by signal processing to separate the pulsatile (oxygenated arterial blood) and nonpulsatile (venous capillary) signal. In this way, the pulse oximeter can estimate arterial SaO_2 with a high degree of accuracy. Pulse oximeters measure SaO_2, and not the more familiar PaO_2. A drop in the SaO_2 with the associated warning drop in pulse oximeter tone is familiar to most clinicians.

Pulse oximetry is not always accurate. At oxygen saturations less than 75%, many (especially older) instruments become increasingly inaccurate. In burns and smoke inhalation injury, the presence of carboxyhemoglobin may cause a pulse oximeter to read falsely high because of the similar light absorption spectra of oxyhemoglobin and carboxyhemoglobin. However, the most common problem with oximetry occurs with a reduction in pulsatile signal brought about by peripheral vasoconstriction caused by hypothermia, low cardiac output, or hypovolemia. This may lead to complete loss of oximeter readings. Finally, movement of the probe can confuse microprocessor algorithms, making pulse oximetry difficult in patients with tremors, seizure, or other repetitive movement disorders.

▶ AIRWAY ANATOMY: ITS IMPORTANCE

A clear mental picture or "gestalt" of upper airway anatomy is an essential cognitive underpinning to emergency airway management skills. This knowledge is important for the following reasons:

A. **Making decisions** Assessment of a patient's airway anatomy is the foundation upon which the airway plan is built. Can the patient be ventilated with bag-mask ventilation (BMV)? Can the patient be intubated by direct laryngoscopy? If difficulty is encountered, can rescue oxygenation occur via an extraglottic device or cricothyrotomy? Based on this assessment, the clinician can decide how to proceed: with a rapid-sequence intubation (RSI), an awake intubation, or primary surgical airway.

B. **Structure and function** Knowledge of airway anatomy and its dynamic changes

facilitates the appropriate performance of airway opening skills and BMV. These skills depend on an understanding of functional airway anatomy and how the tissues behave with the patient in either the awake or obtunded state.

C. **Landmark recognition** A sound three-dimensional appreciation of the laryngeal inlet and its surroundings is critical for optimal laryngoscopy. Anatomic structures adjacent to the glottic opening, such as the epiglottis and paired posterior cartilages help provide a "roadmap" to the cords. In addition, anatomic or pathologic variations in airway anatomy must be understood and anticipated.

D. **Spatial orientation** Particularly when using blind or indirect visual intubation techniques, a clear mental image of the anatomy through which the instrument is traveling is required. Problem solving through intubation with a lightwand or intubating laryngeal mask airway is much easier with a solid appreciation of potential anatomical barriers.

▶ FUNCTIONAL AIRWAY ANATOMY

The Upper Airway

The immediate goal of airway management during resuscitation is to obtain a patent upper airway and ensure adequate oxygenation. The upper airway may be defined as the space extending from the nose and mouth down to the cricoid cartilage, while the lower airway refers to the tracheobronchial tree.

The Nasal Cavity

During normal breathing in the awake state, inspired air travels through, and is humidified by, the nasal cavity. The nasal cavity is bounded laterally by a bony framework which includes the three turbinates (conchae) (Fig. 3–3) and medially by the nasal septum. Septal deviation

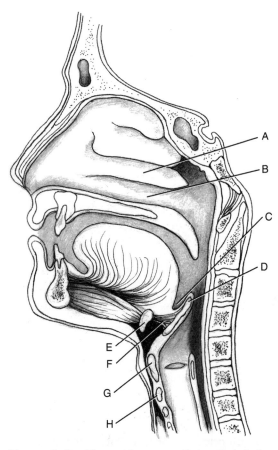

Figure 3–3. Upper airway anatomy: A. Inferior turbinate, B. Major nasal airway, C. Vallecula, D. Epiglottis, E. Hyoid bone, F. Hyoepiglottic ligament, G. Thyroid (laryngeal) cartilage, H. Cricoid cartilage.

occurs commonly, and can impede passage of a nasal endotracheal tube, as can a hypertrophied inferior turbinate. The space between the inferior turbinate and the floor of the nasal cavity, termed the **major nasal airway**,[4] is oriented slightly downward. During an attempted nasal intubation, the tube should therefore be directed straight back and slightly inferiorly. This will help traverse the widest aspect of the nasal airway, beneath the inferior turbinate, while avoiding the thin bone of the more superiorly

located cribriform plate. The nasal cavity is well vascularized, particularly at the anterior inferior aspect of the nasal septum. Many authorities espouse directing an endotracheal tube's bevel toward the septum to minimize the potential for bleeding caused by traumatizing the vascular Kiesselbach plexus. However, published case series suggest that significant bleeding with nasal intubations is less frequent than commonly feared, occurring in under 15% of cases.[5,6]

The Naso- and Oropharynx, and the Mandible

The nasal cavity terminates posteriorly at the level of the end of the nasal septum (the nasal choanae). The space from here to the tip of the soft palate is referred to as the nasopharynx.[4] The oropharynx extends backward from the palatoglossal fold (arching from the lateral aspect of the soft palate to the junction of the anterior two-thirds with the posterior one-third of the tongue[4]), down to the epiglottis. The oro- and nasopharynx are common sites of narrowing or complete airway obstruction in the obtunded patient, as the loss of tone in muscles responsible for maintenance of airway patency allows for posterior movement of soft palate, tongue, and epiglottis. Although classic teaching has been that it is collapse of the tongue against the posterior pharyngeal wall which causes functional airway obstruction in the obtunded patient, in fact, significant airway narrowing or obstruction can occur in one or all of three locations[7–9] (Fig. 3–4 A and B):

- **In the nasopharynx,** as the soft palate meets the posterior pharyngeal wall.
- **In the oropharynx,** as the tongue moves posteriorly to lie against or near the soft palate and posterior pharyngeal wall.
- **In the laryngopharynx,** as the epiglottis moves posteriorly toward the posterior pharyngeal wall.

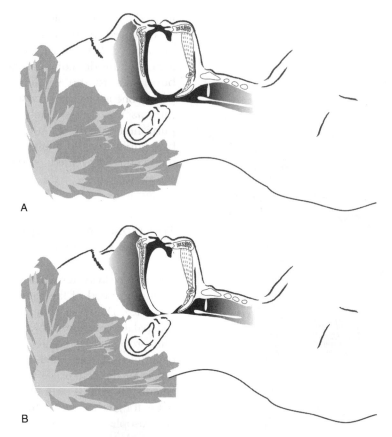

A

B

Figure 3–4 A, B. Sites of airway obstruction in the obtunded patient. A. Patent airway in the awake state. B. In the obtunded state, functional airway obstruction occurs as the soft palate, tongue and epiglottis fall back toward the posterior pharyngeal wall.

The **mandible** figures prominently in alleviating functional airway obstruction. The horseshoe- shaped mandible extends superiorly via two rami to end in the coronoid process and condylar head.[4] The condylar head in turn articulates with the temporal bone at the temporomandibular joint (TMJ), and allows for mouth opening by rotation. In addition, anterior translation of the condyle at the TMJ permits forward movement of the mandible. The latter is crucial for two reasons:

- As the inferior aspect of the tongue is attached to the mandible, anterior translation of the jaw elevates the tongue away from the posterior pharyngeal wall, helping to attain a clear airway in the obtunded patient.

- During laryngoscopy, the laryngoscope blade moves the mandible forward, helping to displace the tongue anteriorly and away from obstructing the line-of-sight view of the laryngeal inlet.

In addition to forward movement of the mandible and tongue, a laryngoscope blade also seeks to compress or displace the tongue into the bony framework of the mandible: this is why individuals with small mandibles (so-called receding chins) can present difficulty with laryngoscopy.

The Laryngopharynx

The laryngopharynx extends from the epiglottis down to the inferior border of the cricoid cartilage. The laryngopharynx can be looked upon as a "tube within a tube," with the circular structure of the larynx located anteriorly within the larger pharyngeal tube. On either side of the larynx, in the pharynx, are the piriform recesses, while the esophagus is located posteriorly (Fig. 3–5). The larynx, which sits at the entrance to the trachea opposite the fourth, fifth, and sixth cervical vertebrae, is a complex box-like structure consisting of multiple articulating cartilages, ligaments, and muscles. The major cartilages involved are the cricoid, thyroid, and epiglottis, together with the smaller paired arytenoid, corniculate, and cuneiform cartilages. Located anteriorly in the midline, the shield-shaped thyroid cartilage is attached by the thyrohyoid membrane to the hyoid bone above, and articulates inferiorly with the cricoid cartilage. The cricoid cartilage is a circular, signet-ring-shaped cartilage which marks the lower border of the laryngeal structure. The hyoid bone and thyroid and cricoid cartilages are all palpable in the anterior neck. The vocal cords attach anteriorly to the inner aspect of the thyroid cartilage, and posteriorly to the arytenoid cartilages, which in turn also articulate with the cricoid cartilage. The cricoid cartilage is significant in airway management for a number of reasons:

A. Because of its rigid nature, application of posterior pressure on the cricoid cartilage can occlude the underlying esophagus, helping to prevent passive regurgitation of gastric contents.

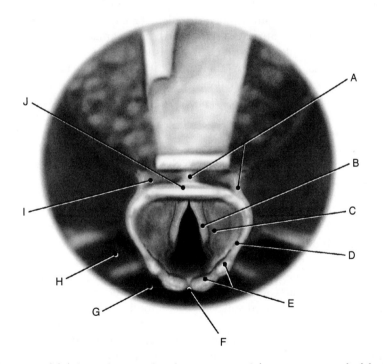

Figure 3–5. Laryngeal inlet anatomy: structures seen at laryngoscopy. A. Median and lateral glossoepiglottic folds, B. Vocal folds (true cords), C. Vestibular folds (false cords), D. Aryepiglottic folds, E. Posterior cartilages, F. Interarytenoid notch, G. Esophagus, H. Piriform recess, I. Vallecula. J. Epiglottis.

B. It is the narrowest point of the airway in the pediatric patient (the glottic opening is narrowest in the adult patient), and can be an area of potential obstruction due to swelling (producing the clinical syndrome pediatricians call croup), or congenital or acquired subglottic stenosis. Such narrowing of the subglottic space may block passage of even a normally sized endotracheal tube (ETT).

C. The cricoid cartilage, together with the thyroid cartilage, is a landmark for locating the cricothyroid membrane, an area of critical importance in performing an emergency surgical airway.

The Laryngeal Inlet

The clinician should be very familiar with the component parts of the laryngeal inlet which are visually presented at laryngoscopy. The paired vocal cords are the "target" for the laryngoscopist, and are identified by their whitish color and triangular orientation. Surrounding the vocal cords, the laryngeal inlet is bordered anteriorly by the epiglottis, laterally by the aryepiglottic folds, and inferiorly by the cuneiform and corniculate tubercles (cartilages), and the interarytenoid notch (Fig. 3–5). The epiglottis projects upward and backward, behind the hyoid bone and base of tongue, and overhangs the laryngeal inlet.[10] The base of the superior surface of the epiglottis is attached to the hyoid bone by the hyoepiglottic ligament (Fig. 3–3), while the inferior surface attaches to the thyroid cartilage via the thyroepiglottic ligament. The overlying mucosa on the upper surface of the epiglottis sweeps forward to join the base of the tongue, with prominences forming the median and paired lateral glossoepiglottic folds. The paired valleys between these folds are called the vallecullae, although both vallecullae are commonly referred to together as the **vallecula** (Fig. 3–3 and 3–5).

To expose the vocal cords, the tip of a curved (e.g., Macintosh) laryngoscope blade can be advanced into the vallecula until it engages the underlying hyoepiglottic ligament. Pressure on this ligament with the blade tip helps evert ("flips up") the epiglottis to achieve a line-of-sight view into the larynx. Attempts to lift the tongue prematurely, before the hyoepiglottic ligament is engaged at the base of the vallecula, will often result in an inadequate view of the glottic inlet. Clinicians preferring straight blade direct laryngoscopy usually elect to place the blade beneath the epiglottis and directly lift it. Either way, the epiglottis is an important landmark in airway management, and should be a source of reassurance, not anxiety. Indeed, it should be actively sought by the laryngoscopist as a guide to the underlying glottic opening.

Originating laterally from each side of the epiglottis toward its base, the aryepiglottic folds form the lateral aspect of the laryngeal inlet by sweeping posteriorly to incorporate the cuneiform and corniculate cartilages. The corniculate cartilages overlie the corresponding arytenoid cartilages, and appear as the characteristic "bumps" (tubercles) posterior to the vocal cords. In practice, many clinicians refer to these prominences as the arytenoids. Confusion can be avoided by referring to these tubercles collectively simply as the posterior cartilages. The underlying arytenoids are anatomic hinges used by laryngeal muscles to open and close the cords. Between and slightly inferior to the paired posterior cartilages lies the interarytenoid notch (Fig. 3–6). With the cords in the abducted position, this notch widens to a ledge of mucosa stretching between the posterior cartilages, but with the cords in a more adducted position, the interarytenoid notch narrows simply to a small vertical line. This notch lies slightly inferior to the posterior cartilages and is important during laryngoscopy because in a restricted view situation, it may be the only landmark identifying the entrance to the glottic opening above.[11]

Posterior to the laryngeal inlet lies the esophagus. It should be noted that the entrance to the upper esophagus is not held open by any rigid

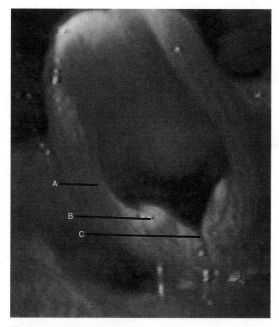

Figure 3–6. Laryngeal inlet anatomy: A. Aryepiglottic fold, B. Posterior cartilages, C. Interarytenoid notch.

structures, and at laryngoscopy is often not seen at all. Conversely, when the esophageal entrance *is* seen, it can look like a dark, (and sometimes inviting) opening. This highlights the importance to the laryngoscopist of knowing the expected landmarks of the laryngeal inlet: the posterior cartilages, aryepiglottic folds and overlying epiglottis flank the glottic opening, and *not* the esophagus!

Airway Axes

In the standard anatomic (military) position, the axis of the oral cavity sits at close to right angles to the axes of the pharynx and trachea. To obtain direct visualization during laryngoscopy, this angle needs to be increased to 180°. The pharyngeal and tracheal axes can be aligned by flexion of the lower cervical spine at the cervicothoracic junction, while alignment

of the oral and pharyngeal/tracheal axes then occurs with extension at the atlantooccipital junction and upper few cervical vertebrae (Fig. 3–7 A, B). Final visualization by line-of-sight is then achieved using the laryngoscope blade to anteriorly lift the mandible and displace the tongue (Fig. 3–8). This alignment of axes by proper positioning before laryngoscopy reduces the need for tongue displacement required during laryngoscopy, which may in turn reduce the amount of force required to expose the cords. Where not contraindicated by C-spine precautions, the airway axes can be aligned before laryngoscopy by placing folded blankets under the extended head to produce the "sniffing position."

The Lower Airway

The trachea extends from the inferior border of the cricoid cartilage to the level of the sixth thoracic vertebra, where it splits into the left and right mainstem bronchus. The trachea is 12 to 15 cm long in the average adult and is composed of C-shaped cartilages joined vertically by fibroelastic tissue and completed posteriorly by the vertical trachealis muscle.[10] The anterior tracheal cartilaginous rings are responsible for the "clicking" sensation transmitted to a clinician's fingers following successful introduction and advancement of a tracheal tube introducer (bougie). The right mainstem bronchus is shorter and more vertical than the left, making it a common location for the tip of an endotracheal tube that has been advanced too far. Avoiding a right mainstem intubation will be aided by situating the ETT no more than 23 cm at the teeth in males and 21 cm in females, reflecting the average teeth-to-carina distance of 27 and 23 cm in the average male and female, respectively.

Surgical Airway Anatomy

One-third of the trachea lies external to the thorax: the first 3–4 tracheal rings lie between

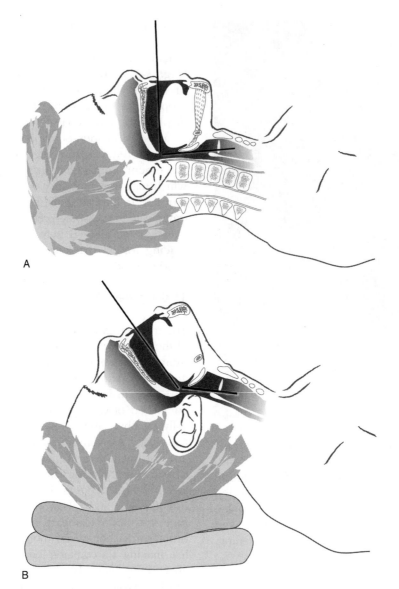

Figure 3–7 A, B. Alignment of oral and pharyngeal/tracheal axes (A) before and (B) after placing the patient in the "sniff" position.

the cricoid and the sternal notch. These rings are the common location for elective tracheotomies. Urgent percutaneous access to the trachea is more commonly achieved through the relatively avascular and easily palpable cricothyroid membrane (Fig. 3–9). Located between the cricoid and thyroid cartilages, the membrane is 22–30 mm wide and 9–10 mm high, in the average adult. This means that the maximal outer diameter of a tube or cannula placed through the cricothyroid membrane, as part of an emergent surgical airway, should be no greater than 8.5 mm (the

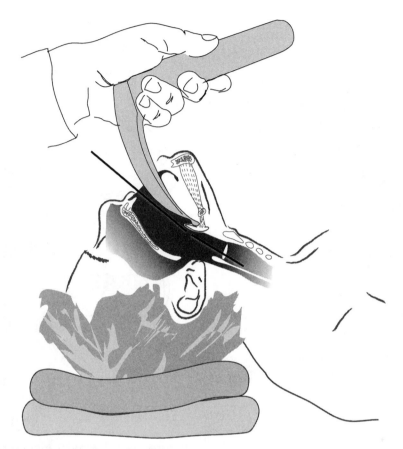

Figure 3–8. Final alignment of the airway axes is achieved through tongue displacement and anterior lift of the mandible using a laryngoscope.

outside diameter [OD] of a #4 tracheostomy tube is 8 mm; the OD of a #6 tracheostomy tube is 10 mm; and a 6.0 ID ETT has an OD of 8.2 mm). The average distance between the midpoint of the cricothyroid membrane and the vocal cords above is only 13 mm. The lower third of the membrane is usually less vascular than the upper third.

Emergency cricothyrotomies are performed after failure to intubate, **in conjunction with** a failure to oxygenate by BMV or extraglottic device. Rarely, airway pathology may mandate a primary cricothyrotomy or tracheotomy. It should be noted that developmentally, the cricoid cartilage initially lies immediately beneath the thyroid cartilage. For this reason, in the younger pediatric patient (i.e., up to age 8), there is no well-defined cricothyroid membrane allowing easy access to the airway.

▶ AIRWAY INNERVATION

Knowledge of the innervation of the airway is important to the airway manager contemplating application of airway anesthesia to facilitate an "awake" intubation. The posterior third of the tongue is innervated primarily by the

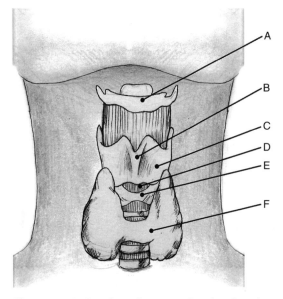

Figure 3–9. Anterior neck landmarks. A. Hyoid bone, B. Laryngeal prominence ("Adam's apple"), C. Thyroid (laryngeal) cartilage, D. Cricothyroid membrane, E. Cricoid cartilage, F. Thyroid gland.

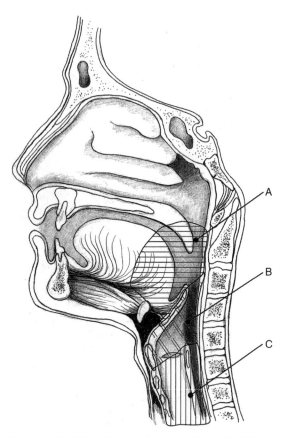

Figure 3–10. Airway innervation. Distributions supplied by A. Glossopharyngeal nerve, B. Superior laryngeal nerve and C. Recurrent laryngeal branches of the vagus nerve.

glossopharyngeal nerve (Fig. 3–10), as are the soft palate and palatoglossal folds. Pressure on these structures can evoke a "gag" response. The glossopharyngeal nerve can be blocked with small volumes of local anesthetic injected at the base of the palatoglossal fold in the mouth, but also responds well to topically applied anesthesia. The internal branch of the superior laryngeal nerve supplies the laryngopharynx, including the inferior aspect of the epiglottis and the larynx above the cords. It can be blocked topically by holding pledgets soaked in local anesthetic solution (e.g., 4% xylocaine) in the piriform recesses. Alternatively, it can be blocked by injecting a small volume of local anesthetic in the proximity of the nerves as they pierce the thyrohyoid membrane, near the lateral aspects of the hyoid bone. Below the cords, sensation is provided by the recurrent laryngeal branch of the vagus nerve.

▶ ABNORMAL AIRWAY ANATOMY

The challenge of airway management is increased when the patient has airway anatomy that differs from the norm. Variations from normal can be classified in two ways:

- Difficulties can be caused by normal anatomic variations such as a small chin, large tongue, high arched palate, or an obese neck.
- Pathologic processes such as airway trauma, inflammation, infection, tumor, or congenital anomaly can create challenges in all aspects of airway management.

Assessing the patient for anatomic variations and pathologic conditions is an important step that must occur during the preparation phase of airway management.

▶ DESCRIBING THE VIEW OBTAINED AT LARYNGOSCOPY

The view of the laryngeal inlet obtained at direct laryngoscopy is commonly recorded using a scale described by Cormack and Lehane[12] (Table 3–1; Fig. 3–11). The Cormack-Lehane (C-L) scale is a widely accepted classification schema for glottic visualization, and will be referred to throughout this book. Other authors have further subdivided the Grade 2 and 3 view[13–15] (Table 3–1; Fig. 3–12). This is clinically relevant in that "easy" Grade 1 and 2A views are approached differently (direct laryngoscopy [DL] alone +/– external laryngeal manipulation) than "restricted" Grade 2B and 3A views (DL plus bougie). "Difficult" Grade 3B and Grade 4 views are managed differently still (e.g., using alternative intubation techniques such as the LMA Fastrach, Trachlight, or indirect fiberoptic devices).

Another classification is the **POGO** score, used to describe the **P**ercentage **O**f **G**lottic **O**pening visualized during laryngoscopy (Fig. 3–13).[16] Its use results in improved interrater reliability[17] in describing laryngeal views compared to the C-L classification. The POGO score is applicable to C-L Grades 1 and 2 situations only, and, while useful to help record exactly how much of the laryngeal inlet was seen at laryngoscopy for charting or data collection purposes, it will not necessarily aid the clinician in making prospective airway management decisions.

▶ THE PEDIATRIC AIRWAY: PHYSIOLOGY AND ANATOMY

The differences between pediatric and adult airway management are often overemphasized to the point of causing undue anxiety in the clinician. This need not be the case. Basic principles of airway assessment and management apply equally to both the pediatric and adult airways. The differences of note between adult and pediatric airways are most pronounced in the first 2 years of life, with similarities outweighing differences thereafter (Fig. 3–14).

Pediatric Airway Anatomic Differences

A summary of significant differences between adults and children follows:

A. The head-to-body size ratio is greater in infants and young children. Optimal airway angulation for laryngoscopy is achieved in infants by placing a towel under the shoulders. Preschoolers are usually in good intubating position when lying flat on a stretcher; older children often require a pillow under their heads to achieve the sniffing position.

B. The infant tongue is large relative to the jaw, and the larynx is more cephalad. In infants, the larynx is at C 2–3 and migrates in the first 5 years to its adult location at C 4–5. This relatively high larynx creates an anatomic relationship sometimes called *glossoptosis* and is usually described by the laryngoscopist as an *anterior larynx*. This requires more tongue displacement during laryngoscopy and explains the relative popularity among pediatric practitioners of straight laryngoscope blades for intubation.

C. Preteen children may have large tonsils (so large that they may meet in the midline). This can interfere with laryngoscopy and may lead to bleeding from laryngoscope trauma.

D. Loose primary teeth may be dislodged and aspirated.

E. From age 1 to 5, the epiglottis is growing faster than the rest of the larynx. It often takes on an unusual appearance (like a tulip), may be longer and more "U" shaped, and is often soft and floppy. It is often

▶ **TABLE 3-1** CORMACK-LEHANE[12] AND COOK MODIFICATION[13] GRADING OF LARYNGEAL INLET STRUCTURES VISIBLE AT LARYNGOSCOPY

Cormack-Lehane[12] Grade	Cormack-Lehane Description	Cook[13] Modification of Cormack Grade	Description of Cook Modified Cormack Grades	Alternative Cook Nomenclature
Grade 1	All or most of the glottic aperture is visible	Grade 1		easy
Grade 2	Only the posterior extremity of the glottis is visible (i.e. the posterior cartilages), visible	Grade 2A	Posterior cords and cartilages visible	
		Grade 2B	Only posterior cartilages visible	restricted
Grade 3	Only the epiglottis can be visualized: no part of the glottic aperture can be seen	Grade 3A	Epiglottis visible and can be lifted	
		Grade 3 B	Epiglottis adherent to posterior pharynx	difficult
Grade 4	Not even the epiglottis can be visualized			

28

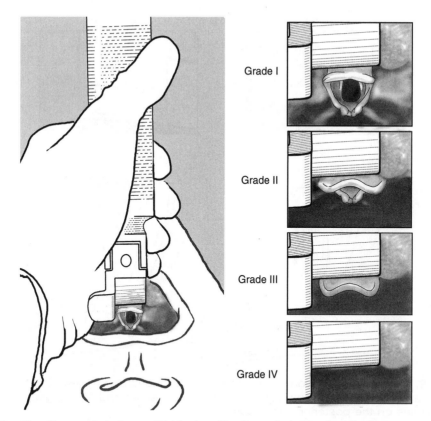

Figure 3–11. The Cormack-Lehane (C-L) classification of glottic visualization.

difficult to evert by placing the blade tip in the vallecula. Pediatric laryngoscopists generally position the laryngoscope blade (curved or straight) posterior to the epiglottis (i.e., picking it up directly) to expose the glottis.

F. Cuffed ETTs are not essential below age 5 because the cricoid ring, the narrowest part of the pediatric airway, can form a reasonably tight fit and seal around the ETT. It is important to demonstrate a small leak around the tube because an occlusive fit may lead to subglottic ischemic injury.

G. The glottic opening is tipped more inferiorly (an adult's is 90° to the line of sight, while a child's is closer to 135°).

H. The small airway is prone to edema and obstruction, especially at the subglottic level.

I. The short trachea often results in right mainstem ETT placement. ETT depth should be age/2 + 12.

J. Once an ETT is placed, moving the head may cause the ETT to migrate up or down. There is a significant risk of right main intubation or inadvertent extubation after tube fixation. Radiographic recheck and confirmation are frequently required.

K. An ETT must be secured with particular care in children. Tonguing can be vigorous in children and small movements can lead to kinking or extubation.

Pediatric Physiologic Differences

Compared to adults, infants and children have a higher minute ventilation, basal O_2 consumption

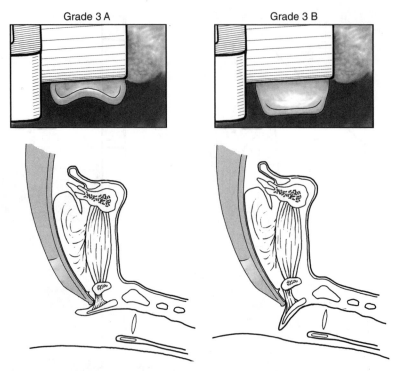

Figure 3–12. Cook's modification of the Cormack-Lehane Grade 3 view: Grade 3A (epiglottis obscures the view of any laryngeal structures, but is elevated) and 3B (epiglottis points posteriorly and/or lies on the posterior pharyngeal wall).

rate and cardiac output. Combined with a lower FRC, this leads to more rapid desaturation during apnea. Infants respond rapidly to hypoxia by dropping the heart rate and raising pulmonary vascular resistance. This in turn leads to a profound drop in cardiac output, and hypotension. Hypoxic bradycardia rarely progresses to true asystole unless hypoxia is prolonged. Although this rapid "death spiral" can be frightening, it can be rapidly reversed with oxygenation and

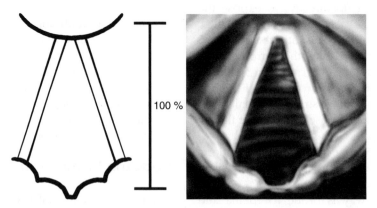

Figure 3–13. Percentage of Glottic Opening (POGO) score.

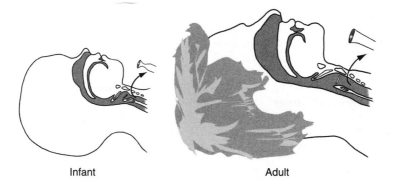

Infant   Adult

Figure 3–14. Pediatric airway anatomy differences are most apparent in the infant and include a relatively large occiput, which places the neck into flexion; a relatively larger tongue, and a more cephalad larynx. Other differences include a longer, "floppier" epiglottis, more 'angled' glottis and a funnel shaped upper airway, narrowest at the cricoid cartilage.

ventilation: atropine and epinephrine are rarely required. The best way to deal with this issue is to prevent it: **the pace of infant intubation sequences must be much faster** than that to which most practitioners are accustomed in their adult practice.

Medication dosing and equipment sizing for the pediatric patient can be addressed by the use of the Broselow tape, with an accompanying dedicated pediatric airway and resuscitation cart.

▶ SUMMARY

A thorough knowledge of airway-related physiology and anatomy is vital for the acute-care clinician. Physiologic considerations dictate the need for preoxygenation and suggest when the patient will be less likely to tolerate difficulty, if encountered, with airway management. Familiarity with airway anatomy is vital for successful direct laryngoscopy, where landmark recognition is instrumental in leading the clinician to the laryngeal inlet. Equally, to be successful with the use of alternative intubation devices, the

clinician must maintain a "mental image" of the airway anatomy through which they pass.

REFERENCES

1. Benumof JL, Dagg R, Benumof R. Critical hemoglobin desaturation will occur before return to an unparalyzed state following 1 mg/kg intravenous succinylcholine. *Anesthesiology.* 1997;87(4):979–982.
2. Mort TC. Preoxygenation in critically ill patients requiring emergency tracheal intubation. *Crit Care Med.* 2005;33(11):2672–2675.
3. Bateman NT, Leach RM. ABC of oxygen. Acute oxygen therapy. *Bmj.* 1998;317(7161):798–801.
4. Morris IR. Functional anatomy of the upper airway. *Emerg Med Clin North Am.* 1988;6(4):639–669.
5. Tintinalli JE, Claffey J. Complications of nasotracheal intubation. *Ann Emerg Med.* 1981;10(3):142–144.
6. Latorre F, Otter W, Kleemann PP, Dick W, Jage J. Cocaine or phenylephrine/lignocaine for nasal fibreoptic intubation? *Eur J Anaesthesiol.* 1996;13(6):577–581.
7. Nandi PR, Charlesworth CH, Taylor SJ, Nunn JF, Dore CJ. Effect of general anaesthesia on the pharynx. *Br J Anaesth.* 1991;66(2):157–162.

8. Shorten GD, Opie NJ, Graziotti P, Morris I, Khangure M. Assessment of upper airway anatomy in awake, sedated and anaesthetised patients using magnetic resonance imaging. *Anaesth Intensive Care.* 1994;22(2):165–169.

9. Hillman DR, Platt PR, Eastwood PR. The upper airway during anaesthesia. *Br J Anaesth.* 2003;91(1): 31–39.

10. Ellis H, Feldman S. *Anatomy for Anaesthetists.* 6th ed. Oxford: Blackwell Scientific Publications; 1993.

11. Levitan RM. *The Airway Cam(TM) Guide to Intubation and Practical Emergency Airway Management.* Wayne, PA: Airway Cam Technologies, Inc. ; 2004.

12. Cormack RS, Lehane J. Difficult tracheal intubation in obstetrics. *Anaesthesia.* 1984;39(11):1105–1111.

13. Cook TM, Nolan JP, Gabbott DA. Cricoid pressure—are two hands better than one? *Anaesthesia.* 1997;52(2):179–180.

14. Cook TM. A new practical classification of laryngeal view. *Anaesthesia.* 2000;55(3):274–279.

15. Yentis SM, Lee DJ. Evaluation of an improved scoring system for the grading of direct laryngoscopy. *Anaesthesia.* 1998;53(11):1041–1044.

16. Levitan RM, Ochroch EA, Kush S, Shofer FS, Hollander JE. Assessment of airway visualization: validation of the percentage of glottic opening (POGO) scale. *Acad Emerg Med.* 1998;5(9): 919–923.

17. O'Shea JK, Pinchalk ME, Wang HE. Reliability of paramedic ratings of laryngoscopic views during endotracheal intubation. *Prehosp Emerg Care.* 2005;9(2):167–171.

CHAPTER 4

Oxygen Delivery Devices and Bag-Mask Ventilation

▶ KEY POINTS

- It is important to avoid inappropriate fixation on endotracheal intubation. Bag-mask ventilation (BMV) may be a critical first step in oxygenating a patient before and/or between intubation attempts.
- The bag-valve mask (BVM) device (manual resuscitator), with a good face-mask seal, may be used passively (without positive pressure ventilation) in the spontaneously breathing patient, to deliver close to 100% oxygen.
- If needed, in the patient still demonstrating respiratory effort, assisted bag-mask ventilation may be performed, timed to deliver a positive pressure breath with the patient's inspiratory effort.
- An adequate jaw thrust, and, where permitted, head extension are the keys to effective BMV.
- Difficult mask ventilation is usually easily resolved by altering technique, including the early use of an oral airway, combined with two-person BMV.
- Predicted difficulty with BMV may significantly impact the decision of how to proceed with an intubation.

▶ INTRODUCTION

Oxygenation and ventilation are key goals of airway management and are commonly achieved by **bag-mask ventilation (BMV),** endotracheal intubation, or both. BMV in particular is a critical airway management skill. In some studies, BMV has been shown to be no less effective than endotracheal intubation or extraglottic device use.[1–3] However, in spite of its importance, formal training in BMV technique is often lacking,[4] with studies showing poor performance and retention of the technique in hospital personnel.[5] This problem can be compounded by the delegation of BMV to a less skilled team member, together with an inappropriate fixation on the more invasive technique of endotracheal intubation. As a potentially life-saving skill, BMV is a critical step in oxygenating a patient before and between intubation attempts. The ability to oxygenate the patient with BMV has very specific airway management implications: in a difficult situation, successful BMV may obviate the need to employ less familiar rescue oxygenation techniques such as extraglottic device placement or cricothyrotomy.

▶ OXYGEN SUPPLY

Indications for instituting oxygen (O_2) therapy appear in Table 4–1. Often taken for granted, the clinician must ensure that the **oxygen supply** is intact and functioning. Assuming oxygen is being supplied without deliberately checking *on each occasion* an airway intervention is undertaken, will eventually result in a patient being managed on room air! Malpositions of the proximal end of oxygen tubing include the following:

- Appropriately attached to the oxygen outlet, but without the oxygen flowmeter being turned on.
- Attached to the neighboring medical air outlet.
- Attached to the suction outlet.
- On the floor.
- Attached to an empty oxygen cylinder.

Oxygen can be supplied via pipeline from a central gas supply to wall- or ceiling-mounted outlets, or from portable cylinders. Oxygen cylinders vary in size from the large tanks carried in ambulances to smaller, more portable tanks used for transport within a hospital or for individual patients.

▶ **TABLE 4–1** INDICATIONS FOR INSTITUTION OF OXYGEN THERAPY.

Cardiac and respiratory arrest
Hypoxemia (PaO_2 <60; SaO_2 <90%)
Systemic hypotension (BP <100 mm Hg systolic)
Low cardiac output and metabolic acidosis (Bicarbonate <18 mmol/l)
Respiratory distress (RR >24/minute in the adult)

Source: Fulmer JD, Snider GL. American College of Chest Physicians (ACCP)—National Heart, Lung, and Blood Institute (NHLBI) Conference on Oxygen Therapy. *Arch Intern Med.* 1984;144:1645–55.

▶ OXYGEN DELIVERY

First-line therapy in managing the acutely ill patient almost always involves oxygen delivery. This may be provided **passively** if the patient has a patent airway and sufficient respiratory effort, or **actively,** via positive pressure ventilation (PPV). PPV in turn can be delivered by BMV, noninvasive positive pressure ventilation (NPPV) or via an extraglottic device or endotracheal tube.

▶ OXYGEN DELIVERY DEVICES— PASSIVE

Oxygen is a drug and needs to be treated with respect, but it rarely causes harm in the acutely ill patient. Where indicated, it should be delivered in precise concentrations. Whenever possible, its use should be monitored with a pulse oximeter. Oxygen delivery devices can be categorized as **low (variable performance)** or **high (fixed performance) flow.** Low flow devices such as nasal cannulae, simple face masks and nonrebreathing face masks deliver oxygen at less than the patient's peak inspiratory flow rate. Inspired oxygen concentration will thus vary with the patient's pattern of breathing. In contrast, high flow devices such as the Venturi face mask deliver oxygen at a rate in excess of the patient's peak inspiratory flow rate, and allow for more precise titration of the inspired oxygen concentration.

Nasal Cannulae

Applied to the nostrils, nasal cannulae can be used to modestly increase the fractional inspired concentration of oxygen (FiO_2). Using the dead space of the nasopharynx as a reservoir for oxygen, the delivered FiO_2 is never precisely known, as it will vary with the patient's minute ventilation, inspiratory flow rate, and oxygen flow rate. While nasal prongs have their use in a patient who is mildly ill, limitation of the maximum deliverable FiO_2 make their use in patients requiring advanced airway support unadvisable. High-flow O_2 delivery by nasal prongs is uncomfortable and quickly dries the nasopharynx.

Simple Face Mask

Encompassing mouth and nose, application of oxygen at 6–10 liters per minute (LPM) through a simple face mask will result in a delivered FiO_2 of 30%–50%. As the patient's peak inspiratory flow exceeds that of the supplied oxygen, dilution of oxygen by room air entrained around the mask edges and through exhalation ports will occur, limiting delivered FiO_2. Exhalation of gas is through these same exhalation ports. There is little control of the actual inspired FiO_2 using this device—it supplements oxygenation, but to a variable degree. Humidification can be added to the setup to maximize patient comfort.

Nonrebreathing Face Mask (NRFM)

Using a similar face-piece to the simple mask, the nonrebreathing face mask (NRFM) increases the delivered FiO_2 with the addition of a reservoir bag and two valves (Fig. 4–1). Supplied oxygen is directed into the reservoir bag (which must be unraveled when taken out of the package). A valve positioned between the mask and the reservoir bag allows 100% O_2 to enter the face mask during patient inspiration, but prevents flow back into the reservoir bag during exhalation. A second one-way valve located over one of the two exhalation ports allows exhalation through the port, while preventing entrainment of room air on inspiration. With a tight mask seal and minimal entrained room air, delivered FiO_2 approaches 80%. It should be noted that supplied oxygen flow for the nonrebreathing face mask must be adjusted so that the reservoir bag never completely collapses (i.e., >10–15 LPM) during the patient's inspiration to minimize room-air entrainment.

In practice, the spontaneously breathing patient receiving face-mask oxygen who is likely to require more advanced airway support should usually have a nonrebreathing face mask applied, unless a high FiO_2 is contraindicated (as with an unmonitored patient with advanced chronic obstructive pulmonary disease [COPD]). Any patient requiring such a high concentration

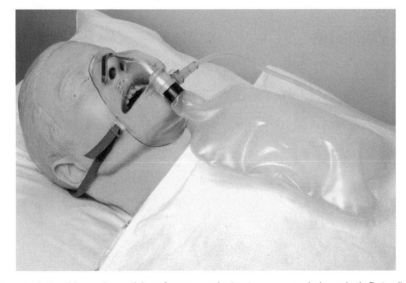

Figure 4–1. Nonrebreathing face mask (note reservoir bag is inflated).

of O_2 should be closely observed and monitored with the anticipation of the need to proceed to endotracheal intubation.

Venturi Mask

Of the devices described in this section, the Venturi mask system allows the most precise control of delivered FiO_2. Using the same cone-shaped oxygen mask as the simple face mask, this system (Fig. 4–2) incorporates a removable Venturi adapter proximal to the oxygen inlet. Wall gas is forced through the Venturi valve, creating a small jet of oxygen within the device. The jet creates a negative pressure around it (the Venturi effect) that entrains room air at a fixed rate, resulting in a predictable mixing of 100% oxygen with room air. The speed of the jet and volume of air entrained is controlled by the size of the hole and rate of oxygen flow controlled at the source, resulting in a predictable delivered concentration of oxygen. As gas is delivered at a rate exceeding the patient's maximum inspiratory flow rate, changes in breathing do not affect the oxygen concentration delivered. With specific oxygen flow rates, different color-coded

Venturi adapters supply an FiO_2 between 24% and 50%. Precise control of FiO_2 may be desired when reliable assessment of the alveolar-arterial (A-a) gradient is needed, or when applying O_2 to certain COPD patients.

▶ OXYGENATION AND VENTILATION SYSTEMS—ACTIVE

Noninvasive Positive Pressure Ventilation

Noninvasive positive pressure ventilation (NPPV) is a method of providing positive pressure ventilatory support via a face mask, nasal mask, or mouthpiece (as opposed to an endotracheal tube) to selected patients with acute ventilatory failure. Required equipment varies from a simple continuous positive airway pressure (CPAP) valve, through purpose-made bilevel devices, to full service intensive care unit (ICU) ventilators. Positive pressure delivery modes also vary, with options extending from simple CPAP to patient-triggered delivery of set volumes or pressures. Bilevel positive airway pressure (BiPAP) ventilation

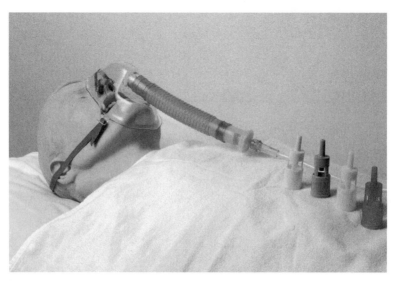

Figure 4–2. Face mask with Venturi adaptors for different inspired oxygen concentrations.

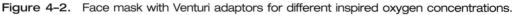

is used to deliver different pressures during inspiration and expiration.

NPPV has been shown to improve outcomes in certain patients with acute hypercapneic ventilatory failure. Certainly, there is strong evidence to support its use in patients with COPD, and to a lesser extent, cardiogenic pulmonary edema.[6,7] Patients with acute respiratory failure from other causes have shown less benefit, to date. Improved outcomes in the COPD and pulmonary edema populations include a reduction in the need for intubation; ICU admissions; length of hospital stay; and mortality.[6,7] Success is more likely in patients who are younger and exhibit an early response to the intervention,[8] and in the subgroup of patients with the following associated parameters: pH >7.25, respiratory rate <30, Glasgow Coma Scale (GCS) >11.[9] Respiratory failure patients *in extremis* require more definitive airway support by way of endotracheal intubation, as patient anxiety and "air hunger" may complicate attempted NPPV delivery.

The Boussignac CPAP System

The Boussignac system (Fig. 4–3) is a newer disposable oxygen delivery device that provides

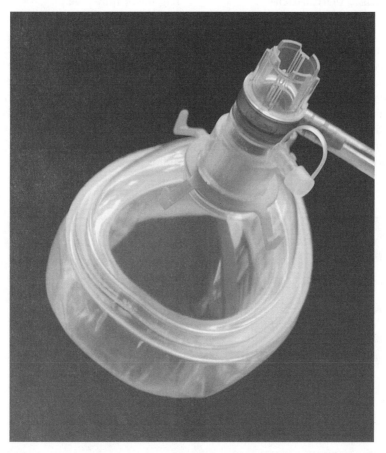

Figure 4–3. The Boussignac continuous positive airway pressure (CPAP) system provides flow dependent CPAP and also allows in-line medication nebulization, and suction access without removal of the mask.

flow-dependent CPAP without the need for a flow generator. A standard O_2 source and flowmeter are used to deliver variable degrees of CPAP according to the flow selected. For example, 10 LPM of oxygen flow provides 2.5–3.0 cm H_2O of CPAP; 15 LPM provides 4.5–5.0 cm H_2O; and 25 LPM provides 8.5–10.0 cm H_2O of CPAP. The delivered FiO_2 will depend on respiratory rate and tidal volume (generally, a minute ventilation <15 LPM delivers 70%–100% FiO_2).[10] A nebulizer can be added to the system for medication administration, and a suction catheter can be passed with the mask in place.

Bag-Valve Mask Ventilation Systems

The bag-valve mask (BVM) ventilation device (Fig. 4–4) is used to manually deliver positive pressure through an applied face mask, extraglottic device or endotracheal tube. The former would be an initial step in an apneic or hypoventilating patient, and is almost always indicated prior to, or during intubation of an ill patient. The clinician should be intimately familiar with the workings of the BVM device, as it has a number of valves, and needs proper assembly to work. Also known as **manual resuscitators,** these devices incorporate a self-inflating bag, a one-way bag inlet valve, and a nonrebreathing patient valve. The patient valve end features a universal connector with a 22-mm outside diameter (OD), which fits standard face masks, and a 15-mm internal diameter (ID) that connects to standard endotracheal tubes, extraglottic devices, and cricothyrotomy or tracheostomy cannulae. An oxygen inlet port is located on the bag inlet valve end to accept the oxygen source tubing. To enable 100% oxygen delivery, oxygen flow must be adjusted to ensure the attached reservoir bag never fully collapses.

The face mask used in conjunction with the manual resuscitator is generally made of rubber or plastic, and may incorporate an inflatable cuff around its margin to better conform to the patient's facial anatomy. The tight seal thus afforded is mandatory when the manual resuscitator is being used for PPV, but is also useful in the spontaneously breathing patient, as the good seal obtained ensures delivery of close to 100% oxygen.

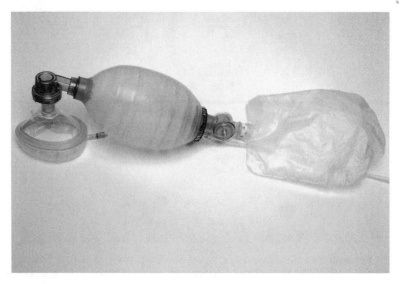

Figure 4–4. Bag-valve mask (BVM) manual resuscitator.

Adult-sized manual resuscitators are supplied with a 1600 mL self-inflating bag; child size 500 mL; and infant 240 mL. The pediatric sized BVM devices may have an additional valve just proximal to the face mask—a pressure limiting or "pop-off" valve. This is calibrated to release applied airway pressure at approximately 40 cm H_2O, to help prevent barotrauma. In clinical situations where there is a recognized airway obstruction that is not readily reversible (e.g., epiglottis, croup, airway edema, severe asthma), the pop-off valve may need to be controlled manually to ensure continued lung inflation.

▶ ADJUNCTS TO BVM DEVICES— OROPHARYNGEAL AND NASOPHARYNGEAL AIRWAYS

Designed to alleviate obstruction caused by posterior relaxation of the tongue against soft palate or the soft palate against the posterior pharynx, both oral and nasal airways help create a patent channel for ventilation. Correctly placed, the distal end of each device should be located beyond the soft palate and base of tongue, just above the epiglottis (Fig. 4–5).

Oropharyngeal Airways

DESCRIPTION

Oropharyngeal airways (OPAs) (Fig. 4–6) help alleviate functional airway obstruction caused by relaxation of the tongue against the soft palate. They are most often used as an adjunct to BMV of an obtunded or unconscious patient. Made of plastic, the component parts are a curved hollow lumen (in the Guedel version), proximal flange which abuts the patient's lips, and proximal bite block which doubles as a color-coded size indicator.

SIZING

OPAs are sized by length in centimeters, and are available in sizes for all ages. Choosing the appropriate size is important, as too long an OPA may precipitate laryngospasm or create obstruction, while if too small, it may be ineffective.[11] Although never formally validated, many clinicians approximate correct OPA length by placing it alongside the patient's cheek: from the corner of the lips, the tip of the OPA should reach the angle of the mandible (Fig. 4–7).[12] A typical adult female will take an 8-cm OPA, and an adult male, 9 or 10 cm.

USE

The OPA should be inserted inverted, (i.e., with its concave surface directed cephalad) and advanced

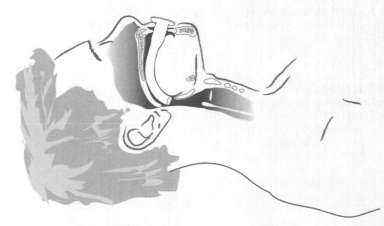

Figure 4–5. The oropharygneal airway (OPA) when correctly placed is positioned behind the tongue and cephalad to the epiglottis.

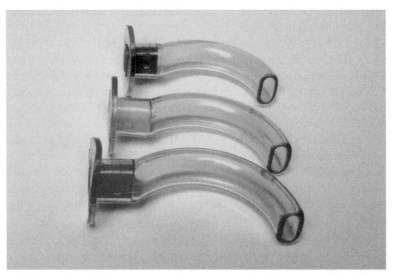

Figure 4–6.   Adult-sized oropharyngeal airways.

until the distal tip will proceed no further in the inverted position. At that point, the OPA is rotated 180°, so that the concavity faces caudad. Advancement continues around the curve of the tongue until fully inserted. Inverted insertion helps avoid worsening obstruction caused by posterior tongue displacement into the hypopharynx during OPA placement. Alternatively, it can be inserted noninverted with a tongue depressor to manage the tongue: this is the preferred technique in infants and younger children, to help avoid trauma to delicate tissues.

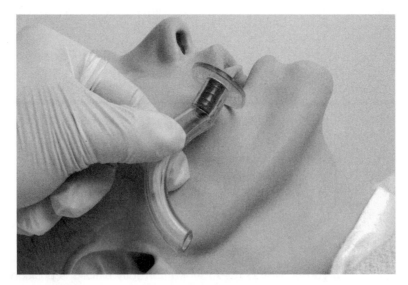

Figure 4–7.   Sizing an oropharyngeal airway on an airway training manikin.

Precautions and Contraindications

OPAs are not well tolerated in the awake or semi-conscious patient with intact airway reflexes, where insertion may stimulate gagging, vomiting and aspiration or laryngospasm. In addition, care must be taken to rule out a foreign body in the oropharynx prior to OPA insertion.

Nasopharyngeal Airways

Description

A nasopharyngeal airway (NPA) may be a useful option when trismus precludes OPA insertion, and may be better tolerated than an OPA in the awake or semiconscious patient with intact airway reflexes. While effective at alleviating functional airway obstruction, downsides to the NPA include transient patient discomfort during insertion and the potential for causing epistaxis. NPAs, also known as "nasal trumpets", are made from soft material such as latex or silicon, have a hollow interior, beveled leading edge, and a proximal flange to abut the patient's nostril (Fig. 4–8).

Sizing

Adult NPAs are generally sized by their internal diameter (ID) in mm. Typical adult sizes for small, medium, and large NPAs are 6, 7, and 8 mm ID, respectively. One commonly used (but non-validated) sizing method is to use an NPA of a length corresponding to the distance from nose tip to the tragus of the ear. A second method, whereby an NPA is used of a diameter equal to that of the patient's fifth finger was not found to functionally correlate well when studied.[13] Sizing based on patient height makes more anatomic sense, resulting in a recommendation for a 6 mm ID NPA for an average adult female and 7 mm for an average male.[14]

Use

The NPA is lubricated and advanced into the patient's nostril, perpendicular to the face, resulting in passage along the floor of the major nasal airway. A slight twisting motion can be used during insertion. If significant resistance is encountered, insertion should be attempted through the other nostril. Insertion continues until the flange of the NPA abuts the nasal ala.

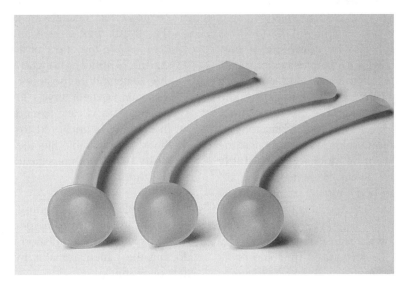

Figure 4–8. Nasopharyngeal airways.

PRECAUTIONS AND CONTRAINDICATIONS

NPA use is *relatively* contraindicated in known bleeding diathesis, including heparinized, warfarinized, or recently thrombolyzed patients, and in suspected cribriform plate fracture. However, this latter directive has been made on the basis of only a few case reports:[15,16] in the head-injured patient, common sense dictates balancing the substantial risk of hypoxemia with the benefits of cautiously obtaining a patent airway, if an oral airway can't be used.

▶ THE INITIAL APPROACH TO THE AIRWAY

Basic Life Support (BLS) teaching mandates assessing the unconscious patient for (a) responsiveness, (b) airway patency, and (c) adequacy of respiratory effort, by looking for chest rise, and listening and feeling for air egress from the patient's mouth and nose.[17] The patient with no evidence of effective gas exchange may or may not still be making respiratory efforts against an obstructed upper airway.

Recognition of the Obstructed Airway

Airway obstruction may be **complete** or **partial.** The patient with a completely obstructed airway will be unable to speak, and as hypoxia ensues, will rapidly lose consciousness and cease breathing. Partial airway obstruction may be **functional,** due to the soft palate, tongue, and epiglottis falling back toward or against the posterior pharynx, or due to **pathologic** changes occurring within the lumen of the airway (e.g., foreign body, tumor, or infection) or externally compressing the airway (e.g., neck hematoma).

The patient with signs of partial airway obstruction may be recognized by some or all of the following signs:

- Snoring inspiratory efforts (with functional airway obstruction) or inspiratory and/or expiratory stridor (with pathologic changes in the area of the glottis).
- Paradoxical breathing: a "rocking" motion of chest and abdomen, whereby the abdomen rises with attempted inspiration, and the chest falls.
- Indrawing above the sternal notch and between the ribs.
- Voice changes.

Response to the Obstructed Airway: Airway Opening Maneuvers

Although the potential causes of airway obstruction are many, the following initial airway clearing maneuvers are appropriate to try in most patients:

- **Head extension** at the atlanto-occipital joint on the neck (omit in the patient where C-spine precautions are in effect). As seen in Figs. 4–9 A and B, as the head is extended, functional obstruction is alleviated as the epiglottis and tongue are elevated off the posterior pharyngeal wall.
- **Jaw lift/thrust**—similar changes but with a greater effect occur with jaw thrust or lift (Fig. 4–10). Figs. 4–11 A and B dramatically demonstrate the effect of a jaw lift in moving the obstructing tongue away from both the palate and the posterior pharyngeal wall to obtain a patent airway in an unconscious patient. This is easy to understand because the tongue is anchored to the mandible—lifting the mandible lifts the tongue.
- **Chin lift**—combines head extension and jaw thrust.

If simple airway opening maneuvers do not result in a return to a spontaneous, unobstructed pattern of ventilation, or even if they do, but the patient remains hypoxic, consider the following:

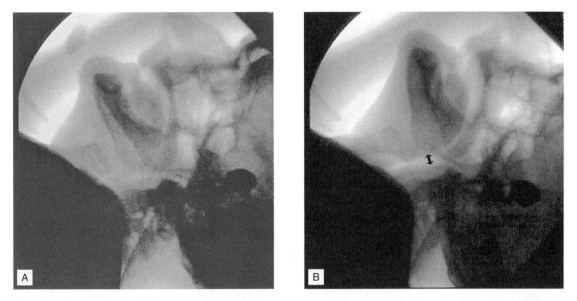

Figures 4–9. Lateral fluoroscopic views of an unconscious patient. In (A), the airway is initially functionally obstructed. With head extension in the same patient, (B), a patent airway (arrow) is created as tongue and epiglottis are elevated away from the posterior pharyngeal wall.

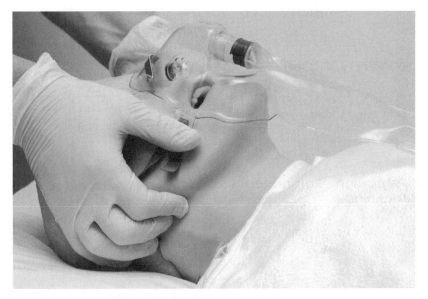

Figure 4–10. A jaw thrust being demonstrated on an airway management trainer.

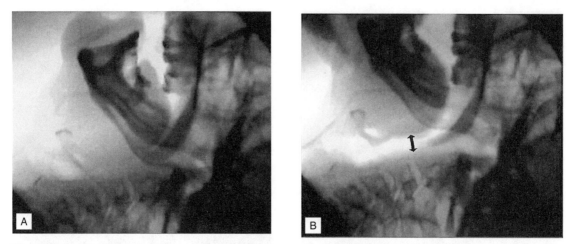

Figures 4–11. Lateral fluoroscopic views of an unconscious patient. (A) The airway is functionally obstructed. (B) With a jaw thrust in the same patient, a widely patent upper airway (arrow) is created.

- Insertion of an oral (if airway reflexes permit) and/or nasal airway.
- Assisted BMV.
- Endotracheal intubation.

Often the clinician will progress through the first two options while preparing for endotracheal intubation.

▶ BAG-MASK VENTILATION

As outlined previously, BMV is a crucial, yet frequently poorly taught skill, which must be mastered by the clinician with acute-care responsibilities.

Bag-Mask Ventilation: Components of Routine Technique

There are three important components to proper BMV technique: mask seal, airway opening, and ventilation.

MASK SEAL

An appropriately sized face mask is attached to the bag-mask device and applied to the patient's face. The lower border of the mask's cuff is first applied to the groove between the lower lip and the chin, after which the mask can be placed down across the nasal bridge. The thumb and index finger of the clinician's hand applies sufficient pressure on the face mask to achieve a good seal (Fig. 4–12). Note, however, that sealing pressure must be achieved *without* excessive downward pressure on the patient's mandible, as this may worsen functional obstruction—rather, the mandible is *lifted* to meet the mask. Small adjustments to the position of the mask on the patient's face (e.g., with small movements to left or right) are made as needed to achieve a seal.

AIRWAY OPENING

The ring and long fingers grasp the bony ridge of the patient's mandible, and, if practical, the fifth finger hooks under the angle of the mandible. These three digits provide counterpressure to the digits applying the mask to the face, but also apply an *upward lift* to the mandible to help perform an airway opening jaw thrust. Note that these three fingers should *not* be placed directly under the patient's chin, as midline pressure under the chin can contribute to airway obstruction. This

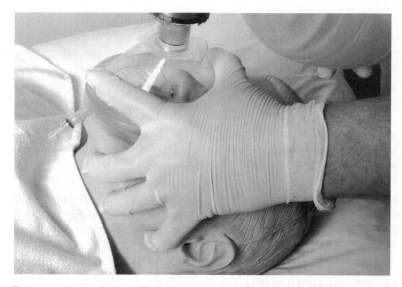

Figure 4–12. Bag-mask ventilation: The thumb and index digits apply pressure to attain a seal of the mask against the patient's face, while the third, fourth, and fifth fingers lift the jaw up into the mask.

latter directive is particularly important in small children and infants. Concomitantly, the entire hand also attempts to keep the head extended (if no C-spine precautions).

VENTILATION

The clinician's opposite hand is free to gently squeeze the self-inflating bag. Volumes should be delivered with attention to the patient's status: if apneic, the patient should be gently ventilated at a rate of 10–15 breaths per minute, at a tidal volume of 5–6 mL/kg, or 500 mL in the average adult.[18] In the patient still demonstrating respiratory effort, assisted BMV should be performed, with timing of the positive pressure breath to the patient's inspiratory effort. If the patient is tachypneic, it will be appropriate to simply deliver an assisted breath with every third or fourth patient inspiration.

Assessing Adequacy of Bag-Mask Ventilation

In "bagging" a patient, the clinician must assess whether the patient is in fact being adequately ventilated. A simple "look, listen, and feel" approach to assessing adequacy of BMV is outlined below:

Look for:
- Chest expansion. This is best assessed by observing the patient's chest immediately below the clavicles. Chest expansion in this location reflects underlying lung expansion, whereas movement of the lower thorax can be apparent simply with gastric insufflation, even in the presence of complete airway obstruction.
- Reservoir bag filling from the O_2 source.
- Improving pulse oximeter reading.
- Improvement in the patient's color.

Listen for:
- Any hiss of escaping air caused by a poorly sealed face mask.
- The pulse oximeter tone, indicative of the SaO_2.

Feel for:
- Compliance of the self-inflating bag. If airway obstruction persists, the bag will be hard to

squeeze. Other intrathoracic pathology, such as bronchospasm or pneumothorax can also cause increased resistance and decreased compliance.

- Leaking air against one's hand from a poorly sealed face mask.

Assessing the efficacy of BMV must continue as long as the patient is being bagged, as it is a very dynamic process. Small adjustments to the position of the mask, degree of head tilt or jaw lift are continuously needed during BMV. Changes in the patient's condition (for example, administered paralytic agents wearing off) or clinician fatigue can also impact BMV effectiveness.

▶ RESPONSE TO DIFFICULT BMV SITUATIONS

With appropriate technique, significant difficulty with BMV is rarely encountered in the absence of airway pathology. The most experienced person present should establish adequate airway opening and initiate and assess ease of BMV. Difficult BMV (DMV) is often defined as the inability to maintain an oxygen saturation above 90% with good technique. DMV requires a staged response. Although one response to a difficult BMV situation is to proceed to intubation, DMV may itself predict difficulty with laryngoscopy and/or intubation.[19] Good BMV skills and an approach to DMV are crucial skills in ensuring oxygenation of a patient prior to, or between laryngoscopy attempts.

A Staged Response to Difficult BMV

A. Reposition the head by performing an exaggerated head tilt/chin lift (if not contraindicated).
B. Perform an aggressive jaw thrust.
C. Insert an oropharyngeal airway (and/or a nasopharyngeal airway).
D. Perform a two-person mask ventilation technique.

E. If cricoid pressure is being applied, ease up on, or release it.
F. Consider a mask change (size or type) if seal is an issue.
G. Rule out foreign body in the airway.
H. Consider a "rescue" ventilation device, for example, an extraglottic device such as an LMA or Combitube.
I. Consider an early attempt at intubation.

Steps A, B, and C, as listed above, should occur almost simultaneously and very early in the DMV situation. DMV is often due simply to the failure to adequately open a functionally obstructed airway. Attempted ventilation against this obstruction results in a leak at the mask/face interface, often resulting in the clinician's attempting to remedy the problem by pushing down harder on the mask to attain a seal. This can worsen an already obstructed airway. Rather, what must occur is a more pronounced jaw *lift* or *thrust,* with resultant airway opening occurring as anterior movement of the mandible elevates the tongue, epiglottis, and soft palate away from the posterior pharyngeal wall. This is best performed with the aid of a second person. Two-person mask ventilation is easy to perform and is often much more effective than one person BMV. As shown in Figs. 4–13, 4–14, and 4–15, the 2-person technique can be performed in a number of ways.[20]

Cricoid pressure can cause difficulty with both BMV and laryngoscopy. Excessive cricoid pressure (as may be applied during a rapid-sequence intubation [RSI]) may distort the airway and result in a partial or even complete obstruction. This is especially true in a young child. If significant difficulty with BMV is encountered during application of cricoid pressure, the assistant should transiently ease (initially by 50%) or release the applied pressure.

It may become apparent once BMV is underway that the chosen mask size is incorrect. This is often the case when initial mask sizing occurred with the patient's dentures in place. Especially with encountered difficulty, the improved seal allowed by an appropriately sized mask makes the change worthwhile.

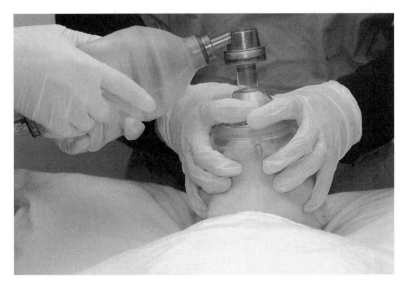

Figure 4-13. Two-person bag-mask ventilation. The primary clinician applies the mask while a second person squeezes the self-inflating bag.

The decision to move to a rescue device such as an LMA or Combitube will depend on the patient's clinical status and whether direct laryngoscopy (DL) has yet been attempted. If there has been no initial attempt at DL, it may be appropriate to proceed with an intubation attempt. If, on the other hand, DMV is encountered in the setting of an already failed attempt at intubation, placement of a rescue ventilation device such as an LMA should be considered. Direct laryngoscopy is also the method of choice to rule out obstructing lesions, including foreign bodies.

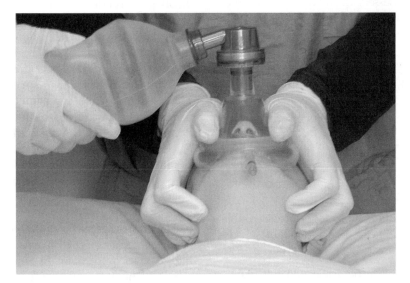

Figure 4-14. Two-person bag-mask ventilation, showing an alternative mask grip for the primary clinician.

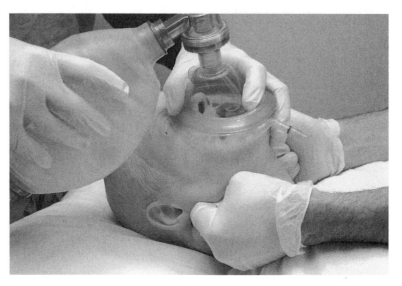

Figure 4-15. Two-person bag-mask ventilation. With this technique, the original clinician continues one-person BMV, while the second person simply performs an aggressive jaw thrust.

▶ PREDICTION OF DIFFICULT BMV

Various patient features are helpful in predicting difficult mask ventilation.[19, 21] As part of the formal airway examination of the patient, these factors should be assessed. The following are features that can create difficulty with BMV—together, they form the simple mnemonic[22] "**BOOTS.**"

Beard: A thick beard can create difficulty in obtaining a good mask seal. Application of water-soluble gel will help to minimize air escaping between hair. Other anatomic variations or patient pathology, such as extreme trauma to the mandible, may also preclude a mask seal.

Obesity: In an obese patient, difficult BMV can be encountered owing to decreased chest wall and diaphragmatic compliance, decreased ability to extend the head, and redundant soft tissue in the pharynx.

Older: Age >55 can be associated with DMV. This is likely multifactorial and may be related to problems of range of motion in the neck and the temporomandibular joint. Age is also associated with loss of teeth and soft tissue elasticity and tone. Placement of an OPA or NPA and a good mask seal will help overcome these problems.

Toothless: The teeth play a role in maintaining facial architecture. In the edentulous patient, tissue collapse in the cheeks allows a leak to occur at the corners of the mouth and makes a good mask seal difficult. "Gathering" the cheek up with the hypothenar aspect of the mask-holding hand while simultaneously tilting the mask a little toward the contralateral side will help. Alternatively, an assistant can be delegated to hold the cheek up against the side of the mask (ideally one size smaller than usual). Early use of an OPA will help. Placement of bunched up gauze in the buccal pouch of the cheeks on either side of the oral airway may help with mask seal by puffing out the cheeks. Some clinicians elect to leave dentures in during BMV to help maintain facial architecture. Neither dentures nor gauze should be left in the intubated patient.

Sounds: A number of conditions associated with abnormal upper and lower airway sounds may cause difficulty with BMV.

A history of **snoring** has been correlated with DMV.[21] As with the obese patient, this may be associated with redundant oropharyngeal tissues. Early placement of an OPA, and maintaining a head-extended position will help.

Stridor is almost always a sign of pathologic airway obstruction and should be considered an ominous sign. Any patient presenting with inspiratory or expiratory stridor should be considered as potentially very difficult or impossible to bag-mask ventilate.

The patient with **"stiff"**, poorly compliant lungs, (often associated with wheezing or rales) will present increased resistance to bag-mask ventilation and requires higher than normal insufflation pressure.

The presence of two or more of the factors presented above significantly increases the potential for DMV.[21] The true incidence of DMV in the emergency department (ED) is not clear but is likely greater than that seen with the elective surgical population. In the operating room, DMV has been reported to occur in up to 5–8% of elective surgical patients.[19, 21] Interestingly, the DMV rate is twice as high (15.5%) in patients who were also described as difficult intubations.[19]

Prediction of difficulty with BMV is an important component of the airway assessment, as BMV remains the "go to" method of gas exchange both before and between intubation attempts. It also represents a vital decision node in airway management in two ways:

A. **Decision making:** Anticipated difficulty with BMV may point to the need for an awake technique for intubation, especially if difficulty with laryngoscopy is also predicted (see Chap. 11).
B. **Defining the failed airway:** In the setting of failed intubation, the inability to maintain the SaO_2 >90% with BMV defines **failed oxygenation,** mandating proceeding with

rescue oxygenation via an extraglottic device or cricothyrotomy (see Chap. 12).

One last implication of predicted difficulty with BMV is the automatic need for an additional assistant, assuming a high probability of requiring a two-person technique.

▶ BMV TIPS AND PEARLS

Ideal Head and Neck Positioning for BMV

Ideally, for BMV, the head and upper neck should be extended[23] (a) to attain a more direct path for the delivered volumes from face to trachea, (b) to maintain longitudinal tension on the lumen of the upper airway[24] and possibly, (c) to increase retrolingual and retropalatal space.[25] When studied, no additional benefit was noted with elevation of the occiput (i.e., the "sniff" position) compared with simple head tilt starting in the neutral position.[23]

Gastric Insufflation

Protracted periods of BMV or poor technique (e.g., delivering breaths during the expiratory phase of the patient's respiratory cycle; not maintaining an adequately open upper airway; or using excessive tidal volumes or positive pressure) can lead to insufflation of the esophagus and stomach. Gastric distention in turn presents two problems:

- It predisposes to regurgitation of gastric contents, potentially leading to aspiration, with its sequellae.
- Particularly in children, but also in adults, massive gastric distention can significantly elevate and interfere with movement of the diaphragm, in turn creating further difficulty with BMV by impacting respiratory system compliance. In extreme cases, gastric rupture can occur.

Gastric insufflation can be avoided by careful attention to delivered tidal volumes, employing the lowest ventilation pressures possible (below 20 cm H_2O), and using airway adjuncts such as the OPA and NPA. Evidence is emerging that especially in the cardiac arrest patient, lower esophageal sphincter pressure decreases rapidly from the normal 20 cm H_2O to as little as 5 cm H_2O, underscoring the need to minimize applied insufflation pressures.[26] Application of cricoid pressure (see below) can also be considered. Although most patients can be adequately oxygenated and ventilated using good, well-timed BMV technique, some gastric insufflation is inevitable. BMV should therefore be viewed as a "bridging" procedure to be used for a limited period of time. If clinically significant gastric distention is suspected, an oro- or nasogastric tube should be passed to decompress the stomach.

Cricoid Pressure and BMV

Posterior pressure on the cricoid cartilage compresses the esophagus between the cartilaginous ring of the cricoid and the body of the C6 vertebra. It is often used to prevent passive regurgitation of gastric contents during rapid-sequence intubation, but can also be considered in the unconscious patient during BMV to reduce inadvertent insufflation of air into the stomach,[27] as discussed above. However, it must be appreciated that cricoid pressure can cause difficulty with BMV,[28, 29] especially if applied at excessive pressures or in an upward direction.[30] If this is suspected, it should be at least transiently released, to determine if that is the cause of difficulty.

"AutoPEEP"

The patient with reactive airways disease experiences air trapping and difficulty with exhalation. In all patients, but particularly those with known or suspected air trapping disease, attention must be paid to allowing sufficient time for exhalation during BMV. Failure to do this may result in a buildup of intrathoracic pressure, which in turn risks both cardiovascular collapse and barotrauma. Pressure may also be alleviated simply by intermittently releasing the seal made by the mask against the face.

Cervical Spine Precautions and BMV

BMV can be performed safely in the patient who is considered at risk for a cervical spine (C-spine) injury, for example, the unconscious trauma patient. However, radiologic studies have shown that movement of the C-spine with BMV is as much or more than that occurring with laryngoscopic endotracheal intubation.[31–34] As such, during BMV, manual in-line neck stabilization (MILNS) should be applied. Head tilt should be omitted: jaw lift is the only airway-opening maneuver that should be used.

The Clinician with Small or Tiring Hands

A one-person technique may be difficult or impossible for the clinician with smaller hands, or a clinician of average stature dealing with a very large patient. In such situations, early use of a two-person technique should be considered.

Laryngospasm

Laryngospasm is a tight and complete adduction of the vocal cords. It sometimes occurs in response to attempted airway manipulation in deeply sedated patients, and may be more common in the pediatric patient. Its effects can be dramatic, with an almost total inability to bag-mask ventilate the patient. If this is suspected, application of CPAP with the BVM device will often help break the spasm: simply continue to apply a tight seal with the mask, while maintaining light but continuous positive pressure on the bag. Severe or recalcitrant cases may require a small dose of skeletal muscle relaxant, for example, succinylcholine 20 mg in the adult patient.

▶ SUMMARY

All clinicians with airway management responsibilities must be able to assess the critically ill patient for airway patency and adequacy of gas exchange. BLS protocols should be followed to open the airway, and if needed, positive-pressure ventilation with BMV instituted. BMV must be learned and practiced, and should not be looked upon as an easy skill. As the clinician becomes familiar with basic BMV, various adjuncts and additions to BMV can be used, such as PEEP and "pop-off" valves, depending on the practice environment. A formal approach should be applied to the difficult BMV situation, and the predictors of difficult BMV appreciated. Faced with ongoing difficulty in performing BMV and/or intubation, the clinician should consider placing an extraglottic device such as a laryngeal mask airway or Combitube.

REFERENCES

1. Dorges V, Wenzel V, Knacke P, Gerlach K. Comparison of different airway management strategies to ventilate apneic, nonpreoxygenated patients. *Crit Care Med.* 2003;31(3):800–804.
2. Gausche M, Lewis RJ, Stratton SJ, et al. Effect of out-of-hospital pediatric endotracheal intubation on survival and neurological outcome: a controlled clinical trial. *JAMA.* 9, 2000;283(6):783–790.
3. Stockinger ZT, McSwain NE, Jr. Prehospital endotracheal intubation for trauma does not improve survival over bag-valve-mask ventilation. *J Trauma.* 2004;56(3):531–536.
4. Stapleton ER. Basic life support cardiopulmonary resuscitation. *Cardiol Clin.* 2002;20(1):1–12.
5. Martin PD, Cyna AM, Hunter WA, et al. Training nursing staff in airway management for resuscitation. A clinical comparison of the facemask and laryngeal mask. *Anaesthesia.* 1993;48(1):33–37.
6. Caples SM, Gay PC. Noninvasive positive pressure ventilation in the intensive care unit: a concise review. *Crit Care Med.* 2005;33(11):2651–2658.
7. Masip J, Roque M, Sanchez B, et al. Noninvasive ventilation in acute cardiogenic pulmonary edema: systematic review and meta-analysis. *JAMA.* 2005;294(24):3124–3130.
8. Mehta S, Hill NS. Noninvasive ventilation. *Am J Respir Crit Care Med.* 2001;163(2):540–577.
9. Confalonieri M, Garuti G, Cattaruzza MS, et al. A chart of failure risk for noninvasive ventilation in patients with COPD exacerbation. *Eur Respir J.* 2005;25(2):348–355.
10. Templier F, Dolveck F, Baer M, et al. Laboratory testing measurement of FIO2 delivered by Boussignac CPAP system with an input of 100% oxygen. *Ann Fr Anesth Reanim.* 2003;22(2):103–107.
11. Gabbott DA, Baskett PJ. Management of the airway and ventilation during resuscitation. *Br J Anaesth.* 1997;79(2):159–171.
12. Levitan R, Ochroch EA. Airway management and direct laryngoscopy. A review and update. *Crit Care Clin.* 2000;16(3):373–388.
13. Roberts K, Porter K. How do you size a nasopharyngeal airway. *Resuscitation.* 2003;56(1):19–23.
14. Stoneham MD. The nasopharyngeal airway. Assessment of position by fibreoptic laryngoscopy. *Anaesthesia.* 1993;48(7):575–580.
15. Muzzi DA, Losasso TJ, Cucchiara RF. Complication from a nasopharyngeal airway in a patient with a basilar skull fracture. *Anesthesiology.* 1991;74(2):366–368.
16. Schade K, Borzotta A, Michaels A. Intracranial malposition of nasopharyngeal airway. *J Trauma.* 2000;49(5):967–968.
17. Part 4: Adult Basic Life Support. *Circulation.* 2005;112(24_suppl):IV19–IV34.
18. Wenzel V, Idris AH, Montgomery WH, et al. Rescue breathing and bag-mask ventilation. *Ann Emerg Med.* 2001;37(4 Suppl):S36–S40.
19. Yildiz TS, Solak M, Toker K. The incidence and risk factors of difficult mask ventilation. *J Anesth.* 2005;19(1):7–11.
20. Davidovic L, LaCovey D, Pitetti RD. Comparison of 1-versus 2-person bag-valve-mask techniques for manikin ventilation of infants and children. *Ann Emerg Med.* 2005;46(1):37–42.
21. Langeron O, Masso E, Huraux C, et al. Prediction of difficult mask ventilation. *Anesthesiology.* 2000;92(5):1229–1236.

22. Walls RM, Murphy M. Identification of the difficult and failed airway. In: Walls RM, ed. *Manual of Emergency Airway Management*. 2nd ed. Philadelphia: Lippincott Willimas and Wilkins; 2004.

23. Morikawa S, Safar P, Decarlo J. Influence of the headjaw position upon upper airway patency. *Anesthesiology*. 1961;22:265–270.

24. Hillman DR, Platt PR, Eastwood PR. The upper airway during anaesthesia. *Br J Anaesth*. 2003;91(1): 31–39.

25. Isono S, Tanaka A, Ishikawa T, et al. Sniffing position improves pharyngeal airway patency in anesthetized patients with obstructive sleep apnea. *Anesthesiology*. 2005;103(3):489–494.

26. Gabrielli A, Wenzel V, Layon AJ, et al. Lower esophageal sphincter pressure measurement during cardiac arrest in humans: potential implications for ventilation of the unprotected airway. *Anesthesiology*. 2005;103(4):897–899.

27. Wenzel V, Idris AH, Dorges V, et al. The respiratory system during resuscitation: a review of the history, risk of infection during assisted ventilation, respiratory mechanics, and ventilation strategies for patients with an unprotected airway. *Resuscitation*. 2001;49(2):123–134.

28. Palmer JHM, Ball DR. The effect of cricoid pressure on the cricoid cartilage and vocal cords: an endoscopic study in anaesthetised patients. *Anaesthesia*. 2000;55(3):263–268.

29. Hocking G, Roberts FL, Thew ME. Airway obstruction with cricoid pressure and lateral tilt. *Anaesthesia*. 2001;56(9):825–828.

30. Hartsilver EL, Vanner RG. Airway obstruction with cricoid pressure. *Anaesthesia*. 2000;55(3):208–11.

31. Brimacombe J, Keller C, Kunzel KH, et al. Cervical spine motion during airway management: a cinefluoroscopic study of the posteriorly destabilized third cervical vertebrae in human cadavers. *Anesth Analg*. 2000;91(5):1274–1278.

32. Aprahamian C, Thompson BM, Finger WA, et al. Experimental cervical spine injury model: evaluation of airway management and splinting techniques. *Ann Emerg Med*. 1984;13(8):584–587.

33. Donaldson WF 3rd, Heil BV, Donaldson VP, et al. The effect of airway maneuvers on the unstable C1-C2 segment. A cadaver study. *Spine*. 1997;22(11): 1215–1218.

34. Hauswald M, Sklar DP, Tandberg D, et al. Cervical spine movement during airway management: cinefluoroscopic appraisal in human cadavers. *Am J Emerg Med*. 1991;9(6):535–538.

CHAPTER 5

Tracheal Intubation by Direct Laryngoscopy

▶ KEY POINTS

- Direct laryngoscopy remains the procedural standard for emergency intubation.
- The clinician should always psychologically prepare for a difficult airway, in an attempt to "anticipate the unanticipated."
- Special attention must be paid to positioning the morbidly obese patient to facilitate direct laryngoscopy.
- Cricoid pressure and external laryngeal manipulation (ELM) are two separate maneuvers done on two separate structures, for different purposes.
- Failure to engage the hyoepiglottic ligament in the vallecula is a probable cause of the novice failing to achieve an adequate view during direct laryngoscopy.
- Head lift, two-handed laryngoscopy and ELM represent *three* ways to use *two* hands on the *first* intubation attempt ("3–2–1").
- Beware the "pseudolarynx," especially in young children.
- A tracheal tube introducer ("bougie") or fiberoptic stylet can be used on the first intubation attempt when "best look" direct laryngoscopy has failed to yield an adequate view.

- Cervical spine immobilization will often lead to an "epiglottis-only," Grade 3 view during direct laryngoscopy.
- To avoid patient morbidity, esophageal intubations must be immediately recognized and corrected.

▶ INTRODUCTION

This chapter will review direct laryngoscopy and intubation, including the initial response to encountered difficulty. *Direct* laryngoscopy (DL) is so named because it results ideally in *direct* line-of-sight visualization of the glottis (Fig. 5–1). While DL is only one method of facilitating definitive airway management, it is still the procedural standard for intubation in emergencies, and as such is deserving of a detailed discussion. Alternative intubation techniques, including blind naso-tracheal intubation, are discussed in later chapters.

▶ PREPARATION FOR ENDOTRACHEAL INTUBATION

The adage that "your first shot is your best shot" is very applicable to laryngoscopy and intubation. Prior to proceeding with any intubation, it is essential that the following preparations have been undertaken:

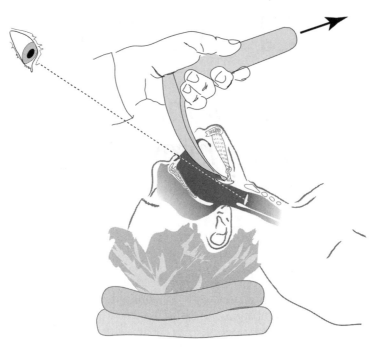

Figure 5–1. Direct laryngoscopy is so-named as it affords a direct line-of-sight view from the clinician's eye to the laryngeal inlet.

A. *Equipment* should be assembled and immediately available for management of either a standard or unanticipated very difficult airway. If possible, this equipment should be prepared prior to the patient's arrival. Ideally, a dedicated airway equipment cart with all the necessary tools, checked daily, should be a fixture in most acute-care areas.

B. The patient and clinician performing the intubation should be **positioned** in the optimal (allowable) position for direct laryngoscopy.

C. The patient has been optimally **preoxygenated.**

D. Large-bore **intravenous (IV) access** has been obtained and a fluid bolus delivered, when appropriate.

E. **Drugs** needed to facilitate airway management are available. Care should be taken to match the drug type and dosage with the patient and any acute or underlying chronic conditions.

F. **Personnel:** Airway management is not a one-person job. *At least* one assistant is necessary to help, guided by specific directions. If problems are anticipated, this should be communicated to the team, and roles assigned before getting started.

▶ EQUIPMENT FOR TRACHEAL INTUBATION

A well-equipped airway cart is not useful unless it is at the bedside and its contents are familiar. The following mnemonic may be helpful to ensure that essential pieces of equipment are immediately available: **STOP "I" "C" BARS.**

Suction—Rigid tonsillar suction is vital, turned on and placed in close proximity to the patient's head. If there is a high likelihood of encountering copious amounts of blood or regurgitated matter, two running suctions are not excessive. The suction tubing must be connected to an appropriate wall unit. The rigid suction catheter should be checked to see if it has a thumb port that must be occluded to work effectively.

Tubes—An appropriately sized endotracheal tube (ETT, e.g., adult female 7.0; adult male 8.0 internal diameter, [ID]) is prepared, as well as a tube a half or full size smaller. Rarely is a larger tube size required in an adult patient. A 10 cc syringe is attached to the pilot line, and the cuff integrity checked by fully inflating, then deflating it. The ETT tip can be lubricated with 2% lidocaine jelly or other water soluble lubricant. For all emergency intubations, a lubricated stylet should be inserted into the ETT. If a curved Macintosh blade is used, the stylet curve should not exceed the default curvature of the ETT. Alternatively, and in particular for a straight blade, a "straight to cuff" shape will be beneficial, whereby the tube is styletted straight, with a 25–35° upward bend placed just proximal to the cuff[1] (Fig. 5–2). For pediatric patients, the Broselow tape can be consulted for appropriate ETT sizing.

Oxygen and positive pressure—A manual resuscitator with oxygen reservoir bag, attached to high flow O_2 should be available. As the only source of positive pressure ventilation, this device should be checked by occluding the patient end with a finger and squeezing the self-inflating bag, feeling for the positive pressure thus developed. The reservoir bag should be distended.

Pharmacology—All the drugs that could possibly be needed should be drawn up *and labeled*. This may include drugs needed for topical airway anesthesia, IV sedation, or rapid-sequence intubation (RSI), including induction agent and muscle relaxant. The armamentarium should always include an agent to treat postintubation hypotension—merely instituting positive pressure ventilation can interfere with venous return and

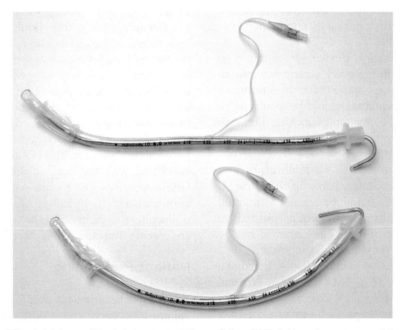

Figure 5–2. "Straight to cuff" stylet preparation of the ETT (above) compared to natural curve (below).

cause hypotension, particularly in the volume-depleted patient.

Intravenous access—Good IV access (ideally 18G or larger) should be in situ, free-flowing and not on a pump. It is rare that a patient will not benefit from a fluid bolus of 10–20 mL/kg prior to intubation.

Connect to monitors and **C**onfirmation—During intubation, the patient should ideally be monitored with an electrocardiogram (ECG) tracing, noninvasive blood pressure cuff (cycling at intervals of no longer than 3 minutes), and a pulse oximeter. In addition, objective means for confirming tracheal location of the ETT should be available, for example, capnometry and/or an esophageal detector device.

Blades and **B**ougie—The laryngoscope should be checked for bright light intensity. Several blades should be available. The #3 Macintosh (curved) blade will be useful as a default blade, with the #4 for larger males. To those familiar with it, a straight blade (e.g., Miller, Phillips, or Wisconsin) can be a useful primary or alternative blade. A tracheal tube introducer (**bougie**) should be within easy reach during *all* emergency intubation attempts.

Alternative intubation device—In addition to the bougie, during every emergency intubation attempt, equipment for an alternative intubation technique should be available for immediate use. Examples include the LMA Fastrach™ (Intubating Laryngeal Mask Airway [ILMA]), fiberoptic optical stylet, or Trachlight. These devices all require preparation by someone familiar with their use. If the patient is being bag-mask ventilated with difficulty in between intubation attempts, the primary clinician will not be available to prepare this equipment.

Rescue oxygenation technique—A Laryngeal Mask Airway (e.g., LMA Classic™, ProSeal, Supreme, or Fastrach), Combitube, or other extraglottic device is useful as a rescue oxygenation tool. One such device should be sized for the patient and within arm's reach

for the infrequent failed intubation or failed oxygenation (Chap. 12) situation.

Surgical (i.e., cricothyrotomy) technique—For most intubations, simply knowing the equipment's location and how to use it is adequate preparation. However, for anticipated very difficult situations, it may be appropriate to have this equipment out and opened: a component of the so-called "double set-up".

▶ POSITIONING FOR LARYNGOSCOPY AND INTUBATION

The clinician should be optimally positioned before an intubation attempt, as should the patient.

Clinician Positioning

Comparisons of the posture of experienced and novice laryngoscopists have observed the following: experienced clinicians stand further back, with straighter backs and arms,[2] and hold the laryngoscope closer to the base of the blade[3] (Fig. 5–3). During direct laryngoscopy, the laryngoscopist's arm should be only modestly flexed at the elbow and adducted, and not bent at right angles and abducted. Better mechanical advantage is then developed by the application of a more in-line axial force through the arm to the handle of the laryngoscope. Once a view of the laryngeal inlet is obtained, some clinicians elect to keep the arm adducted against the trunk for additional support. This position of the arm is consistent with the optimal distance from the laryngoscopist's eye to the patient's glottis of approximately 16–18 inches. Attention to clinician positioning may help deliver favorable mechanical and visual advantage during laryngoscopy.

Patient Positioning

Three aspects of patient positioning are crucial. Failure to observe these positioning principles may make obtaining a good view at laryngoscopy more difficult.

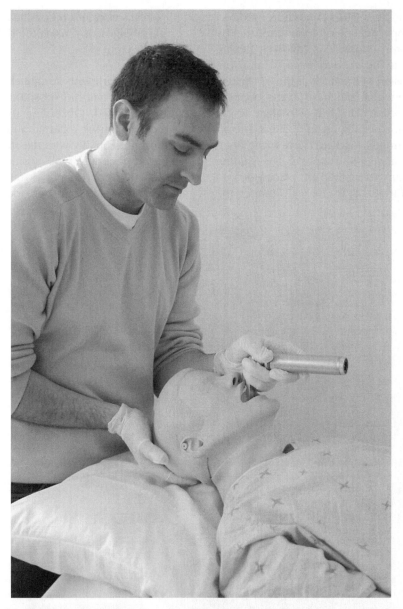

Figure 5–3. Clinician positioning during direct laryngoscopy: relatively straight back; modestly flexed, adducted elbow, and a grip on the laryngoscope handle close to the blade.

A. **"Up-down,"** referring to stretcher height. Often overlooked, the patient should be at the appropriate height—with the middle of the patient's head at the level of the clinician's belt buckle.

B. **"North-south"**: the patient's head should be positioned as close as possible to the upper ("north") end of the stretcher.

C. **"Sniff,"** that is, head and neck positioning. Classic teaching suggests placing the head and neck in the "sniffing" position for direct laryngoscopy. When not contraindicated by C-spine precautions, this involves flexing the neck at the cervico-thoracic junction, with extension of the neck at the upper few cervical vertebrae and head at the occipito-cervical junction. This will help align airway axes, in turn helping attain a direct line-of-sight view from the clinician's eye to the laryngeal inlet (Fig. 3–8, Chap. 3). The sniffing position can be attained by placing folded blankets (about 4"/8 cm high) under the patient's occiput and/or lifting the head during laryngoscopy, using the right hand under the occiput.

The axis alignment sought by placing the patient in the sniffing position can be externally referenced. Observing the patient from the side, when the external auditory meatus is lined up horizontally with the sternal notch, the patient is generally well positioned for laryngoscopy in a good "sniff" position (Figs. 5–4 A and B). This same "ear-to-sternum" positioning

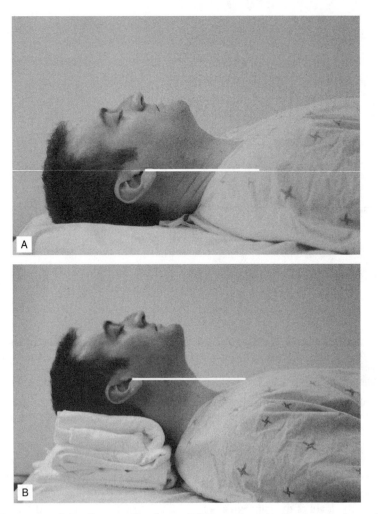

Figures 5–4. In contrast to the positioning of the patient in the neutral position (A), a line drawn from the external auditory meatus to the patient's sternum ("ear to sternum" line) will give a rough indication of good positioning for direct laryngoscopy (B).

is also key to positioning the morbidly obese patient[4] (see next section). While some recent publications have suggested that cervicothoracic flexion is not a necessary component of optimal positioning for laryngoscopy,[5–7] other studies challenge this contention by suggesting the utility of a head lift[8,9] in improving laryngeal view.

▶ POSITIONING IN SPECIAL SITUATIONS

C-Spine Precautions

In the patient requiring C-spine precautions, the sniff position is not an option. DL under these conditions will be more difficult, with an expected incidence of blind, Grade 3 views (no part of the glottis visible) of 20%–25%[10] with application of manual in-line neck stabilization (MILNS). The incidence of Grade 3 views increases to 50% or more[10, 11] with a cervical collar applied. For this reason, during attempts at laryngoscopy and intubation, MILNS should be substituted for the cervical collar, as the latter increases difficulty by also interfering with mouth opening. Note that the function of in-line stabilization is as a reminder to the laryngoscopist to minimize movement, not necessarily to preclude any movement whatsoever.

Morbid Obesity

Airway management in the morbidly obese patient can be difficult in terms of bag-mask ventilation (BMV), laryngoscopy and intubation, as well as cricothyrotomy. In this population, unless the patient is well positioned, during laryngoscopy, the handle of the laryngoscope may abut the chest wall. Specially made short handles can be used in this situation but are usually unnecessary when the patient is properly positioned. Such positioning can be attained by building a ramp with folded blankets (Fig. 5–5). Five to seven folded blankets are placed under the occiput, 3–5 under the shoulders, and 1–3 under the scapulae. This will elevate the face above the chest wall and eliminate the concern of the handle hitting the chest. During "ramping," the unsupported arms are allowed to fall to the side, taking with them additional soft tissue from the anterior chest. These benefits cannot be accomplished by simply raising the head of the bed, nor by just lifting the head of the obese patient at laryngoscopy. Ramping is required in the morbidly obese patient to achieve the previously mentioned "ear to sternum" positioning[4] (Fig. 5–6 A and B).

Pregnancy

The patient in advanced stages of pregnancy must be positioned with a right hip wedge.

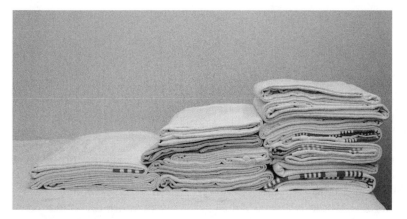

Figure 5–5. A "ramp" created with folded blankets for positioning a morbidly obese patient prior to laryngoscopy.

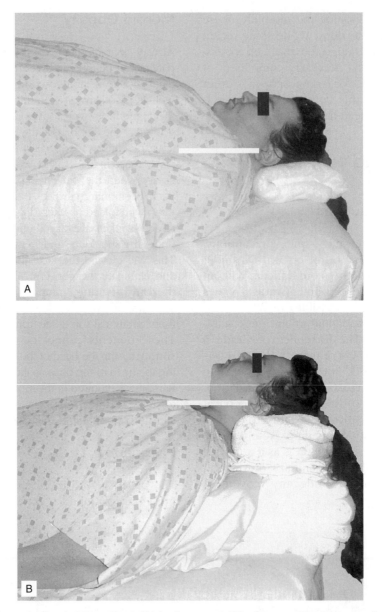

Figure 5–6. A morbidly obese patient (A) before and (B) after positioning on a "ramp" of folded blankets. Note the "ear-sternum" line before and after.

Tipping the gravid uterus to the left will help avoid compression of the aorta and inferior vena cava, which can otherwise cause supine hypotension syndrome. There is also a higher incidence of difficult laryngoscopy and intubation in the obstetrical population,[12] and pregnant patients in the second and third trimesters should be considered at high risk for passive regurgitation.

Both morbidly obese and third trimester pregnant patients have a limited functional residual capacity, and can be expected to desaturate quickly when rendered apneic, for example, during an RSI.

The Patient in Extreme Respiratory Distress

The acutely dyspneic patient will not tolerate the supine position. If an awake intubation is planned, the patient can be intubated in the sitting or semisitting position using DL or other intubation technique. In this situation, the clinician may need to be positioned on a chair at the patient's head (Fig. 5–7). If an RSI is planned, the patient will need to be in the sitting position until loss of consciousness occurs with the induction agent.

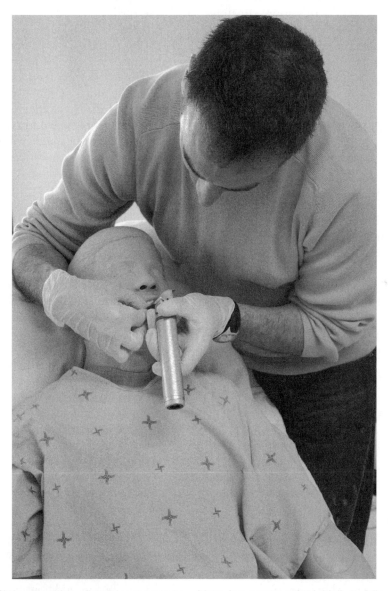

Figure 5–7. Sitting position direct laryngoscopy. Note laryngoscopist initially guiding laryngoscope blade with fingers of right hand.

The Pediatric Patient

The neonate, with its large head and occiput relative to the thorax, will often end up with the neck excessively flexed, if placed supine on a table. This is the one situation in which a folded towel may need to be placed under the shoulders, to *decrease* lower C-spine flexion to the same degree that is needed in the adult. The toddler and young child (to approximately age six) will be well-positioned merely placed with the head flat on a table. Above age six, positioning with the usual towel or folded blanket under the occiput will be needed.

▶ PREOXYGENATION

During the preparation phase, the patient should receive as close to 100% O_2 as possible. Holding a manual resuscitator (supplying O_2 at 15 L/min, with a functioning O_2 reservoir system) firmly on the face is ideal. If the patient's spontaneous ventilations are felt to be inadequate, timed inspiratory assisted ventilation may be required. Obviously, in the apneic patient, positive pressure ventilation will be needed. **Preoxygenation is a vitally important step. Unintentionally omitting this step puts the patient at risk of profound hypoxemia during attempted intubation.**

▶ DIRECT LARYNGOSCOPY

Laryngoscopes and Blades

The laryngoscope used for DL consists of a blade and handle: the handle houses the power supply and sometimes the light source. Generally the laryngoscope blade snaps on to the top of a handle. Rotating the blade to a position 90° to the handle activates the illumination supply, which is delivered toward the tip of the blade. Some blades have a distal bulb-on-blade design, while others transmit light from a bulb located in the handle to the blade tip via a fiberoptic bundle. A fiberoptic laryngoscope with a rechargeable battery system is likely the most dependable and has the potential to provide the brightest lighting. Blades can be reusable or disposable. Disposable blades are made of plastic or steel. As the most important piece of intubation equipment, the laryngoscope should be of reliable quality.

Familiar to many clinicians, the **Macintosh** blade (Fig. 5–8) is curved, designed to partially conform to the shape of the tongue. It is most often used by placing the blade tip in the vallecula, at the junction of the base of the tongue and origin of the epiglottis. As the blade tip is pressed into this space and lifted, pressure on the hyoepiglottic ligament will help indirectly lift the epiglottis anteriorly, exposing the underlying glottic opening. A size 3 Macintosh blade will be appropriate in the majority of adult patients, although in larger patients, especially those with long necks, a Macintosh 4 blade may be needed. Also note that curved blades can be used to directly "pick up" or elevate the epiglottis.

Straight laryngoscope blades (Fig. 5–9) such as the **Miller, Phillips,** or **Wisconsin** are designed primarily to displace the tongue to the left and directly elevate the epiglottis, thus exposing the vocal cords. Often used as the blades of choice in pediatric patients, they can also be useful in the adult patient with an "anterior" larynx, small mandible, large tongue, or prominent central incisors.[13] Many straight blade aficionados prefer its use by a **paraglossal** approach, whereby the blade is placed alongside the tongue, on its right. This approach has been shown to be effective in some situations where curved blade laryngoscopy had failed.[14]

Finally, specialty blades exist to help in difficult situations. The **McCoy blade,** also known as the **levering tip** or **CLM (Corazelli-London-McCoy)** blade, has the basic shape of the Macintosh, but in addition, features a levering

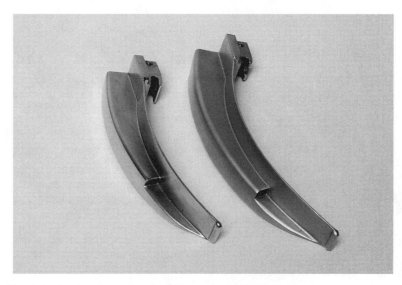

Figure 5–8. Macintosh size 3 and 4 (adult) curved blades.

distal tip. When an activating lever is depressed toward the laryngoscope handle (Figs. 5–10 A and B), the blade tip levers upward, helping to elevate the epiglottis (Figs. 5–11 A and B).

The literature suggests it may be useful in converting Grade 3 views to 2 or better, particularly when caused by applied manual in-line stabilization.[15–18]

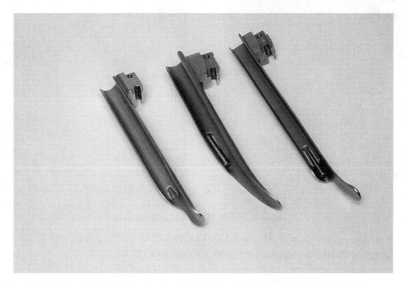

Figure 5–9. From left to right, Wisconsin, Phillips, and Miller straight blades.

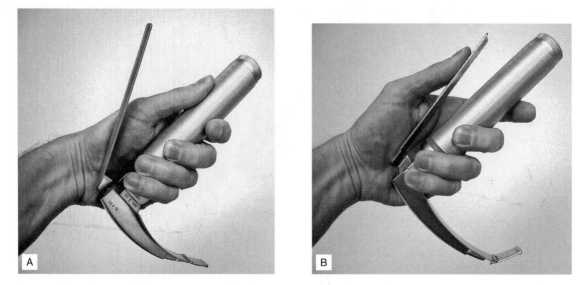

Figure 5–10.   A, B The McCoy (CLM) blade, (A) in the neutral and (B) partially activated positions.

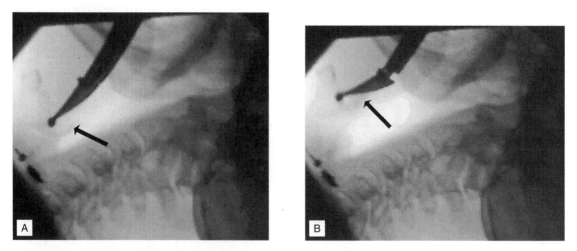

Figure 5–11.   Fluoroscopic images of the McCoy blade (A) before and (B) after partial blade tip activation (the arrow in both images points to the epiglottis).

Direct Laryngoscopy Technique: General Comments

In performing DL, a few points are noteworthy:

A. To successfully perform direct laryngoscopy, the clinician must be very familiar with the anatomy of the oropharynx and laryngeal inlet (reviewed in Chapter 3). A sound knowledge of the anatomy will help the clinician obtain an optimal view during laryngoscope blade placement.

B. As emphasized earlier, the patient *and* the clinician should be properly positioned, with the stretcher elevated, the patient at the head of the bed and the head and neck in the sniff position (if not contraindicated). Optimal positioning should be undertaken prior to the first attempt at laryngoscopy, and not deferred until difficulty has already been encountered.

C. A cross-finger "scissor" technique is useful to help open the mouth for initial blade insertion: the thumb pushes the mandible/lower teeth caudad to open the mouth, while the index finger crosses over the thumb to provide counterpressure on the maxilla/upper teeth (Fig. 5–12).

D. The laryngoscope handle should be held close to the blade. Better mechanical advantage will result and there will be less tendency to lever back with the scope.

E. Following initial blade insertion, the clinician's right hand can be placed under the patient's occiput: with this hand concomitantly lifting the head, additional lower neck flexion and head extension can be undertaken, (i.e., exaggerated "sniff"), often helping to expose the cords during laryngoscopy.

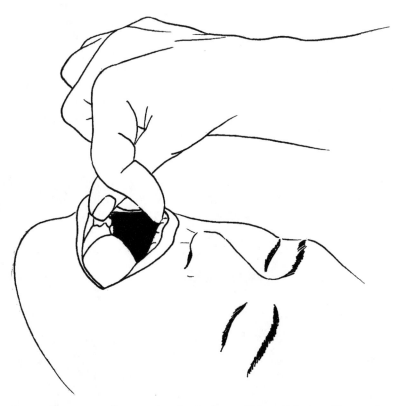

Figure 5–12. Cross-finger mouth opening technique. This will help with oropharyngeal airway, extraglottic device, and laryngoscope blade insertion.

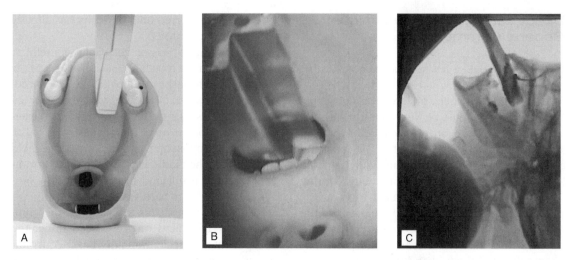

Figure 5–13. Direct laryngoscopy: Initial blade insertion—(A) on a model, (B) in a human subject, and (C) under fluoroscopy.

Direct Laryngoscopy Technique: Curved/Macintosh Blade

The laryngoscope handle is held in the left hand. Dentures, if present, should be removed. The patient's mouth is opened with the right hand, using the previously described cross-finger technique. The blade should be inserted on the right side of the tongue (Figs. 5–13 A, B, and C) and is advanced to its base. This should happen **slowly** and deliberately, taking time to identify anatomy at the blade tip—with adequate preoxygenation, there is no rush. This "identify-as-you-go" technique will help avoid placing the blade too far, an error commonly committed by the novice clinician. As the base of the tongue is approached, some traction is exerted along the long axis of the laryngoscope handle (Figure 5–1) to start compressing the tongue (Figs. 5–14 A, B and C).

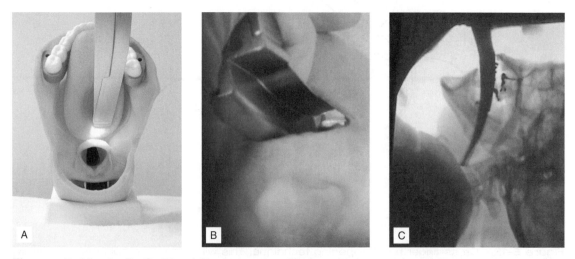

Figures 5–14. A, B, C. Direct laryngoscopy: Blade advancement and tongue compression, looking for landmarks—(A) on a model, (B) in a human subject, and (C) under fluoroscopy.

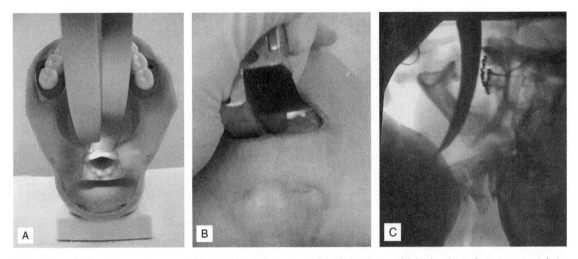

Figures 5–15. Direct laryngoscopy: Identification of epiglottis and blade tip advancement into vallecula—(A) on a model, (B) in a human subject, and (C) under fluoroscopy.

A view of the epiglottis is sought: it is an important landmark, needed to guide subsequent blade placement. After the epiglottis is identified, the tip of the blade is advanced into the vallecula (the space at the junction of the base of the tongue and the origin of the epiglottis, Figs. 5–15 A, B, and C). Once the blade is placed fully into the vallecula, the blade tip is centered, by moving it to the left. This will further displace the tongue to the left. With the blade tip now seated in the vallecula, additional lift can be applied along the longitudinal axis of the laryngoscope handle (Figs. 5–16 A and B). **The handle should generally not**

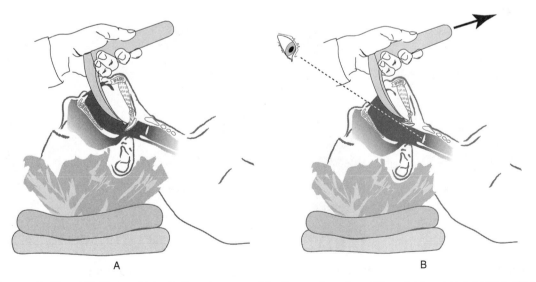

Figure 5–16. (A) Curved blade tip placement in the vallecula, with subsequent traction along the long axis of the laryngoscope handle (B), indicated by the arrow. Note the resultant indirect elevation of the epiglottis.

exceed an angle of about 30° to the floor. Thus lifting forward along the handle's axis has two effects: (a) it will further compress the tongue out of the way into the submandibular space, and (b) the blade tip will place pressure on the underlying hyoepiglottic ligament, in turn helping to lift the epiglottis, revealing the vocal cords beneath (Figs. 5–17 A, B and C). It should be noted that if a chosen blade is too short to successfully contact the hyoepiglottic ligament at the junction of the tongue base and epiglottis, the epiglottis may not move up and out of the way (Figs. 5–18 A and B). If this is suspected, a longer blade should be used. Failure to engage the hyoepiglottic ligament in the vallecula is a probable cause of the novice failing to achieve an adequate view during direct laryngoscopy. Conversely, too long a blade can occasionally trap and downfold the epiglottis, artificially creating a Grade 3 view.

The laryngoscope should never be levered back while attempting to attain a view at laryngoscopy. This puts the upper teeth at risk of damage, and also decreases the space available for initial tube passage through the mouth.

Direct Laryngoscopy Technique: Straight Blade

The straight blade is often used to displace the tongue laterally, followed by direct lifting of the epiglottis to expose the larynx (Fig. 5–19). Using this "paraglossal," or alongside-the-tongue approach, the blade is inserted from the right side of the mouth (Fig. 5–20) and advanced along the right margin of the tongue. With the tongue displaced to the left, the jaw is lifted by traction along the axis of the laryngoscope handle. Two schools of thought exist about subsequent glottic exposure: one suggests advancing the blade as far as it will go (i.e., down the upper esophagus), then withdrawing until the cords "pop" into view, while the other espouses an "identify as you go" method, as is the case with curved blade placement. With this latter technique, once the epiglottis is identified, the blade tip is "scooped" beneath the epiglottis to achieve its direct elevation (Fig. 5–21).

The view of the cords at the blade tip with straight blade laryngoscopy is often combined with a restricted space at the right lateral corner

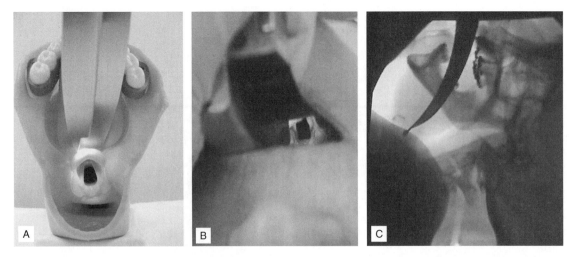

Figure 5–17. Direct laryngoscopy: Blade lift together with caudad pressure on hyoepiglottic ligament to elevate epiglottis and expose underlying laryngeal inlet—(A) on a model, (B) in a human subject, and (C) by fluoroscopy.

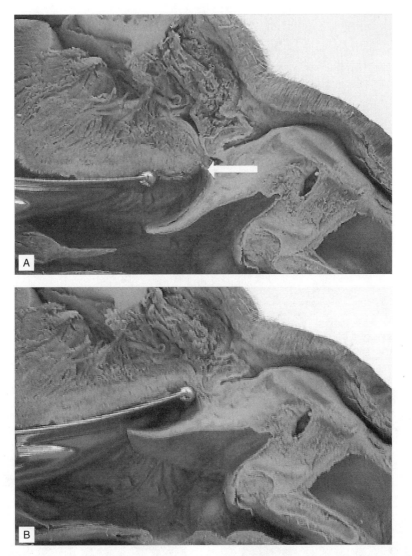

Figure 5-18. A, B. (A) Failure to advance the blade tip completely into the vallecula (arrow) results in no contact with the hyoepiglottic ligament, with resultant failure to indirectly lift the epiglottis. (B) With the blade tip correctly located in the vallecula, contact with the hyoepiglottic ligament results in good indirect lifting of the epiglottis.

of the mouth. Passage of the ETT under these circumstances may obscure the view of the cords. This may be overcome by having an assistant apply lateral traction to the lip at the corner of the mouth, thus creating room for ETT passage from the right. Alternatively, prior passage of a bougie may help to overcome this restriction at the proximal position of the blade. For primary passage of a styletted ETT, the distal tube should be bent upward just proximal to the cuff by no more than 35°, as more acute angulation is associated with difficult tube passage.[1]

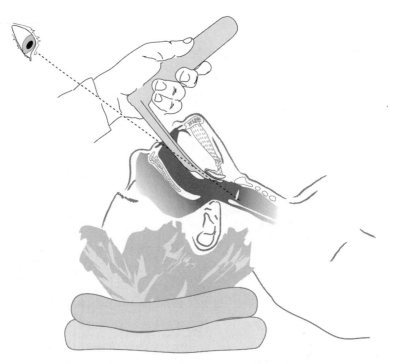

Figure 5–19. Straight blade laryngoscopy with the epiglottis being directly lifted to allow direct visualization of the glottis.

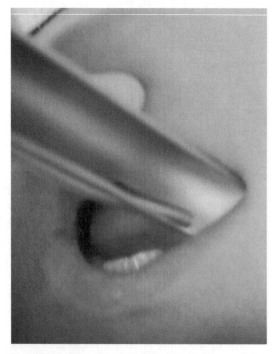

Figure 5–20. Straight blade insertion at the right side of the mouth as part of a paraglossal approach to direct laryngoscopy.

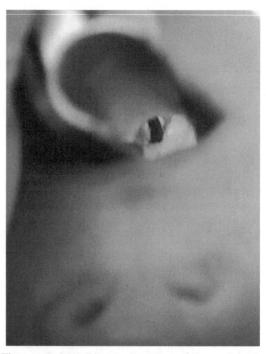

Figure 5–21. Direct elevation of the epiglottis using the Phillips straight blade for a paraglossal approach to direct laryngoscopy.

▶ PASSING THE ENDOTRACHEAL TUBE (ETT)

The prepared tube, with lubricated stylet in place, should be passed by an assistant to the clinician's open right hand, thereby avoiding the need to interrupt direct visualization of cords. With curved blade use, the ETT should be placed from the right side of the patient's mouth, with its concavity initially facing to the right ("three o'clock"), to avoid obscuring the view of the cords. As the tip of the tube approaches the cords, the ETT is rotated counterclockwise (to the "12 o'clock" position), naturally bringing its tip anterior. When using a straight blade, the tube is passed from the extreme right, with the distal ETT tip pointed back toward the midline laryngeal inlet. In the spontaneously breathing patient, the tube should be passed during inspiration to avoid trauma to the cords. **Remember that one of the most important signs of a properly placed tube is to watch it go through the cords** (Fig. 5–22). Tube passage should occur slowly enough to be able to satisfactorily visually confirm it has indeed passed between the cords. The tube should be advanced to about 21 cm at the teeth. Once positioned, the tube is held with one hand, the laryngoscope removed, and the cuff inflated with 5–8 mL of air. The syringe is detached and the stylet removed from the tube (if not already done). Objective confirmation of the correct (endotracheal) location of the ETT should then be undertaken, and positive pressure ventilation (PPV) instituted at a controlled rate.

Note that occasionally, in the confusion surrounding intubation, the ETT cuff is not inflated. This may result in the failure of typical objective and subjective signs of endotracheal intubation, including end-tidal carbon dioxide ($ETCO_2$) detection, chest rise, and breath sounds with positive pressure. Conversely, cuff overinflation is also undesirable and can be avoided by seeking the "minimum-leak" pressure after the tube position has been confirmed. This is done during PPV by gradually withdrawing air from the cuff, one milliliter (mL) at a time, until a leak is heard: at that point, the cuff is reinflated by one additional mL. This maneuver will help avoid excessive cuff pressure with resultant ischemia of the tracheal mucosa.

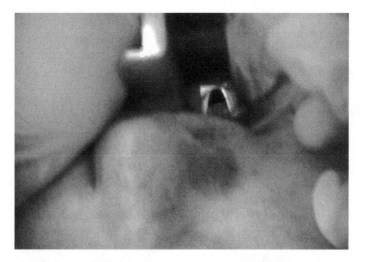

Figure 5–22. Visualization of the ETT being passed between the cords, from the right side of the mouth.

Although the authors advocate the use of a stylet for every intubation, the applied curve should not be exaggerated (i.e., "hockey-sticked") for either curved or straight blade use. This excessive bend, commonly advocated, was historically used to help intubate the poorly visualized larynx. The authors contend that other techniques and adjuncts (i.e., head lift, external laryngeal manipulation [ELM], bougie, or fiberoptic stylet) deal more effectively with the poorly visualized larynx. Furthermore, the use of a hockey-stick type bend may lead to difficulty with forward tube passage down the trachea,[1] as the ETT tip may get caught anteriorly on the cricoid or a tracheal cartilaginous ring.

▶ CONFIRMATION OF ETT LOCATION

Following intubation, confirmation of the tracheal location of the ETT is obviously vital. Unrecognized esophageal intubations still occur, sometimes with lethal results. In general, it can be said that there are **objective**[19] and more **subjective** means of confirming ETT location. For every intubation, at least **two objective criteria** of ETT location should be met.

Objective Methods of Confirming Endotracheal Tube Location

Observing the ETT Go Through the Cords

If the ETT is visualized going between the cords (Fig. 5–22), it must be in the correct place. A few additional comments on this otherwise simplistic statement are in order:

- This is such an important confirmatory sign that the ETT should be placed slowly and deliberately, allowing time to consciously confirm that the ETT is indeed visible between the cords.
- This is the reason the ETT should be inserted from the right side of the mouth—to

allow ongoing visualization of the cords during ETT placement.
- If intubation has been undertaken in the face of a poorly visualized glottic opening, applying downward (posterior) pressure on the ETT while continuing to apply an upward lift on the laryngoscope (the "Ford maneuver") may sometimes allow visualization of posterior elements of the larynx.
- Beware the "pseudolarynx," especially in young children. When strong upward traction is exerted on the tip of a long blade, the esophageal opening can become elongated. As the stretched mucosa becomes ischemic, the lateral walls of this opening can become "blanched," potentially looking like true or false cords to the inexperienced clinician. This point underscores the necessity of being very familiar with the anatomy of the laryngeal inlet, from the pearly white appearance and shape of the cords superiorly, to the expected paired posterior cartilages framing the inlet inferiorly.

End-Tidal Carbon Dioxide (ETCO$_2$) Detection

ETCO$_2$ detection to confirm endotracheal intubation has rapidly become a standard of care in emergency airway management. The technique provides a simple and inexpensive method of confirming correct endotracheal, as opposed to esophageal tube placement. A disposable CO$_2$ detector is simply placed in-line at the ETT connector (in the patient with a cardiac output). The presence of exhaled CO$_2$ will be indicated by a change in color, for example, from purple to yellow (Fig. 5–23).

Continuously reading capnographs are being used increasingly in out-of-operating room (OR) environments, using infrared spectrometry to measure and display carbon dioxide concentration in inspired and expired gas. This enables monitoring of mechanical ventilation and procedural sedation. Under normal circumstances, gas

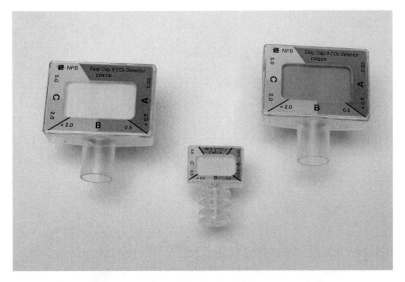

Figure 5-23. Easy Cap II colorimetric end-tidal CO_2 detection will result in a color change from purple to yellow. A pediatric version is available for patients <15 kg.

sampled at the end of expiration (the $ETCO_2$) closely approximates the arterial pCO_2. The combination of pulse oximetry with capnography can non-invasively provide the near-equivalent of real-time arterial blood-gas analysis.

However, like oximetry, capnography has important limitations. Of particular significance in the emergency intubation is the observation that profound shock (or cardiac arrest) may lead to significant pulmonary hypoperfusion and reduced (or absent) CO_2 delivery from tissue to lung. This obviously limits the utility of capnography to confirm endotracheal intubation in arrested patients. However, capnography is not completely useless during resuscitation: it has been shown to be an effective early indicator of the return of circulation after successful resuscitation from cardiac arrest.

$ETCO_2$ DETECTION EFFECTIVENESS

False positive readings (i.e., tube in esophagus, yet color change still occurs) can occur in three situations: (a) CO_2 has been washed in to the esophagus during previous bag-mask ventilation; (b) the patient has ingested carbonated beverages; or (c) the patient has ingested sodium bicarbonate–containing antacids, which, combined with stomach hydrochloric acid, can result in CO_2 release.[20] However, in all of these situations, rapid washout of CO_2 should occur: hence the recommendation to only attach the $ETCO_2$ detector after several breaths have already been delivered (the "six-breath rule"), to help improve sensitivity and specificity.

Esophageal Detector Devices

The principle behind esophageal detector device (EDD) use is that the esophagus collapses when a negative pressure is applied to its lumen, whereas the trachea does not.[21] EDDs come in two forms:

- A 60 cc catheter-tipped (Toomey) syringe can be used. Normally used for aspirating or irrigating foley catheters or nasogastric tubes, the tip of such a syringe can be forced into the end of the ETT connector after intubation (Fig. 5–24). The syringe plunger is aspirated and released. If the plunger stays out, there is no negative pressure, implying

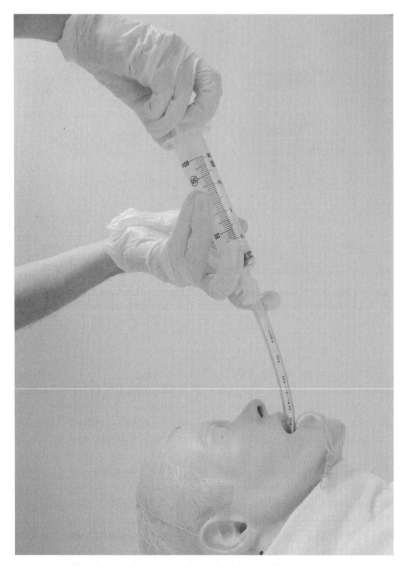

Figure 5–24. A Toomey syringe used as an esophageal detector device.

it has aspirated air out of the tracheal air-space and the tube is correctly sited. If the plunger slides back to near its original position, the ETT is in the esophagus. In the latter situation, the esophagus has collapsed around the ETT tip with aspiration, creating a vacuum. Purpose-made syringes with 15 mm connectors for easy ETT attachment are available commercially, at greater cost.

- A second type of EDD uses a rubber bulb proximally on a syringe (akin to and sometimes called a "turkey baster"), which returns to inflated conformation spontaneously after being squeezed. The bulb is squeezed and the device attached to the ETT. If it refills quickly (with air from the tracheal airspace), the ETT is in the trachea. If it stays depressed or refills slowly, the ETT is in the esophagus.

EDD Effectiveness

Esophageal detector devices have been shown to be very sensitive and specific, at least in healthy patients.[22] They should be considered a good choice to help objectively confirm correct ETT placement in the arrested patient, where $ETCO_2$ detectors may be unreliable. False negative results (i.e., tube is in trachea, syringe does not easily aspirate, or bulb fails to inflate) may occur with a tube obstructed with mucus or secretions; with severe bronchospasm; in the morbidly obese patient; and in other conditions, such as pulmonary edema, which cause markedly decreased dead space.[20] While still accurate in detecting esophageal intubation after intentional moderate gastric insufflation, the EDD may fail after massive gastric insufflation.[22] This suggests that in contrast to the "6-breath rule" for the $ETCO_2$ detector, an EDD should be used before any further ventilation occurs through a newly placed ETT.

Visualization of Tracheal Rings

Visualization of tracheal cartilaginous rings, and/or carina through the ETT with a flexible fiberoptic bronchoscope, or semimalleable fiberoptic stylet can be considered a fourth objective sign of tracheal intubation (Fig. 5–25).

Subjective (Clinical) Signs of Tracheal Intubation

Clinical signs of successful tracheal intubation have been classically relied upon to confirm tracheal ETT location in out-of-OR intubations. While these signs should still be sought, they should complement the objective signs as delineated above, and not be substituted for them.

- **Chest Auscultation.** Although the chest should be observed for expansion and auscultated following intubation, generally speaking, this should not be relied upon to confirm endotracheal intubation.[23] For example, in the scenario where a patient has been intubated via an "awake" technique using topical airway anesthesia, the spontaneously breathing patient may continue to have breath sounds and chest expansion, even in face of an esophageal intubation. Auscultation is obviously still

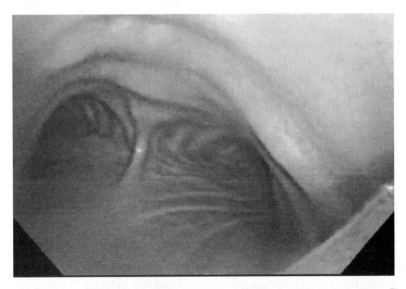

Figure 5–25. Tracheal cartilaginous rings and the carina, as seen though a fiberoptic bronchoscope passed down an endotracheal tube.

useful, as long as this limitation is appreciated, but should be used mainly to rule out right mainstem intubation or previously missed pneumothorax.

- **Increasing oxygen saturation.** In a well preoxygenated patient, oxygen desaturation following apnea can take up to 8 minutes. In addition, slow processors in some older pulse oximeters take a while to react to and indicate increasing (or decreasing) oxygen saturation.

- **BVM device compliance.** After intubation, if the initial compliance of the BVM bag is poor (i.e., it is hard to squeeze), an esophageal intubation should be suspected. Note that significant bronchospasm can create the same effect with a correctly sited ETT, however.

- **Vapor or misting** on the inside of the ETT on expiration. This is **not** a reliable sign of tracheal intubation, as ETT misting can also occur with esophageal tube placement.[24,25]

- **The patient can no longer speak.** If the patient was groaning before intubation and is still groaning after intubation, the tube is probably misplaced! With a tracheally placed ETT, with cuff inflated, vocalization cannot occur.

- **Auscultation over the stomach.** If sounds are heard coincident with delivery of positive pressure ventilation on auscultation of the epigastrium, esophageal intubation should be suspected. The suggestion by some to leave the esophageal ETT in situ during a reintubation attempt may be impractical, as it crowds the oral cavity and, more importantly, precludes optimal oxygenation/ ventilation by mask between attempts.

- **Heart rate and BP normalize.** A hypoxic patient may become hyper- or hypotensive and initially tachycardic. Bradycardia occurs as a later sign of profound hypoxia in adults, although earlier in children. Such continued worsening of vital signs suggests an esophageal intubation.

- **Chest x-ray.** An anterior-posterior portable chest x-ray will not distinguish trachea from esophagus. It may be useful to confirm correct depth of the ETT and to rule out pneumothorax or other chest pathology.

To reiterate, while the clinical signs are good to see, and should be sought, correct positioning of the ETT in the trachea should always be with **two** of the **objective** signs, for example, visualization of tube between cords and either $ETCO_2$ detection (with perfusing rhythm), or an esophageal detector device (patient in cardiac arrest).

▶ DIFFICULT DIRECT LARYNGOSCOPY

The remainder of this chapter discusses the initial response to difficult direct laryngoscopy. Note that difficult *laryngoscopy* does not always imply difficult tracheal *intubation*: even with no view of the glottic opening visible, a bougie may allow easy first-attempt intubation with blind passage beneath the epiglottis. Conversely, difficult intubation can still occur with a full view of the cords, as may be the case in a patient with subglottic stenosis.

Defining Difficult Laryngoscopy

DL usually results in visualization of all, or at least part of the glottic opening. Simply put, difficult laryngoscopy refers to the Cormack Grade 3 or 4 view,[26] where the view of the glottic opening is obscured (Fig. 3–11, Chap. 3).

Response to Difficult Direct Laryngoscopy

Maximizing the chances of **first pass success** at DL and intubation is important since, as discussed in Chap. 12, patient morbidity and mortality climbs with multiple attempts at emergency intubation.[27] As such, the clinician should always perform optimal DL on the first attempt, with the expectation of obtaining a good view, using all the components of "best look" laryngoscopy. These components, some of which have already been discussed, are reviewed below and summarized in Table 5–1.

Patient Positioning
- Stretcher at the correct height; patient at head of stretcher.
- Patient is in sniff position, if not contraindicated.

Clinician Positioning
- Clinician is positioned with a relatively straight back, and a slightly flexed, adducted laryngoscopy arm.
- Laryngoscope is held towards the blade.

▶ **TABLE 5–1** COMPONENTS OF "BEST LOOK" LARYNGOSCOPY

- **Patient positioning optimized**: patient at head of bed; stretcher height good; ear-sternum line optimized unless contraindicated.
- **Optimal muscle relaxation** has occurred, if used.
- **Laryngoscopist's positioning optimized**: Laryngoscope held towards blade; back straight, arm modestly flexed and adducted +/- stabilized on trunk.
- **Appropriate blade tip location**: With indirect epiglottis lift, blade tip in vallecula is contacting hyoepiglottic ligament.
- **Appropriate laryngoscope lift**: along axis of the handle. Use second hand if needed.
- **Head lift**: Use right hand to lift head (if not contraindicated) during laryngoscopy.
- **ELM/BURP**: to bring the laryngeal inlet into view.
- Consider whether **cricoid pressure** is adversely affecting the view.
- **Use adjunct to DL**, e.g., bougie (tracheal tube introducer) or fiberoptic stylet.

Muscle Relaxant
If an RSI technique is in use, the muscle relaxant should have had time to onset. Inexperienced clinicians sometimes fail to wait the 45–60 seconds required for full effect from an intubating dose of skeletal muscle relaxant.

Epiglottis Control
The epiglottis must be identified and controlled, with advancement of the curved blade tip fully into the vallecula, or by direct lifting.

Appropriate Laryngoscope Lift
Forward traction should be applied along the long axis of the laryngoscope handle. With the left hand already holding the base of the laryngoscope handle, if necessary, the right hand can be placed further up the handle (Fig. 5–26). This two-handed approach, although rarely needed, helps in applying the appropriate lifting force, and tends to promote traction in the appropriate direction, along the long axis of the laryngoscope handle, thus decreasing any tendency to lever the laryngoscope. Once the view of the glottic opening is attained, the left arm can be adducted against the clinician's trunk to help maintain a lifting force long enough to place the ETT with the right hand. Alternatively, an assistant's hand placed under the head can help maintain the view during ETT placement.

Head Lift
Performing a **head lift** during laryngoscopy, when not contraindicated by C-spine precautions, may improve the view of the laryngeal inlet.[8,9] During laryngoscopy, the clinician's right hand is placed under the occiput and lifts the head upwards, keeping the face parallel to the floor (Fig. 5–27). This increases lower neck flexion, while also increasing extension of the head and the upper C-spine, resulting in a more pronounced "sniffing" position. Indeed, it can be thought of as "customizing" patient head and neck positioning to exactly that needed for an optimal view. Once this optimal view has been obtained, an assistant's hand replaces the

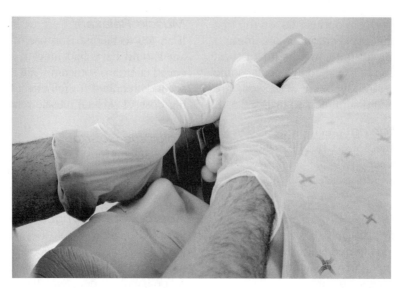

Figure 5-26. Direct laryngoscopy with a second hand aiding the lift along the long axis of the laryngoscope handle.

clinician's under the occiput, freeing up the clinician's right hand to place the endotracheal tube. Head lift, and/or assisted traction on the laryngoscope handle with a second hand, may help in situations where the clinician of lesser stature is faced with intubating a larger patient.

External Laryngeal Manipulation (ELM) or "BURP"

Posterior and cephalad pressure applied to the thyroid (synonymous with laryngeal) cartilage during DL will often improve glottic exposure. This maneuver is referred to as BURP[28]

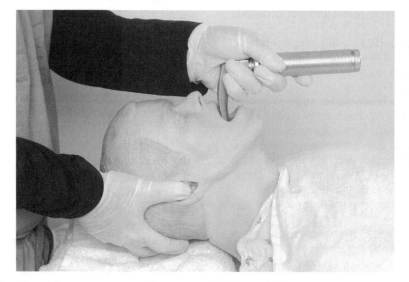

Figure 5-27. Direct laryngoscopy with concomitant head lift.

(**b**ackward, **u**pward and to the laryngoscopist's **r**ight **p**ressure) or ELM. ELM represents a less prescribed manipulation of the thyroid cartilage, still aimed at bringing the glottic inlet into view (Fig. 5–28). This highly effective maneuver should be a reflex response whenever a poor view is obtained at laryngoscopy.

The initial attempt at ELM should be done by the clinician, who gets immediate feedback on its effectiveness. If ELM is deemed beneficial, an assistant will then have to reproduce the effect while the clinician places the endotracheal tube. The clinician may need to verbally or manually guide the assistant's fingers on the thyroid cartilage, until the optimal view is reproduced.

ELM EFFECTIVENESS

It should be noted that confusion exists in the minds of some about the function of cricoid pressure or Sellick's maneuver (done to prevent passive regurgitation of stomach contents), and ELM (done to improve the view of the laryngeal inlet at laryngoscopy). **Cricoid pressure and ELM are two separate maneuvers, applied to two separate structures, for different purposes.** Excessive cricoid pressure, or the combination of ELM with cricoid pressure, may in fact worsen the view during laryngoscopy.[32–34] When faced with a Grade 3 or 4 view at DL (e.g., during an RSI), cricoid pressure can be transiently eased or released to see if the view improves.

Several studies looking at the efficacy of ELM/BURP [29–32] concluded that ELM improved the laryngoscopic view by one whole grade in most patients initially rated Grade 2 or 3. Of interest, in two studies, *all* patients presenting a Grade 3 (epiglottis only) view were converted to Grade 1 or 2 with ELM.[29, 31] These manipulations were effective with both curved and straight blade laryngoscopy.[31] This literature strongly supports the use of this maneuver during any laryngoscopy where a suboptimal view is obtained.

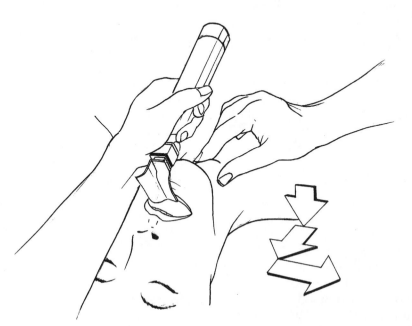

Figure 5–28. External Laryngeal Manipulation (ELM), or Backward, Upward to the Right Pressure ("BURP") to help expose the cords at direct laryngoscopy.

Note that the strategies outlined in (E) and (F) and (G) above represent *three* ways to use *two* hands on the *first* attempt ("3–2–1"), and reflect the concept of DL being a two-handed procedure.

Use of an Adjunct to Direct Laryngoscopy

Use of a tracheal tube introducer (bougie) or fiberoptic stylet can also be undertaken during the first attempt at direct laryngoscopy, when faced with an obscured view despite optimal technique. These devices are discussed in more detail in the following sections.

Consideration of a Change of Blade Type, Length, or Location

For a second attempt at DL, a blade change can be considered, if it is likely to help.

▶ ADJUNCTS TO DIRECT LARYNGOSCOPY: THE TRACHEAL TUBE INTRODUCER (BOUGIE)

If optimal laryngoscopy with head lift or ELM has failed to yield a good view of the glottic opening, the **tracheal tube introducer** (also known as the gum elastic bougie, Eschmann stylet, or simply the bougie) can be a valuable adjunct to DL. It can be beneficial in the following situations:

- **Grade 3 (epiglottis only) view:** A bougie can be used to gently blindly access the trachea, with subsequent tube passage over it.
- **Poor Grade 2 view:** When only the posterior cartilages or interarytenoid notch are visible, tube passage can still be difficult. Prior passage of the bougie above the cartilages will help ease tube passage.
- **As a general intubation aid:** For example, a bougie may help address difficult tube passage with straight blade use due to restricted space at the corner of the mouth.

Although many clinicians are adept at blindly "hooking" a styletted ETT under the epiglottis in the Grade 3 situation, use of the bougie holds the following advantages:

- Relative to the size of the glottic opening, the bougie is smaller in diameter than an ETT, increasing chances of successful blind tracheal access.
- Following blind passage, tactile feedback is transmitted from the bougie to the clinician's fingers, helping to indicate successful tracheal access before tube passage (discussed in more detail below).
- Most importantly, when compared directly to blind placement of a styletted ETT in the grade 3 situation, success using the bougie is significantly higher.[35]

Bougie Description

Made in different disposable and reusable versions by multiple manufacturers, bougies are approximately 60–70 cm long, accept a 5.5 or 6.0 mm ID or larger ETT, and have a distal upward-bending coudé tip (Fig. 5–29). Most have markings on the shaft indicating 10 cm distances. Many users advocate creating additional temporary curvature by bending the distal third of the bougie in a circle, to bring the tip into contact with the 30 cm marker just before use.[36]

Strictly speaking, the gum elastic bougie is none of those things: the reusable version is (latex free) woven polyester; it is not elastic, nor is it a dilating bougie![37] While a better term is the tracheal tube introducer, the bougie terminology will be retained in this narrative as it remains the commonly used name.

Bougie Use

If a Grade 3 view is encountered, persistent after ELM and head lift, the bougie is picked up,

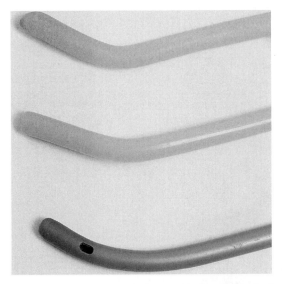

Figure 5–29. The distal coudé tip, angled at 35°, of various brands of single- and multiuse bougie.

and holding it at around the 20-cm mark, it is gently placed via the corner of the mouth and advanced towards the midline beneath the epiglottis, seeking to keep its tip in contact with the undersurface of the epiglottis (Figs. 5–30 and 5–31). Often a slight "pop" will be felt as it advances through the glottic opening, whereupon it is further advanced. Two tactile phenomena can then be sought to confirm that endotracheal, and not esophageal placement, has been achieved.

- Firstly, once the bougie tip has passed through the cords and is being advanced down the trachea, a fine **"click-click" sensation** may often (>90% of the time)[38] be appreciated, as the tip runs over the tracheal cartilaginous rings. Experience suggests, however, that this sensation can vary considerably from patient to patient, from nothing more than a feeling of fine sandpaper in some, to a fairly overt click-click in others. No such sensation is generally obtained if advancing down the esophagus.

- The second sign suggesting tracheal placement of the bougie is that with continued advancement, **resistance will be encountered as it "holds up" in a small distal airway.** This holdup will occur at about the 30 cm mark (plus or minus 5 cm in the adult)

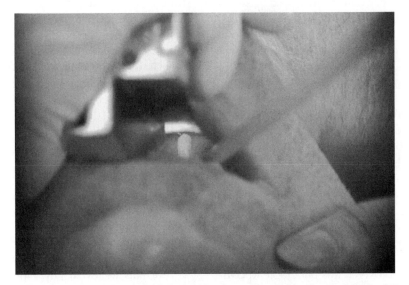

Figure 5–30. Placement of the angled tip of the bougie under the epiglottis into the trachea.

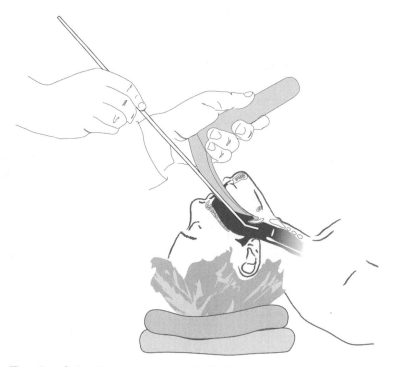

Figure 5–31. The tip of the bougie is placed blindly beneath the epiglottis, keeping its tip midline and anterior.

(Fig. 5–32) and is a consistent finding if the bougie is correctly placed in the trachea.[38] If the bougie can still be advanced at 40 cm or more, it is most likely in esophagus. Bougie hold-up, if sought, should be done gently in order to avoid trauma to the lower bronchi, and should probably be avoided if the clinician already suspects successful tracheal access based on tracheal clicks.

- Softer, **third and fourth** signs of successful tracheal access are coughing or bucking in the incompletely paralyzed patient, and a slight tendency for the bougie to twist clockwise in the clinician's fingers as it hits carina and heads down the right mainstem bronchus.

Once the bougie is suspected to have been successfully placed in the trachea, the ETT can then be advanced over it. It is preferable to **continue performing laryngoscopy** as the ETT is advanced over the bougie (Fig. 5–33), to help control the tongue, elevate the epiglottis, and straighten the axes. Once the tube has been placed in the trachea, the laryngoscope blade is removed and, while holding the ETT firmly, the bougie is removed. Note that if successfully used in a Grade 3 situation, one of the "gold standards" of endotracheal placement will be lacking: having visualized the ETT passing through the cords. Thus, $ETCO_2$ and/or EDD confirmation of ETT placement is even more vital.

Bougie Troubleshooting

Although bougie use is most often straightforward, a few problems can be encountered:

A. **Failure to access the trachea**. The situation where the epiglottis has been elevated, but fails to reveal any aspect of the glottis (so-called Grade 3A, Fig. 3–12, Chap. 3) is

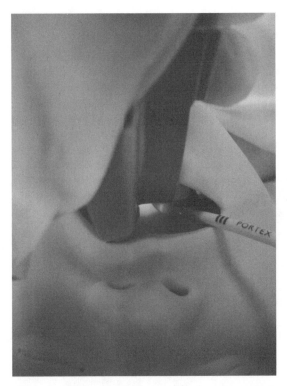

Figure 5-32. As the bougie is advanced, obtaining a tactile sensation from tracheal rings and a holdup close to the 30 cm marking (arrow) suggests successful tracheal access.

ideal for bougie use. However, occasionally the bougie tip fails to slip easily through the cords. While continuing optimal laryngoscopy, the bougie should be rotated slightly to left or right, while maintaining gentle forward pressure. This will help the tip slip off the right or left true or false vocal fold or away from the anterior commissure. Successful tracheal access following these maneuvers is often heralded by a slight "popping" sensation, as the bougie slides off the obstructing structure and advances through the cords.

B. **Posteriorly directed epiglottis**. In situations where the epiglottis fails to lift at all with laryngoscopy, and is pointed downwards (Grade 3B, Fig. 3–12, Chap. 3) or is sitting on the posterior pharyngeal wall, bougie use may be less successful. In this situation, the epiglottis can be directly elevated with a longer curved blade, or a straight blade, whereupon the bougie can be used. Alternatively, the tip of some of the newer, stiffer, single-use bougies can be used to directly lift the epiglottis, to enable a brief view of posterior cartilages and to confirm that the bougie has been advanced above them.

C. **Failure to advance the tube over the tracheally placed bougie.** Occasionally, the tube fails to pass easily over the bougie and through the cords. Most often this is due to the leading edge of the ETT's bevel catching up on the right vocal fold. Three maneuvers will help avoid this occurrence:

- Ongoing laryngoscopy during tube passage over the bougie.[39]
- **A counterclockwise rotation of the ETT** by 90° during tube passage.[39] Experienced laryngoscopists often do this routinely during bougie-aided intubation, to rotate the leading edge of the bevel away from the right vocal fold.
- Use of a smaller ETT (half or a full size less than usual).

Bougie Effectiveness

ROUTINE AND DIFFICULT AIRWAY MANAGEMENT

The bougie is a valuable adjunct. In the authors' experience with the device, patients presenting Grade 3 laryngoscopic views are routinely intubated on the first attempt with the bougie. In a published series studying 100 patients with simulated Grade 3 laryngoscopies, bougie use resulted in a 96% successful intubation rate after two attempts, in contrast to the 66% success rate attained with attempted blind placement of a styletted endotracheal tube.[35] A second study reported on bougie use as part of a predefined algorithm for elective surgical patients presenting with an unanticipated difficult airway. In this

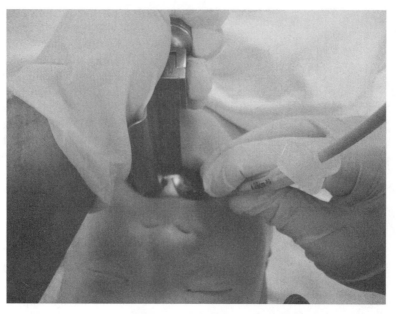

Figure 5–33. The endotracheal tube is railroaded over the bougie during ongoing laryngoscopy (to help control tongue and epiglottis).

population, bougie use resulted in a 90% intubation success rate by the second attempt.[40] Successful use of the bougie has also been reported in the prehospital environment,[41] although with a lower success rate. Bougie use during rapid-sequence intubation with applied cricoid pressure has been shown to facilitate successful tube placement in restricted view situations.[42] Finally, a number of case reports and series document the bougie's successful use in the difficult airway.[38, 39, 43, 44] It should be noted that the bougie may not be well tolerated in the "awake" or lightly sedated patient: it is most appropriately used during an RSI or in a deeply obtunded patient.

C-Spine Precautions

The bougie may be helpful during intubation by DL with applied manual MILNS. Movement of the C-spine can be minimized by seeking to obtain no more than a view of the posterior cartilages at laryngoscopy, placing the bougie above them, then passing the tube. At least one study has demonstrated a higher success rate with bougie-aided, compared to simple DL in the C-spine precaution situation.[45]

The bougie is an effective, inexpensive, and simple-to-use adjunct to direct laryngoscopy. The authors believe there should be a "bougie on the chest" prior to **all** emergency intubations, to facilitate quick ETT placement in difficult situations.

▶ ADJUNCTS TO DIRECT LARYNGOSCOPY: FIBEROPTIC STYLETS

Semirigid fiberoptic stylets incorporate a fiberoptic bundle allowing indirect visualization via a proximal eyepiece. The ETT is ensleeved over the fiberoptic stylet, and the distal end of the stylet is positioned at the leading edge of the ETT. Faced with a Grade 3 view at laryngoscopy, the fiberoptic stylet/ETT assembly can be placed beneath the tip of the epiglottis during ongoing laryngoscopy, whereupon a view of the cords is sought through the instrument's eyepiece. The ETT is then advanced through the cords under indirect vision. In experienced hands, fiberoptic stylets may be particularly useful in Grade 3B or -4 views, where bougie use is less successful. As the price of these devices continues to drop, fiberoptic stylets may become a more common adjunct for use in difficult, and even routine, attempts at direct laryngoscopy. Further information on their use and effectiveness appears in Chap. 6.

▶ CHANGING THE BLADE

Note that the above maneuvers can all be performed during the first or second attempt at laryngoscopy. Between attempts, the patient should be reoxygenated by BMV to ensure that a failed oxygenation situation does not exist. For a second or subsequent attempt, a **blade change** can be considered, although it should only be done with a specific objective in mind.

Changing to a Longer Blade

Changing to a longer blade may be appropriate in a long-necked individual, or when attempting to directly pick up a long, floppy epiglottis. In addition, if the curved blade in use is too short to be fully advanced into the vallecula, and thus fails to contact the underlying hyoepiglottic ligament (Figs. 5–18 A and B), the epiglottis may not elevate up and out of the way. One hint that this may be the case is when direct laryngoscopy, with the appropriate lift, fails to mobilize the epiglottis at all. Faced with this finding, a change to a longer blade can be considered.

Changing to a Different Type of Blade

A change to a different blade type can be considered by the clinician skilled in its use, particularly if there's a good chance it will help. Changing to a straight blade may be particularly

useful in the situation in which a posteriorly pointing or long epiglottis is encountered. As previously reviewed, the levering tip (McCoy/ CLM) blade may help in Grade 3 situations, especially those caused by C-spine precautions.

Changing the Same Blade's Tip to a Different Location

Although the dogma is pervasive that one must directly elevate (i.e., "pick up") the epiglottis with the straight blade and indirectly lift it (tip placement in the vallecula) with the curved blade, one should feel free to do whatever works. For example, a long curved blade can be used to directly elevate the epiglottis.

▶ POSTINTUBATION CARE AND COMPLICATIONS

Care

After tube placement, the cuff should be inflated and the stylet removed. Endotracheal placement should be confirmed by objective means, as discussed above. Cricoid pressure, if applied, can then be released. Clinical signs such as chest rise, breath sound auscultation, and oxygen saturation should also be assessed. **Vital signs should be reassessed**, especially the **blood pressure**. The tube should be secured, initially with the clinician's hand, and subsequently with tape, tie, or a commercial fixation device. If twill tie is used, care must be taken to ensure the ties are not excessively tight around the patient's neck, particularly in the head-injured patient. Use of a bite block should be considered, to avoid the patient's biting down and occluding the tube. A chest x-ray should be obtained, not to determine success of intubation, but to locate the tube in relation to the carina, and as part of patient assessment. Paralysis may be initiated, or continued after intubation, if indicated, with one of several agents used in conjunction with an appropriate sedative-hypnotic and narcotic analgesic. Finally, ETT cuff pressure can be adjusted to the "minimum leak" position.

Complications of Endotracheal Intubation

Although everyone breathes a sigh of relief after the ETT is placed and its correct position has been confirmed, problems can still be encountered:

- **Esophageal intubation.** To avoid patient morbidity, esophageal intubations must be immediately recognized and corrected. The topic has been reviewed above.
- **Accidental extubation.** There are many documented instances of morbidity and mortality attributable to accidental extubation. This aspect of airway management is particularly relevant in the emergency patient, as numerous transfers will occur following intubation (e.g., to diagnostic imaging, the OR, intensive care unit (ICU), or interfacility transfer): classically a time of high risk for accidental extubation. Tube ties, or commercially available products for securing the tube are preferred, as blood, sweat, and regurgitated matter may make tape a less effective option.
- **Endobronchial intubation.** Observation and auscultation of the chest will help rule out endobronchial intubation, as will a chest x-ray. The printed numbers on the side of the ETT should be observed to ensure the tube is not positioned too deep in the patient, prior to fixation.
- **High airway pressures.** High airway pressures encountered after intubation may be due to ETT, or patient factors. Tube factors include occlusion by thick secretions, pulmonary edema, blood, or vomitus. A suction catheter can be passed to help assess tube patency, or preferably, the tube should be changed, if occlusion is suspected. Patient factors are numerous and include esophageal or endobronchial intubation, bronchospasm, and pneumo/hemothorax.

- **Hypotension**. Postintubation hypotension can be caused by administered medications, relief of high sympathetic tone, or the institution of positive pressure ventilation, especially in the volume depleted patient. Special mention should be made of **auto-PEEP**. If adequate time is not allowed for expiration, especially in the patient with air-trapping pathology (e.g., bronchospasm, COPD) resulting "breath stacking" (increased intrathoracic pressure; decreased venous return) can rapidly result in cardiovascular collapse.

▶ DIRECT LARYNGOSCOPY EFFECTIVENESS

ROUTINE AND DIFFICULT AIRWAY MANAGEMENT

Published data suggests that successful laryngeal exposure using DL occurs in all but 2%–8% of cases in elective surgical populations.[12] Of the cases where no aspect of the laryngeal inlet can be identified, most are Grade 3 (epiglottis only) views, and as outlined above, can be successfully dealt with using the bougie.

SKILLS ACQUISITION

DL has a significant learning curve. Studies suggest that the learning curve flattens after about 50 laryngoscopies have been performed.[46–48] Instructional videos on laryngeal anatomy delivered as part of a training program have been shown to improve success rates in novices.[49] Training using human patient simulators has also been shown to be effective for novices learning to perform DL and intubation.[50] Such studies suggest that in time, well-designed programs combining both multimedia presentations and patient simulators may improve the subsequent learning curve of DL on human subjects.

C-SPINE PRECAUTIONS

Cervical spine injury is present in approximately 2% of blunt trauma victims: this risk trebles in patients with a GCS of 8 or less.[51–53] In the at-risk patient, C-spine precautions should be observed. That being said, the risk of iatrogenic spinal cord injury during DL is extraordinarily low.[54] As previously stated, application of manual in-line stabilization can be expected to increase difficulty with direct laryngoscopy. Although alternative intubation techniques such as rigid or flexible fiberscopes have been espoused as being preferable to DL in this setting, no evidence exists demonstrating a superior clinical outcome with their use over direct laryngoscopy.[53] Carefully performed DL for intubation of the at-risk blunt trauma victim is considered acceptable practice and within the standard of care.[53,54] Use of the levering tip blade[15–17] and/or exposure of no more than the posterior cartilages at laryngoscopy, followed by a bougie-assisted intubation[45] may help minimize difficulty and movement.

▶ PEDIATRIC INTUBATION

The greatest impediment to successful intubation in the pediatric population is the anxiety of the clinician. Compared to the general adult emergency department population, intubation in children, although less frequently required, is usually easier. Principles of DL in pediatric patients are similar to those in the adult. Preparation is also similar, aided by sizing choices made with reference to the Broselow tape or a chart. Generally, an ETT one-half size larger and smaller than the expected size should be immediately available. Although classically, uncuffed tubes have been used in the smaller child, this directive may change with time. Positioning issues have been previously discussed. Preoxygenation may be difficult in the uncooperative child, but should always be attempted.

While many clinicians espouse routine use of the straight blade in the young child due to the frequent occurrence of a long, floppy epiglottis, other experienced clinicians use the curved blade for all ages in the pediatric population. Again, familiarity with the chosen technique and the destination airway anatomy are key.

Pediatric ETCO$_2$ detectors are available and should be used.

In terms of response to difficult DL, the principles discussed above are equally applicable to the pediatric patient. Repositioning the head may help, as may external laryngeal manipulation (in the neonate this latter maneuver can be done with the fifth finger of the hand holding the laryngoscope!). Pediatric bougies accommodating a minimum ETT size of 3.5 mm ID are available.

The pediatric population have relatively high oxygen consumptions and as such may desaturate quickly during attempts at intubation. On the other hand, as mentioned earlier, they tend to be quite easy to bag-mask ventilate.

▶ PREDICTORS OF DIFFICULT DIRECT LARYNGOSCOPY

As is the case with bag-mask ventilation, there are anatomic predictors of difficult direct laryngoscopy, and a quick assessment of these factors should be undertaken before proceeding. Although it has been pointed out that the emergency patient requiring intubation will still need intubation whether or not difficulty has been predicted, we contend that an airway exam should be undertaken for the following reasons:

- Predictors of difficulty may point to the ideal approach to the intubation.
- Predicted difficulty mandates additional preparation: extra help should be sought, and adjuncts to direct laryngoscopy as well as alternative intubation devices and rescue oxygenation equipment must be immediately available.

Numerous studies have attempted to correlate laryngoscopic grade with external anatomic features.[55–59] Most studies conclude that examination of more than one feature will increase the chances of predicting difficulty.[56, 60–62] However, it should be stressed that even with a detailed air-way exam, not all patients presenting difficult laryngoscopy will be predicted in advance. The airway examination, while sensitive, is not specific, and has a low positive predictive value.[12] In addition, it may not be possible, or practical, to perform many of these assessment techniques in the patient requiring emergency intubation.[63]

Anatomic Factors Important to Direct Laryngoscopy

A simple diagram (Fig. 5–34) from Cormack and Lehane's paper[26] illustrates many of the anatomic features needed for ease of attaining a direct line-of-sight view of the glottic opening. Arrow 1 in Fig. 5–34 indicates that an anteriorly and/or superiorly positioned larynx will hide the glottic opening behind the tongue and epiglottis, creating more difficulty. Arrow 2 shows how prominent upper incisors create difficulty, and also indirectly reflects mouth opening as a factor. Arrow 3 in Fig. 5–34 illustrates that a prominent

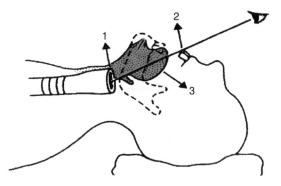

Figure 5–34. The anatomic obstacles to attaining a direct line-of-sight view of the glottic opening. Arrow 1: An anteriorly and/or superiorly positioned larynx. Arrow 2: Prominent upper incisors and limited mouth opening. Arrow 3: A prominent tongue. (*From Cormack[26], with permission.*)

tongue will create difficulty in obtaining line-of-sight view of the larynx. The laryngoscope blade functions to displace and/or compress the tongue into the submandibular space and also helps lift the jaw anteriorly. Thus, laryngoscopy may be predicted to be difficult both in the patient with a hypoplastic mandible, as little space is available into which to compress the tongue, as well as in a patient with poor jaw mobility.

The importance of head and neck positioning on lining up the oral and pharyngeal/tracheal has been addressed in Chap. 3. Figs. 3–7 A and B help illustrate the effect of introducing the "sniff" position (head extension, lower neck flexion) in helping to create line-of-sight visualization of the glottis. Such positioning moves the axes towards closer alignment, but not totally: the laryngoscope blade then completes the job by lifting the jaw anteriorly and displacing the tongue into the submandibular space, enabling direct line-of-sight visualization.

"MMAP"ing the Airway

The foregoing anatomic considerations can be used to deduce predictors of difficult laryngoscopy. The mnemonic[64] MMAP can be used as a reminder of these predictors:

M: **Mallampati** classification
M: **Measurements (3–3–1)**
A: **A-O** (Atlanto-Occipital) extension—ability to extend the head and flex the lower neck
P: **Pathology**: any evidence of pathologic airway obstruction which may create difficulty with laryngoscopy

A. **Mallampati Class.** Assessment of the Mallampati class requires an awake, sitting, cooperative, patient (e.g., the patient in respiratory distress or about to receive procedural sedation). The patient should be asked for maximum mouth opening, and to extrude the tongue without phonating.[65]

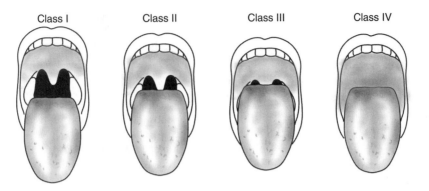

Figure 5–35. Mallampati classes I–IV.

The class obtained is dependent on what structures can be seen (Fig. 5–35). This test reflects both mouth opening and the relative prominence of the tongue in the oropharynx: as discussed above, difficulty displacing or compressing the tongue out of the way at laryngoscopy can increase difficulty. Mallampati originally described 3 views, however, a modified classification describing 4 views is more commonly cited.[66] Class I and II are generally correlated with easy direct laryngoscopy, while III and IV are more suggestive of difficulty.[66] This assessment is often not possible in the patient requiring emergency airway management.

B. **Measurements.** The **3–3–1** measurements can be used to assess other aspects of the patient's airway anatomy.

- **Thyromental span**: Ideally **3 fingerbreadths** should fit under the patient's chin between the superior border of the thyroid cartilage and the mentum of the chin. Fewer than three (of the patient's own fingers) can portend difficulty with laryngoscopy, due to an inadequate space into which to compress the tongue with the laryngoscope blade.
- **Mouth opening**: The patient should also **have 3 fingerbreadths** of mouth opening. Adequate mouth opening is needed for blade insertion and rotation into the pharynx.

- **Jaw protrusion:** Anterior jaw protrusion occurs during direct laryngoscopy, helping move the tongue and epiglottis anteriorly and out of the line-of-sight. Jaw protrusion can be assessed at the bedside by asking the cooperative patient to move the lower teeth in front of the upper teeth. At least **1 cm of jaw protrusion** is desirable. Alternatively, the upper lip bite test can be used. The patient is asked to cover the upper lip with the bottom incisors. This has been shown to provide additional information but, alone, the inability to do this cannot reliably predict difficult laryngoscopy.[67,68]

C. **Atlanto-Occipital extension.** In the absence of C-spine precautions, the patient's ability to flex the neck at the cervico-thoracic junction and extend the head at the atlanto-occipital junction should be assessed. Obviously, this step should be omitted in the patient with C-spine precautions, and assumed to be one factor that makes laryngoscopy in this patient population more difficult.

D. **Pathology.** Airway obstruction as a pathologic condition deserves special mention. The patient with pathologic airway obstruction may be difficult to intubate, even with external anatomic features otherwise suggesting an easy intubation. Airway obstruction can result from medical (e.g., angioedema, airway infections, tumors) or traumatic (e.g., burns, penetrating or blunt neck trauma) conditions. Under such circumstances, concern exists over not knowing what the glottis will look like at direct laryngoscopy: whether normal structures will be identifiable, or in the expected location. There is also concern that patient compensation related to muscle tone, intact reflexes, and positioning may be the only factors preventing complete obstruction. Such patients can be identified, (a) by history, and (b) by inspiratory stridor, loudest (on auscultation) at the larynx. Strong consideration should be given to securing the airway using an awake technique in these situations, when feasible. Significant upper airway pathology is a relative contraindication to RSI.

► SUMMARY

Most intubations in emergencies are performed using direct laryngoscopy. DL retains the advantage of direct visualization of the laryngeal inlet, with immediate confirmation of tube passage through the cords in many cases, and the ability to evaluate the oropharynx for foreign material in the same setting. DL is a core skill to the acute-care clinician. Done properly, with a knowledgeable appreciation of the anatomy, it will be successful most of the time. However, as with BMV, having a good approach to difficult laryngoscopy, predicted or not, is also needed. Finally, even though its utility may be limited in the emergency setting, an airway exam looking for predictors of difficult laryngoscopic intubation is still warranted to help determine the best approach to the intubation, and to anticipate the need for help and preparation of additional equipment.

REFERENCES

1. Levitan RM, Pisaturo JT, Kinkle WC, et al. Stylet bend angles and tracheal tube passage using a straight-to-cuff shape. *Acad Emerg Med.* 2006;13(12): 1255–1258.

2. Walker JD. Posture used by anaesthetists during laryngoscopy. *Br J Anaesth.* 2002;89(5):772–774.

3. Matthews AJ, Johnson CJ, Goodman NW. Body posture during simulated tracheal intubation. *Anaesthesia.* 1998;53(4):331–334.

4. Collins JS, Lemmens HJ, Brodsky JB, et al. Laryngoscopy and morbid obesity: a comparison of the "sniff" and "ramped" positions. *Obes Surg.* 2004;14(9):1171–1175.

5. Adnet F, Baillard C, Borron SW, et al. Randomized study comparing the "sniffing position" with simple head extension for laryngoscopic view in elective surgery patients. *Anesthesiology.* 2001;95(4): 836–841.

6. Adnet F, Borron SW, Lapostolle F, et al. The three axis alignment theory and the "sniffing position": perpetuation of an anatomic myth? *Anesthesiology.* 1999;91(6):1964–1965.

7. Hirsch NP, Smith GB, Adnet F. Historical perspective of the "sniffing position". *Anesthesiology.* 2000;93(5):1366–1367.

8. Levitan RM, Mechem CC, Ochroch EA, et al. Head-elevated laryngoscopy position: improving laryngeal exposure during laryngoscopy by increasing head elevation. *Ann Emerg Med.* 2003;41(3): 322–330.

9. Hochman, II, Zeitels SM, Heaton JT. Analysis of the forces and position required for direct laryngoscopic exposure of the anterior vocal folds. *Ann Otol Rhinol Laryngol.* 1999;108(8):715–724.

10. Heath KJ. The effect of laryngoscopy of different cervical spine immobilisation techniques. *Anaesthesia.* 1994;49(10):843–845.

11. MacQuarrie K, Hung OR, Law JA. Tracheal intubation using Bullard laryngoscope for patients with a simulated difficult airway. *Can J Anaesth.* 1999;46(8):760–765.

12. Crosby ET, Cooper RM, Douglas MJ, et al. The unanticipated difficult airway with recommendations for management. *Can J Anaesth.* 1998;45(8):757–776.

13. Benumof JL. Difficult laryngoscopy: obtaining the best view. *Can J Anaesth.* 1994;41(5 Pt 1):361–365.

14. Henderson JJ. The use of paraglossal straight blade laryngoscopy in difficult tracheal intubation. *Anaesthesia.* 1997;52(6):552–560.

15. Uchida T, Hikawa Y, Saito Y, et al. The McCoy levering laryngoscope in patients with limited neck extension. *Can J Anaesth.* 1997;44(6):674–676.

16. Gabbott DA. Laryngoscopy using the McCoy laryngoscope after application of a cervical collar. *Anaesthesia.* 1996;51(9):812–814.

17. Laurent SC, de Melo AE, Alexander-Williams JM. The use of the McCoy laryngoscope in patients with simulated cervical spine injuries. *Anaesthesia.* 1996;51(1):74–75.

18. Bilgin H, Bozkurt M. Tracheal intubation using the ILMA, C-Trach or McCoy laryngoscope in patients with simulated cervical spine injury. *Anaesthesia.* 2006;61(7):685–691.

19. ACEP. Verification of endotracheal tube placement. *Ann Emerg Med.* 2002;40(5):551–552.

20. Salem MR. Verification of endotracheal tube position. *Anesthesiol Clin North America.* 2001;19(4):813–839.

21. Donahue PL. The oesophageal detector device. An assessment of accuracy and ease of use by paramedics. *Anaesthesia.* 1994;49(10):863–865.

22. Andres AH, Langenstein H. The esophageal detector device is unreliable when the stomach has been ventilated. *Anesthesiology.* 1999;91(2):566–568.

23. Cooper GM, McClure JH. Maternal deaths from anaesthesia. An extract from Why Mothers Die 2000–2002, the Confidential Enquiries into Maternal Deaths in the United Kingdom: Chapter 9: Anaesthesia. *Br J Anaesth.* 2005;94(4):417–423.

24. Kelly JJ, Eynon CA, Kaplan JL, et al. Use of tube condensation as an indicator of endotracheal tube placement. *Ann Emerg Med.* 1998;31(5):575–578.

25. Angelotti T, Weiss EL, Lemmens HJ, et al. Verification of endotracheal tube placement by prehospital providers: is a portable fiberoptic bronchoscope of value? *Air Med J.* 2006;25(2):74–78; discussion 78–80.

26. Cormack RS, Lehane J. Difficult tracheal intubation in obstetrics. *Anaesthesia.* 1984;39(11):1105–1111.

27. Mort TC. Emergency tracheal intubation: complications associated with repeated laryngoscopic attempts. *Anesth Analg.* 2004;99(2):607–613.

28. Knill RL. Difficult laryngoscopy made easy with a "BURP". *Can J Anaesth.* 1993;40(3):279–282.

29. Takahata O, Kubota M, Mamiya K, et al. The efficacy of the "BURP" maneuver during a difficult laryngoscopy. *Anesth Analg.* 1997;84(2):419–421.

30. Ochroch EA, Levitan RM. A videographic analysis of laryngeal exposure comparing the articulating laryngoscope and external laryngeal manipulation. *Anesth Analg.* 2001;92(1):267–270.

31. Benumof JL, Cooper SD. Quantitative improvement in laryngoscopic view by optimal external laryngeal manipulation. *J Clin Anesth.* 1996;8(2):136–140.

32. Levitan RM, Kinkle WC, Levin WJ, et al. Laryngeal view during laryngoscopy: a randomized trial comparing cricoid pressure, backward–upward–rightward pressure, and bimanual laryngoscopy. *Ann Emerg Med.* 2006;47(6):548–555.

33. Haslam N, Parker L, Duggan JE. Effect of cricoid pressure on the view at laryngoscopy. *Anaesthesia.* 2005;60(1):41–47.

34. Snider DD, Clarke D, Finucane BT. The "BURP" maneuver worsens the glottic view when applied in combination with cricoid pressure. *Can J Anaesth.* 2005;52(1):100–104.

35. Gataure PS, Vaughan RS, Latto IP. Simulated difficult intubation. Comparison of the gum elastic bougie and the stylet. *Anaesthesia.* 1996;51(10):935–938.

36. Hodzovic I, Wilkes AR, Latto IP. To shape or not to shape...simulated bougie-assisted difficult intubation in a manikin. *Anaesthesia.* 2003;58(8):792–797.

37. Viswanathan S, Campbell C, Wood DG, et al. The Eschmann Tracheal Tube Introducer. (Gum elastic bougie). *Anesthesiol Rev.* 1992;19(6):29–34.

38. Kidd JF, Dyson A, Latto IP. Successful difficult intubation. Use of the gum elastic bougie. *Anaesthesia.* 1988;43(6):437–438.

39. Dogra S, Falconer R, Latto IP. Successful difficult intubation. Tracheal tube placement over a gum-elastic bougie. *Anaesthesia.* 1990;45(9):774–776.

40. Combes X, Le Roux B, Suen P, et al. Unanticipated difficult airway in anesthetized patients: prospective validation of a management algorithm. *Anesthesiology.* 2004;100(5):1146–1150.

41. Jabre P, Combes X, Leroux B, et al. Use of gum elastic bougie for prehospital difficult intubation. *Am J Emerg Med.* 2005;23(4):552–555.

42. Noguchi T, Koga K, Shiga Y, et al. The gum elastic bougie eases tracheal intubation while applying cricoid pressure compared to a stylet. *Can J Anaesth.* 2003;50(7):712–717.

43. Morton G, Chileshe B, Baxter P. Gum elastic bougie in the hole technique. *Anaesthesia.* 2002;57(10):1037–1038.

44. Combes X, Dumerat M, Dhonneur G. Emergency gum elastic bougie-assisted tracheal intubation in four patients with upper airway distortion. *Can J Anaesth.* 2004;51(10):1022–1024.

45. Nolan JP, Wilson ME. Orotracheal intubation in patients with potential cervical spine injuries. An indication for the gum elastic bougie. *Anaesthesia.* 1993;48(7):630–633.

46. Charuluxananan S, Kyokong O, Somboonviboon W, et al. Learning manual skills in spinal anesthesia and orotracheal intubation: is there any recommended number of cases for anesthesia residency training program? *J Med Assoc Thai.* 2001;84 Suppl 1:S251–255.

47. Konrad C, Schupfer G, Wietlisbach M, et al. Learning manual skills in anesthesiology: Is there a recommended number of cases for anesthetic procedures? *Anesth Analg.* 1998;86(3):635–639.

48. Mulcaster JT, Mills J, Hung OR, et al. Laryngoscopic intubation: learning and performance. *Anesthesiology.* 2003;98(1):23–27.

49. Levitan RM, Goldman TS, Bryan DA, et al. Training with video imaging improves the initial intubation success rates of paramedic trainees in an operating room setting. *Ann Emerg Med.* 2001;37(1): 46–50.

50. Hall RE, Plant JR, Bands CJ, et al. Human patient simulation is effective for teaching paramedic students endotracheal intubation. *Acad Emerg Med.* 2005;12(9):850–855.

51. Holly LT, Kelly DF, Counelis GJ, et al. Cervical spine trauma associated with moderate and severe head injury: incidence, risk factors, and injury characteristics. *J Neurosurg.* 2002;96(3 Suppl):285–291.

52. Demetriades D, Charalambides K, Chahwan S, et al. Nonskeletal cervical spine injuries: epidemiology and diagnostic pitfalls. *J Trauma.* 2000;48(4): 724–727.

53. Crosby ET. Airway management in adults after cervical spine trauma. *Anesthesiology.* 2006;104(6): 1293–1318.

54. Manoach S, Paladino L. Manual In-Line Stabilization for Acute Airway Management of Suspected Cervical Spine Injury: Historical Review and Current Questions. *Ann Emerg Med.* 2007.

55. Oates JD, Macleod AD, Oates PD, et al. Comparison of two methods for predicting difficult intubation. *Br J Anaesth.* 1991;66(3):305–309.

56. Reed MJ, Dunn MJ, McKeown DW. Can an airway assessment score predict difficulty at intubation in the emergency department? *Emerg Med J.* 2005;22(2):99–102.

57. Rocke DA, Murray WB, Rout CC, et al. Relative risk analysis of factors associated with difficult intubation in obstetric anesthesia. *Anesthesiology.* 1992;77(1):67–73.

58. Rose DK, Cohen MM. The airway: problems and predictions in 18,500 patients. *Can J Anaesth.* 1994;41(5 Pt 1):372–383.

59. Tse JC, Rimm EB, Hussain A. Predicting difficult endotracheal intubation in surgical patients scheduled for general anesthesia: a prospective blind study. *Anesth Analg.* 1995;81(2):254–258.

60. Arne J, Descoins P, Fusciardi J, et al. Preoperative assessment for difficult intubation in general and ENT surgery: predictive value of a clinical multivariate risk index. *Br J Anaesth.* 1998;80(2): 140–146.

61. el-Ganzouri AR, McCarthy RJ, Tuman KJ, et al. Preoperative airway assessment: predictive value of a multivariate risk index. *Anesth Analg.* 1996;82(6): 1197–1204.

62. Saghaei M, Safavi MR. Prediction of prolonged laryngoscopy. *Anaesthesia.* 2001;56(12):1198–1201.

63. Levitan RM, Everett WW, Ochroch EA. Limitations of difficult airway prediction in patients intubated in the emergency department. *Ann Emerg Med.* 2004;44(4):307–313.

64. Walls RM, Murphy M. Identification of the difficult and failed airway. In: Walls RM, ed. *Manual of Emergency Airway Management.* 2nd ed. Philadelphia: Lippincott Willimas and Wilkins; 2004;70–81.

65. Mallampati SR, Gatt SP, Gugino LD, et al. A clinical sign to predict difficult tracheal intubation: a prospective study. *Can Anaesth Soc J.* 1985; 32(4):429–434.

66. Samsoon GL, Young JR. Difficult tracheal intubation: a retrospective study. *Anaesthesia.* 1987;42(5): 487–490.

67. Eberhart LH, Arndt C, Cierpka T, et al. The reliability and validity of the upper lip bite test compared with the Mallampati classification to predict difficult laryngoscopy: an external prospective evaluation. *Anesth Analg.* 2005;101(1):284–289.

68. Khan ZH, Kashfi A, Ebrahimkhani E. A comparison of the upper lip bite test (a simple new technique) with modified Mallampati classification in predicting difficulty in endotracheal intubation: a prospective blinded study. *Anesth Analg.* 2003;96(2):595–599.

CHAPTER 6

Alternative Intubation Techniques

▶ **KEY POINTS**

- Repeated direct laryngoscopy (DL) attempts can lead to increasing upper airway trauma, and ultimately to a situation where mask ventilation may also be difficult or impossible.
- If 'best look' laryngoscopy, including use of an adjunct such as the bougie, or possibly a blade change, has failed after one or two attempts, it is reasonable to switch to an alternative intubation technique.
- As an alternative intubating technique, the LMA Fastrach™ has an advantage in that it can also be used to oxygenate and ventilate the patient.
- Lightwand (e.g. Trachlight™) use is not limited by blood and secretions in the airway. However, consistent successful use requires experience.
- Fiberoptic stylets can be used on their own as true 'alternative intubation' instruments, or can be used as adjuncts to direct laryngoscopy.
- Navigation of any fiberoptic instrument through the airway is contingent on advancing the device through a patent airway lumen.
- Videolaryngoscopy provides views of the glottic opening which are often superior to those obtained with conventional direct laryngoscopy.

▶ **INTRODUCTION TO ALTERNATIVE INTUBATION DEVICES AND TECHNIQUES**

Difficult tracheal intubation may be defined as any of:

A. More than two attempts made with the same laryngoscope blade.
B. A change in blade or use of an adjunct (e.g., the bougie) is required.
C. Use of an alternative intubation technique.[1]

An appropriate response to anticipated difficult tracheal intubation requires forethought and planning. However, not all difficult intubation situations can be or are predicted beforehand: some patients with *no* anatomic features suggestive of difficult laryngoscopy and intubation may still be challenging. Faced with difficult laryngoscopy, it is *not* acceptable in contemporary practice to repeatedly attempt to blindly pass an endotracheal tube under the epiglottis, hoping it will pass. Evidence of increased morbidity with multiple attempts at laryngoscopy is mounting, especially with three or more attempts.[2] The anatomic or pathologic conditions rendering direct laryngoscopy difficult (e.g., poor neck mobility, limited jaw opening, or prominent upper teeth) will not improve over time. Rather, repeated attempts can cause increasing airway trauma, with bleeding, edema, or laryngospasm ultimately leading to a situation where mask ventilation may also be difficult or impossible. If "best look" laryngoscopy, including use of adjuncts such as the bougie, and possibly a blade change, have failed after one or two attempts, it is preferable to switch to an **alternative intubation technique**. Alternative intubation devices tend to conform better to anatomic axes of the airway, and will often permit easier tracheal intubation in patients who otherwise present significant difficulty with direct laryngoscopy. Before proceeding to an alternative intubation technique, ease of bag-mask ventilation (BMV) should be assessed and the patient reoxygenated, as necessary.

A number of good alternative intubating tools and techniques exist. The clinician should become familiar with one, or possibly two such

techniques. Many devices presented in this chapter are available at reasonable cost, have favorable learning curves, and some published evidence. The decision of which device to acquire should also take into account the opportunity to practice in the controlled setting of the operating room (OR). Collaboration with local anesthesiologists in choosing a device already in use in the OR will facilitate skill maintenance opportunities.

Both the **Laryngeal Mask Airway (LMA) Fastrach**™, also known as the **intubating laryngeal mask airway** (LMA North America Inc., San Diego, CA, Fig. 6–1) and the **Trachlight** lighted stylet (Laerdal Medical Corp, Wappingers Falls, NY, Fig. 6–2) have an extensive history of use in the OR setting and have reasonable supporting evidence as effective difficult airway tools.[3,4] A third class of alternative

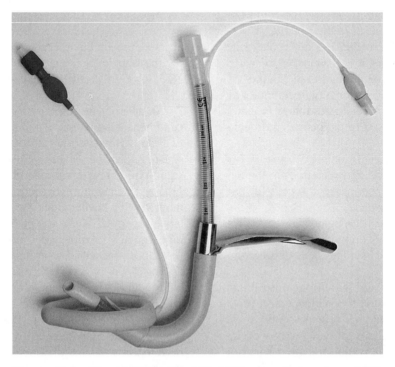

Figure 6–1. The LMA Fastrach™. (With permission from LMA North America Inc.).

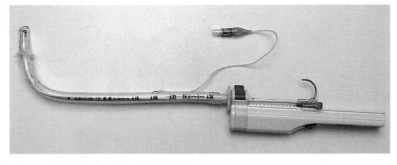

Figure 6-2. The Trachlight.

intubation device is the rigid or flexible fiberoptic instrument. To date, skill requirements and cost have limited the use of these latter instruments for out-of-OR emergency intubations. However, more affordable options in this category are emerging in the form of portable semirigid fiberoptic stylets (e.g., the **Levitan FPS** scope and the **Shikani Optical Stylet**, [SOS], Clarus Medical, St. Paul, MN, Fig. 6–3). In addition, video-based instruments such as the **Glidescope** (Verathon Medical [Canada], Burnaby, BC, Fig. 6–4) are gaining in popularity and are increasingly being used as alternative intubation devices out of the OR.

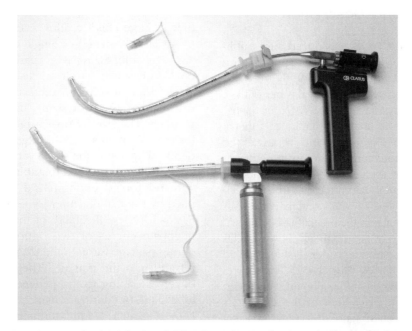

Figure 6-3. The Seeing Optical Stylet, SOS (above) attached to dedicated lightsource and the Levitan FPS optical stylet (below) attached to a "Greenline" handle. Both have an endotracheal tube preloaded for use.

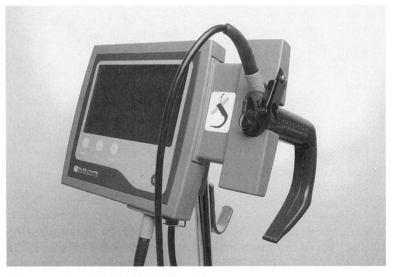

Figure 6–4. Glidescope video system.

► LMA FASTRACH™

LMA Fastrach™ Description

The LMA Fastrach™ was introduced after publication of numerous case reports describing fiberoptic-aided intubation through the LMA Classic™, using small endotracheal tubes (ETTs). One obvious advantage of the LMA Fastrach™ as an alternative intubating technique is that it can be used to oxygenate and ventilate the patient, either between intubation attempts or used as a rescue oxygenation device.[5] Indeed, for a given volume of air in the cuff, there is evidence that it provides a better seal than the LMA Classic™.[4] It is similar to the original LMA Classic™ in the appearance of the distal cuff, however differs in having a shorter, wider, L-shaped rigid stainless steel barrel (Fig. 6–5). The barrel attaches to a guiding handle, allowing for device insertion without placement of the clinician's fingers into the patient's mouth. A prominence at the junction of the mask and barrel is designed to direct the ETT centrally. The LMA Fastrach™ also has a stiff bar lying across the mask aperture,

designed to elevate the epiglottis up and away from the path of the advancing ETT.

At present, the LMA Fastrach™ is available only in large child to adult sizes, equivalent to LMA Classic™ sizes 3–5. Single-use versions are also available. Sizing is generally inscribed on the LMA Fastrach™ itself, and listed on the packaging. Alternatively, a manufacturer's reference card can be used for sizing and cuff inflation volumes. The size 3 LMA-Fastrach™ is designed for use in patients of 30–50 kg; size 4, patients of 50–70 kg, while the size 5 is used for patients above 70 kg. Dedicated reusable, silicon-based, wire reinforced endotracheal tubes are supplied by the manufacturer for use with the LMA Fastrach™. The flexibility of these tubes helps negotiate curves of two opposing directions during passage through the LMA Fastrach™ barrel and into the patient.[4] They also feature a bevel extending to the midline, to discourage tube hang-up during advancement. Although LMA Fastrach™ intubation has also been described using well-lubricated standard ETTs (up to size 8.0) advanced in a reverse curve direction,[6,7] their use is not recommended by

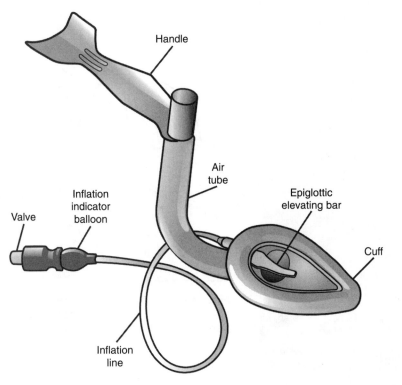

Figure 6–5. LMA Fastrach™. (With permission LMA North America).

the manufacturer, out of concern of possible laryngeal trauma.

LMA Fastrach™ Preparation

Selection of the appropriately-sized LMA Fastrach™ is important, as incorrect mask sizing may impact both ease of ventilation and success of blind intubation.[8] As with the LMA Classic™ (see Chap. 7), insertion of the Fastrach is with the *cuff fully deflated* (Fig. 6–6). The posterior aspect of the cuff should be well lubricated with a water-soluble lubricant. The tube inlet and outlet of the Fastrach airway barrel should also be well lubricated, as should the endotracheal tube itself. Clinical experience suggests lubrication of the airway barrel is even more crucial for the disposable versions.

LMA Fastrach™ Use

The LMA Fastrach™ is used with the head and neck in the neutral position. The following steps are undertaken.

Fastrach™ Insertion and Positioning

A. The LMA Fastrach™ is inserted into the patient's mouth so that the lubricated posterior aspect of the mask tip is flat against the hard palate (Fig. 6–7).

B. The mask is then carefully rotated down into the pharynx, maintaining pressure against the hard palate and posterior pharyngeal wall (Fig. 6–8).

C. Once seated in the pharynx, the cuff is inflated with a volume of air sufficient to

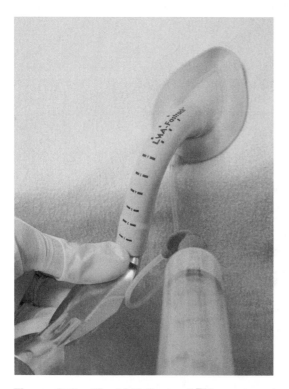

Figure 6–6. The LMA Fastrach™ is prepared for insertion by posterior lubrication and fully deflating its cuff while pressing down on a flat surface. (With permission from LMA North America).

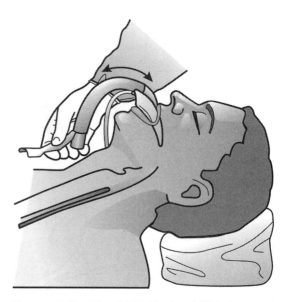

Figure 6–7. The LMA Fastrach™ is inserted and advanced along the hard palate. (With permission LMA North America).

achieve a good seal (or else [size of mask − 1] × 10).

D. At this point, many clinicians routinely perform an "up-down" maneuver, whereby the inflated mask is rotated back out of the patient by 6 cm, a jaw lift performed, and the mask readvanced 6 cm. This maneuver will help release an epiglottis which may have been downfolded during the initial insertion (Fig. 6–9).

E. The Fastrach is then attached to the manual resuscitator device, ventilation is assessed, and the patient reoxygenated (Fig. 6–10).

F. The next step is to seek the position of best ventilation. While manually ventilating the

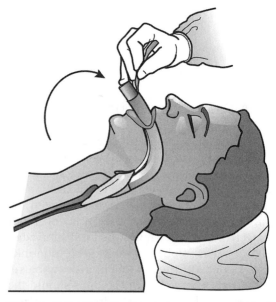

Figure 6–8. The Fastrach has been rotated down into the pharynx. (With permission LMA North America).

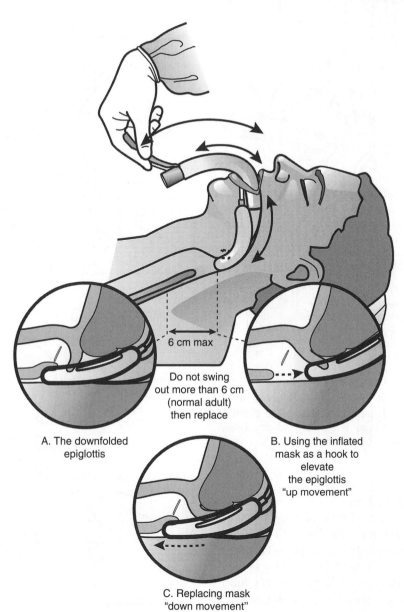

6 cm max

Do not swing
out more than 6 cm
(normal adult)
then replace

A. The downfolded
epiglottis

B. Using the inflated
mask as a hook to
elevate
the epiglottis
"up movement"

C. Replacing mask
"down movement"

Figure 6–9. An "up-down" maneuver is performed to relieve potential obstruction by a down folded epiglottis. A jaw lift is performed and the inflated mask is rotated back out of the patient by 6 cm, then readvanced 6 cm. (With permission LMA North America).

patient, the LMA Fastrach™ is manipulated forward or backward in 1-cm increments until the position at which maximal chest rise occurs with minimal leak (at applied pressures of 20–25 cm H_2O). This step, the first of the two-step **Chandy maneuver**, is helpful in assuring the mask is placed in optimal position for subsequent tube passage.

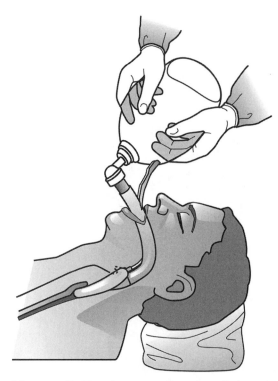

Figure 6–10. A manual resuscitator is attached to the Fastrach, seeking the point of maximum chest rise with ventilation. (With permission LMA North America).

Fastrach Intubation

A. The silicone-based tube is marked with a vertical black line which should face posteriorly toward the clinician: this orients the distal end of the ETT correctly to facilitate passage through the cords. The lubricated ETT is inserted through the Fastrach airway barrel. At 15-cm (indicated by a transverse line on the supplied tube, (Fig. 6–11 A, arrow) the distal end of the tube has reached the epiglottic elevating bar. As the ETT exits the Fastrach barrel and raises the epiglottic elevating bar, some resistance will be encountered: however, the resistance should decrease by the time the tube has been advanced 1.5-cm beyond the transverse line.

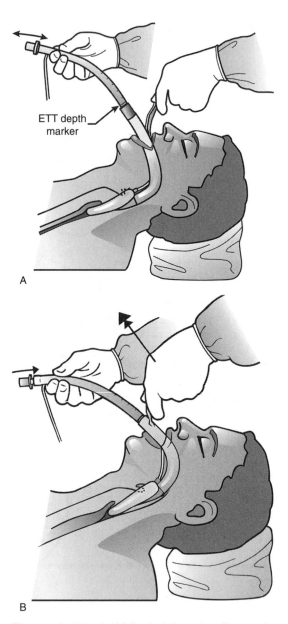

Figure 6–11. A While holding the Fastrach, the dedicated ETT is advanced, with vertical black line facing posteriorly, until the transverse black line on the ETT (arrow) is about to enter into the Fastrach barrel. B At this point, the Fastrach handle (and entire mask) should be lifted vertically (the second step of the "Chandy maneuver," to help apply the Fastrach to the glottic opening and optimize tube delivery. (With permission LMA North America).

B. At this point, the Fastrach handle (and entire mask) should be lifted vertically (the second step of the Chandy maneuver, Fig. 6–11 B), to help increase seal pressure and ensure optimal alignment of the axes of the trachea and the ETT. Most often, the tube passes easily into the trachea. After intubation, objective (i.e., end-tidal CO_2, or an esophageal detector device) signs of endotracheal placement of the ETT are sought, together with clinical confirmation.

Fastrach Removal

A. After confirmation of successful intubation, the LMA Fastrach™ itself can be removed. However, in a difficult airway situation, where the LMA Fastrach™ has been successfully used as a "plan B" alternative intubation device, if the clinician is unfamiliar with the mask removal process, it can be left in place until more experienced personnel are available for its removal. However, if the mask is left in-situ following successful intubation, its cuff should be deflated, arrangements should be made for its timely removal (e.g., within 4 hours), and the patient should be kept well sedated.

B. To remove the LMA Fastrach™, the mask cuff is deflated, and a stabilizer rod (supplied with the Fastrach) is placed at the proximal end of the reinforced ETT (after removing the 15-mm ETT connector) to keep the tube in place as the Fastrach is pulled back. As the mask is withdrawn, once the ETT is visible issuing distally from the mask, the tube is grasped and stabilized as mask removal is completed. The ETT's 15 mm connector is then reinserted, and ventilation of the patient is resumed. It should be noted that the ETT cuff may remain inflated at all times during this process. Fastrach mask removal is somewhat finicky, and should be done by an experienced user.

LMA Fastrach™ Troubleshooting

Maneuvers to help prevent and respond to difficulty with tube passage in the face of apparent good LMA Fastrach™ positioning have been described. These include the following.

Prevention

As already discussed, three maneuvers to help prevent difficult tube passage are (a) withdrawing and reinserting the inflated mask 6 cm (possibly releasing a down-folded obstructing epiglottis); (b) finding the minimum leak position of best ventilation of the mask before attempting intubation; and (c) vertically lifting the mask during attempted tube passage.

Response

If resistance to ETT passage occurs in spite of the above maneuvers, a change of mask size may be needed. This will be indicated by noting where resistance to ETT advancement is encountered, with reference to the transverse 15-cm black line on the ETT.

- A *larger mask* may be needed if resistance to ETT advancement is encountered about 3-cm beyond the transverse line. In this situation, the epiglottic elevating bar may be too proximal to contact and elevate the epiglottis. The tube may be impacting the vallecula, above the epiglottis.
- A *smaller mask* may be indicated if resistance is encountered just millimeters beyond the transverse line. In this situation, the epiglottic elevating bar may be jammed too far distally, behind the posterior cartilages.

Combination Use with Other Devices

Intubation through the LMA Fastrach™ can be facilitated with adjuvant use of the Trachlight[9] (with the internal wire stylet removed), or flexible fiberoptic devices.

Relative contraindications to blind intubation through the LMA Fastrach™ include a known foreign body in the upper airway or trachea; upper airway or upper esophageal pathology; traumatic tracheal disruption, and significant upper airway infection. However, indirect visualization using flexible fiberoptic devices may allow LMA Fastrach™-guided intubation in some airway pathology situations.

LMA Fastrach Effectiveness

ROUTINE AND DIFFICULT AIRWAY MANAGEMENT

After almost a decade of clinical use and study, the LMA Fastrach™ is supported by substantial narrative in the literature. Many case reports and case series attest to its effectiveness in difficult airway situations in both the emergency department (ED)[10,11] and the OR.[7,12] Successful Fastrach mask insertion and ventilation occurs in over 95% of cases and subsequent blind intubation succeeds in around 90% of cases.[4] There is no significant difference in overall or first attempt intubation success rates between patients with normal or abnormal airway anatomy.[4] Using the lightwand as a guide to facilitate LMA Fastrach™ intubation significantly increases overall, and first-attempt success rate.[4]

LMA Fastrach™ facilitated intubation has been successfully described in a number of case series of awake (topically anesthetized) patients,[13,14] and in one series of morbidly obese patients (with a 96% success rate).[15]

SKILLS ACQUISITION

A high rate of success in achieving LMA Fastrach™ insertion and ventilation has been reported in the hands of novice users: a 98% overall success rate, 81–96% on the first attempt.[4] Compared to the LMA Classic™, a higher rate of successful ventilation has been reported with the LMA Fastrach™.[16] Despite the high reported success rates, as is the case with many airway devices, inexperience with the LMA Fastrach™ use is associated with failure to intubate.[17]

C-SPINE PRECAUTIONS

Radiographic studies have shown a small amount of movement of the upper C-spine during LMA

Fastrach™ insertion, of unknown clinical significance.[4] In-line immobilization, the presence of a cervical collar, and cricoid pressure all appear to adversely affect LMA Fastrach™ insertion, ventilation, and blind intubation success rates.[4]

▶ THE AIRQ AND AIRQ REUSABLE

A second extraglottic device which can be used for both ventilation and intubation is the AirQ (Mercury Medical, Clearwater, FL, Fig. 6–12). The AirQ is available in disposable (AirQ) and reusable (AirQ Reusable, formerly known as the Cookgas Intubating Laryngeal Airway [ILA]) formats. The AirQ is available in sizes for use in patients weighing 10 kg and up. The reusable version is autoclavable, can be used up to 40 times, and is designed for use with regular ETTs of size 5.0–8.5 mm ID. To date the manufacturer's instructions advise tracheal intubation through the AirQ with adjunctive use of a flexible or semirigid fiberscope, tracheal tube introducer, airway exchange catheter, or lighted stylet. A dedicated removal stylet is available to help stabilize the ETT in the patient as the mask is removed following intubation. The disposable AirQ is available in four color-coded sizes.

▶ THE LIGHTWAND (E.G., TRACHLIGHT)

Trachlight Description

Lightwand use takes advantage of soft tissue transillumination in the neck, together with the anterior location of the trachea relative to the esophagus. Placed at or through the glottic opening based on an initial "educated guess" as to its position, the operator will see a well-defined, circumscribed, transilluminated glow just below the thyroid cartilage as the endotracheal tube-bearing lighted stylet emerges through the cords and below the cartilage (Fig. 6–13). In contrast, if the lighted stylet has been placed in the esophagus, a diffuse, minimal, or no glow will be seen.

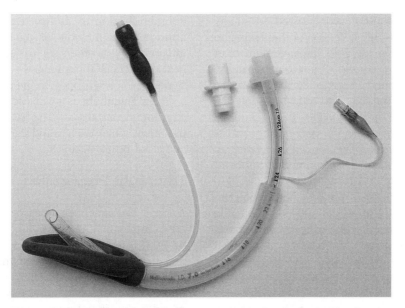

Figure 6–12. The AirQ Reusable (formerly known as the Cookgas Intubating Laryngeal Airway) Courtesy of Mercury Medical, Clearwater, FL.

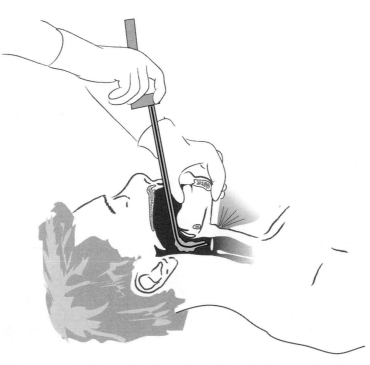

Figure 6–13. With correct initial positioning of the Trachlight, a well-defined, circumscribed transilluminated glow is seen in the anterior neck.

While lightwands have existed for many decades, the Trachlight version of the lightwand represents a considerable improvement over earlier versions. It consists of a reusable, battery-powered handle and a separate flexible wand. The wand, with a distal light and retractable internal wire stylet for rigidity, attaches to longitudinal grooves on the handle, via a connector on its proximal end. This connector can be moved up or down the handle to accommodate tubes of different lengths. A locking clamp on the handle secures a standard endotracheal tube connector. The internal stylet, housed within the wand, allows initially for sufficient stiffness to shape the wand to the needed 90° bend, but can be withdrawn once the trachea is accessed, rendering the tube pliable for easy advancement.

The lightwand requires minimal mouth opening and is actually ideally used with the head and neck in the neutral position. Its successful use is not limited by blood and secretions in the airway. However, as with the LMA Fastrach, it should be appreciated that as a blind technique, the presence of pathologic abnormalities in the airway represents a relative contraindication to its use. Examples of such abnormalities include laryngeal infectious or inflammatory disorders such as epiglottitis; laryngeal or tracheal abnormalities such as polyps or tumors; or foreign body in the airway.[18]

The Trachlight is available in adult, pediatric, and neonatal sizes. The handle is a multiple-use item, while each wand can be resterilized and used up to 10 times.

Trachlight Preparation

A small endotracheal tube should be chosen, for example, 6.5–7.0 mm ID for an adult female, or 7.0–7.5 mm ID for adult male patients. Cutting the endotracheal tube at the 27-cm mark and then replacing the ETT connector will improve control of the device, yet leave plenty of tube external to the patient's mouth for securing. Good lubrication with a silicone- or water-based lubricant should be applied to the outside of the wand as well as the internal stylet. The internal stylet is then advanced as far as it can go into the wand by snapping it into place in its U-shaped housing (Fig. 6–14). The wand should be connected to the grooves on the

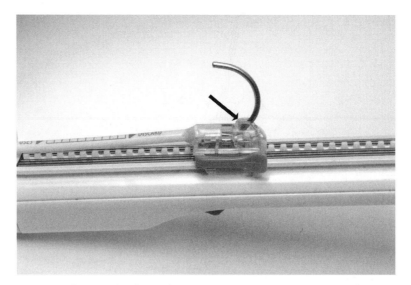

Figure 6–14. The U-shaped housing (arrow) in to which the Trachlight's internal stylet must be snapped.

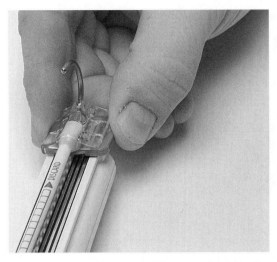

Figure 6–15. The wand is attached to the rail on the Trachlight handle.

handle by depressing a release arm on its proximal end (Fig. 6–15), and the light turned on and checked. The ETT should be loaded on to the Trachlight wand by pushing the ETT's 15-mm connector into the locking clamp on the handle, and closing the clamp lever (Fig. 6–16).

By pressing the release arm on the wand connector (Fig. 6–17), the distal light tip of the wand is advanced to a position just proximal to the bevel of the ETT (Fig. 6–18). The ETT/wand assembly is then bent acutely to an angle of 90° at the level of the indicator (the "bend here") mark on the wand (Fig. 6–19). The light source should again be checked. The light will begin blinking after 30 seconds to minimize heat generation, although this can also be taken as a reminder to reoxygenate the patient.

Trachlight Use

With any blind technique, the operator should maintain a mental image of the anatomy through which the device is traveling, and the Trachlight is no exception. The Trachlight is used with the supine patient's head in a neutral position.[19] A jaw lift is performed with the clinician's non-dominant hand to elevate the tongue and epiglottis away from the posterior pharynx, allowing clear passage for lightwand advancement

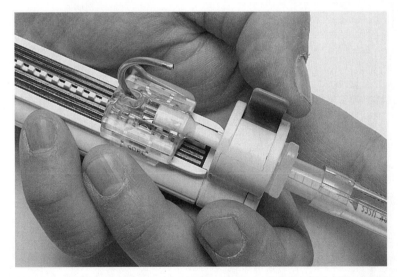

Figure 6–16. The clamp lever which secures the endotracheal tube's 15-mm connector to the Trachlight handle.

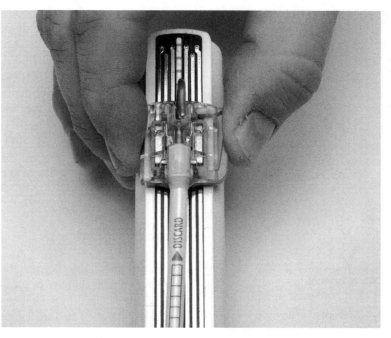

Figure 6–17. Depressing the release arm on the wand allows its movement up and down the Trachlight handle rail, needed to position the wand tip at the end of the ETT.

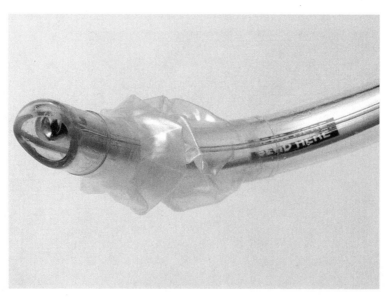

Figure 6–18. The Trachlight tip is placed just proximal to the bevel of the ETT by moving it up or down the handle rail.

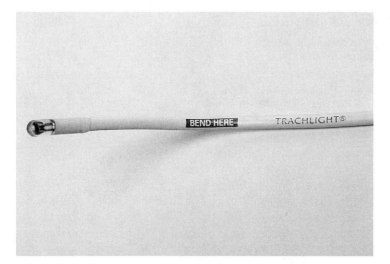

Figure 6–19. "Bend here" marking on the Trachlight shaft, indicating the location to place an acute 90° bend.

(Figure 6–20 A and B). The assembled Trachlight is inserted from the side of the mouth (Figure 6–21), and rotated medially to an upright position in the midline (Figure 6–22), so that the distal end ends up in the hypopharynx. This initial insertion technique helps maintain the 90° bend in the ETT/wand. The Trachlight is then lifted slightly and advanced in the midline, seeking a bright, circumscribed glow just below the laryngeal prominence.

Once the glow is obtained, the internal wire stylet is retracted 6–10 cm (not removed entirely), and the entire ETT/wand assembly is advanced (Figures 6–23 A and B). During

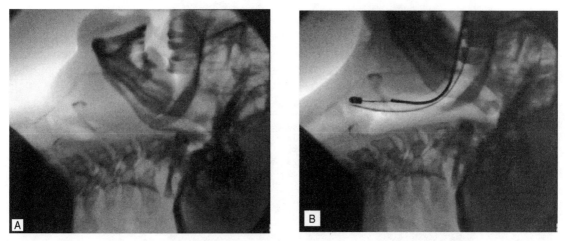

Figure 6–20. **A.** Lateral fluoroscopic view of the airway in an obtunded patient. **B.** In the same patient, a jaw lift allows for free passage of the Trachlight through an unobstructed lumen.

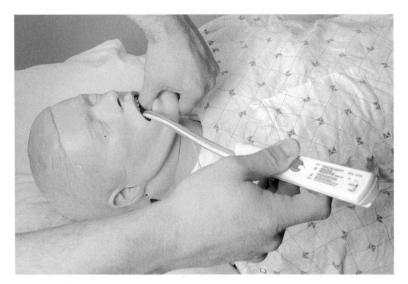

Figure 6–21. Trachlight insertion is with a jaw lift, from the side of the mouth.

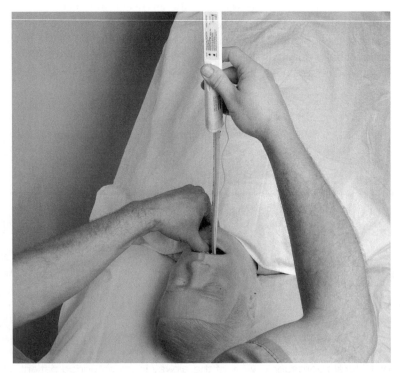

Figure 6–22. Still holding a jaw lift, the Trachlight is rotated upright in the midline.

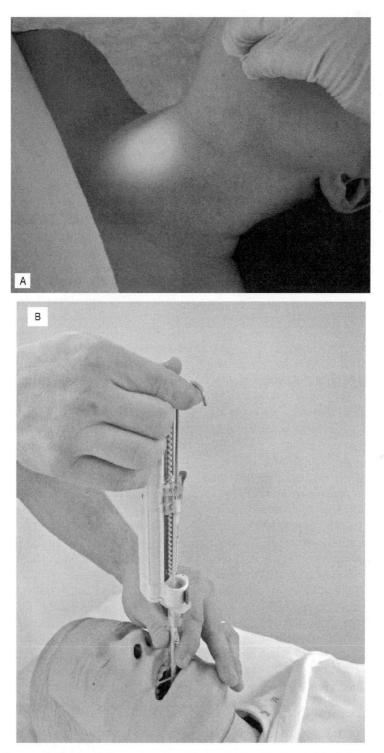

Figure 6–23. Once a bright, midline glow is obtained (A), the Trachlight's internal wire stylet is withdrawn (B), and the tube/wand assembly is advanced.

advancement, the glow will visibly travel caudad in the anterior neck: once at or just below the sternal notch, the tube can be assumed to be properly positioned.[20,21] The locking clamp is then released and the Trachlight is withdrawn from the firmly held endotracheal tube. Endotracheal location should be confirmed with capnography.

Trachlight Troubleshooting

Failure to obtain a glow in the appropriate midline location suggests malpositioning. It should be confirmed that the wire stylet is well-seated in its U-shaped housing proximally, as lateral directional control of the ETT tip will otherwise be lost. If too posterior (esophageal), there will be minimal or no glow appreciable, and the tip of the stylet should be redirected more anteriorly, either by lifting up on the entire device, or rocking it slightly backwards. Too lateral a tip location is suggested by a glow off the midline, lateral to the thyroid cartilage. Minor left/right repositioning should be attempted. In fact, as the tip of the lightwand is rotated slightly from left to right, often a "flash" of light may be seen proceeding down the trachea as the light tip sweeps across the laryngeal inlet. This will help orient the clinician to the location of the cords and trachea.

Occasionally, difficulty with tube passage may be encountered after obtaining the correct circumscribed glow in the midline of the neck: the tube fails to advance as the internal wire stylet is withdrawn. This occurs as the leading edge of the tube abuts anterior or lateral tracheal wall, where it may be impinging on a cartilaginous ring. In these circumstances, the entire Trachlight/tube assembly can be transiently rotated to the right, such that the Trachlight handle ends up almost parallel to the floor. This will often release the "hang-up", allowing for forward passage of the tube. This phenomenon will be encountered less often if the tube is (a) loaded "inverted" (with the tube's concavity facing opposite the bend of the wand) and (b) softened in warm water before use.[22]

The Trachlight can be used in ambient room lighting, although this obviously varies with the brightness of the lighting and patient neck soft tissue thickness. One published series reported successful use in ambient lighting in 88% of cases.[23] However, if difficulty is encountered (or anticipated) in perceiving a glow, room lighting should be reduced.[19,24] Trachlight use in the presence of cricoid pressure, as would be applied during a rapid-sequence intubation (RSI), has been reported to take longer, and have a lower first attempt success rate,[25] although successful Trachlight use is higher in patients who are paralyzed.[26] Combination use of the lightwand to facilitate intubation via the LMA Classic™,[27] LMA Fastrach™,[9] and direct laryngoscopy[28,29] has been reported to good effect. In one of these studies, the lightwand was used as an adjunct to direct laryngoscopy in 350 patients with simulated Grade 3 views: 78% of patients were successfully intubated on the first, and all by the third attempt.[28] Lightwand-facilitated nasotracheal intubation is also well described and effective in experienced hands.[19,30,31]

Trachlight Effectiveness

ROUTINE AND DIFFICULT AIRWAY MANAGEMENT

In experienced hands, the Trachlight is very effective. One of the largest published series on Trachlight intubation in routine surgical patients reported a 98% success rate, most on the first attempt. In contrast to direct laryngoscopy, time to intubation and success with the Trachlight in this series was not correlated with any of the usual anatomic predictors of difficult intubation.[23] A second study by the same group in patients with predictors or a history of difficult laryngoscopy documented a 99% intubation success rate with the Trachlight.[3]

SKILLS ACQUISITION

Manikin[32,33] and human[34] studies using novice personnel have generally shown a higher success rate with direct laryngoscopy, compared to Trachlight use. One other study using anesthesia personnel unfamiliar with the Trachlight showed a significantly higher success rate in the final 10 of 30 Trachlight intubations.[35] Realistically, the Trachlight is a device requiring experience for consistently successful use, and should be chosen as a primary alternative intubation technique by clinicians having the opportunity to become familiar with its use, for example, in the elective setting of the OR.

C-SPINE PRECAUTIONS

The Trachlight is an attractive choice for the intubation of a patient with C-spine precautions, as it is ideally used with the head and neck in the neutral position.[18,19] Two studies[36,37] comparing Trachlight use with direct laryngoscopy, one with applied in-line stabilization, have shown less C-spine movement with Trachlight use. When compared with the LMA Fastrach™ in patients with applied in-line stabilization, the Trachlight resulted in faster intubation times and a higher success rate.[38]

▶ FIBEROPTIC STYLETS

Designed for use from within an ensleeved endotracheal tube, fiberoptic stylets allow indirect visualization through a proximal eyepiece, via a fiberoptic bundle. These devices can be used on their own as true "alternative intubation" instruments, or can be used as adjuncts to direct laryngoscopy. Compared to flexible fiberoptic devices, fiberoptic stylets are relatively easy to use, portable, more robust, and significantly less expensive. Published literature on the use of these tools is limited, but growing as user experience increases.

Fiberoptic Stylet Description

Two examples of fiberoptic stylet are the **Shikani Optical Stylet** (SOS) and **Levitan FPS Scope** (Clarus Medical LLC, Minneapolis, MN). The SOS is a semirigid stylet containing fiberoptic illumination and viewing bundles, which connects to a handle containing a halogen light source (Fig. 6–3). An adapter is also available enabling its use with a regular laryngoscope handle. Attached to the stylet is a sliding "tube-stop" connector which accepts the proximal end of an endotracheal tube. This connector also has a removable attachment which allows connection to oxygen tubing. The SOS is available in one adult and one pediatric size.

Manufactured by the same company as the SOS, the Levitan FPS ("First Pass Success") scope features a similar semimalleable optical stylet and fixed-focus eyepiece. As a shorter and simpler version of the SOS, it was designed primarily to serve as an adjunct to direct laryngoscopy. A precut tube is loaded on the stylet and seated proximally in a fixed fitting that accepts the ETT's 15-mm connector. A small hole in the side of this fitting allows for the application of (low-flow) oxygen down the ETT via a removable connector.[39] The factory shape of the stylet includes a distal 35° bend to facilitate its use as an adjunct to direct laryngoscopy (DL). Power is supplied from any "Greenline" compatible handle or a separate light-emitting diode light source. Cleaning is similar to that required for a laryngoscope blade. The reduced number of fiberoptic bundles in the Levitan FPS scope has helped lower manufacturing costs, while not compromising image quality.

Other examples of fiberoptic optical stylets exist. The **Bonfils Retromolar Intubation Endoscope** (Karl Storz Endoscopy, Culver City, CA) is available in adult and pediatric sizes, and features a fixed 40° anterior distal curvature. It is supplied in a battery-powered portable version as well as with an integrated coupling for video-based use via a dedicated Airway Management Trolley. Also from Karl Storz, the **Brambrinck Intubation Endoscope** is designed specifically for pediatric use. The **StyletScope** (FSS, Nihon Kohden Corp., Tokyo, Japan) has a lever adjacent to its proximal handle, activation of which results in variable anterior flexion of the distal stylet (with its ensleeved tube), to angles of up to 75°. The **Foley Airway Stylet** (FAST, Clarus Medical LLC, Minneapolis, MN) is a flexible optical stylet, compatible with the SOS handle, designed specifically to visually aid LMA Fastrach™ intubation.

Fiberoptic Stylet Preparation

When using a fiberoptic stylet (or other alternative intubation device) in a difficult airway situation, the use of a slightly smaller ETT may facilitate endotracheal intubation. The tube is loaded over the stylet, with its proximal 15-mm connector placed snugly in the movable tube holder (SOS and Bonfils) or fixed (Levitan FPS) proximal ETT fitting (Fig. 6–24). In the case of the SOS and Bonfils stylets, the tube holder is adjusted up or down the stylet shaft to locate the tip of the stylet 1-cm proximal to the end of the ETT, while with the Levitan FPS, a loaded ETT cut to the appropriate length (27.5 cm) should automatically result in the appropriate stylet tip location within the ETT. This positioning allows the tip of the device to be slightly recessed within the distal end of the ETT, protecting it from secretions and minimizing the potential for loss of view from the instrument abutting mucosal tissue.

The distal end of the fiberoptic stylet should be bent (semimalleable scopes only) according to the planned method of use: for use as an adjunct to direct laryngoscopy, it should have 35–40° of anterior angulation just proximal to the ETT cuff. If stand-alone use is planned, the angle should be increased to 60–75° for a midline approach, or left at 35–40° for an over-the-molar approach.

An antifogging agent can be applied to the distal end of the stylet, or it may be heated by placement in a bottle of warm water. One of these antifogging maneuvers should ideally be undertaken, otherwise placement of a cold instrument in a patient will result in a view obscured by fogging.

Fiberoptic Stylet Use

Fiberoptic Stylet Use as an Adjunct to Direct Laryngoscopy

A fiberoptic stylet prepared with an ensleeved tube can be used if difficulty is encountered

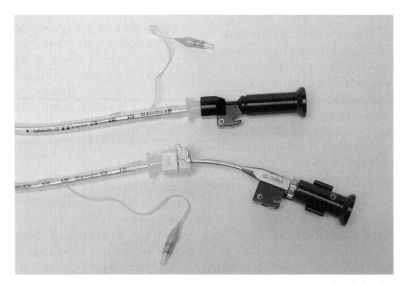

Figure 6–24. Proximal tube stops for Shikani SOS (above) and Levitan FPS (below).

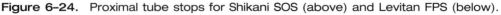

with direct laryngoscopy. If a Cormack Grade 3 (epiglottis only) view persists despite "best look" laryngoscopy, while retaining that view with ongoing laryngoscopy, the tip of the scope/tube assembly is placed, *under direct vision,* close to, but slightly below and away from the tip of the epiglottis ("tip-to-tip," Fig. 6–25 A).[39] This position can be retained by resting the tube gently against the upper teeth while the clinician then transfers from direct vision to indirect fiberoptic visualization through the scope eyepiece. Once the glottic opening has been identified, the ETT/scope assembly is advanced through the cords. During this advancement, to conform to the axis of the trachea, the proximal (eyepiece) end of the scope will have to be gradually rotated downward. After the trachea has been accessed, the laryngoscope can be removed. *While visualization through the eyepiece is maintained,* the left hand can now be used to slide the ETT away from the tube holder housing, and further on down the trachea. Alter-

natively, the laryngoscope can be maintained in position while a briefed assistant advances the ETT off the stylet. Once the ETT is placed, the fiberoptic stylet is withdrawn from the tube by forward rotation. After cuff inflation, the position of the ETT is confirmed with a second objective method.

In the very rare situation in which a Cormack Grade 4 (no identifiable structures) view is obtained at direct laryngoscopy, the fiberoptic stylet/tube assembly can be advanced along the laryngoscope blade, using the blade as a guide until the epiglottis is visualized through the eyepiece. Appropriate maneuvers are then performed to advance the tube beneath the epiglottis and through the cords.

To attain and maintain skills with the device, some clinicians have espoused the use of optical stylets with every intubation attempt[39]: if the cords are easily visualized with direct laryngoscopy, the tube can be advanced in regular fashion with the fiberoptic stylet acting as a

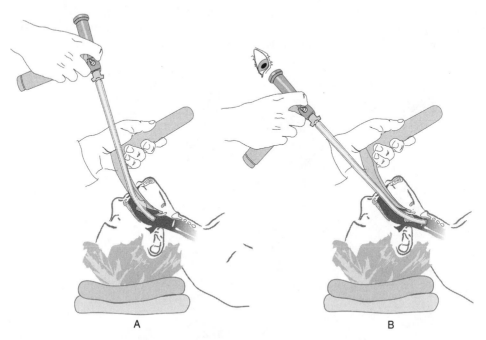

A   B

Figure 6–25. The Levitan FPS is placed under direct vision with aid of a laryngoscope. Once the scope's distal tip is positioned under the tip of the epiglottis (A), visualization of the glottic inlet is sought through the eyepiece and the instrument then advanced through the cords (B).

standard malleable stylet, but if a Grade 3 or worse view is obtained, the fiberoptic stylet/tube assembly can be used to aid indirect visualization of, and passage through the glottic opening, as described above.

Stand-Alone Fiberoptic Stylet Use

Fiberoptic stylets can also be used on their own. With such stand-alone use, the distal curvature of semimalleable versions should be increased for the midline approach, as mentioned above. The scope should be antifogged and the patient's oropharynx suctioned. While performing a jaw lift (Fig. 6–26) with the nondominant hand, the scope is inserted either in the midline over the tongue or via a more lateral approach, over the molars. A midline insertion will involve the clinician's significantly bending over the patient to access the scope's eyepiece (Figure 6–27). Anatomic landmarks are then sought as the scope is advanced: uvula, base of tongue, then epiglottis and cords with a midline approach, or epiglottis then cords with an over-the-molar approach. The tube/stylet assembly can be gently advanced through the cords, at which point

the tube is further advanced off the stylet down the trachea.

Awake Intubation Using a Fiberoptic Stylet

Fiberoptic stylets may be used in the sitting, cooperative patient for an awake tracheal intubation, using a face-to-face approach.[40] Following appropriate application of topical airway anesthesia (Chap. 8), gentle tongue traction is applied by an assistant. The stylet with preloaded ETT is guided through the mouth in the midline, and advanced behind the tongue, until its tip disappears. At this point, the long axis of the scope will be parallel to the floor. The clinician then looks through the proximal eyepiece and seeks the anatomic landmark of the epiglottis, leading to the glottic opening. In the stand-alone manner described earlier, the distal tip of the tube/ stylet assembly is navigated to and through the glottic opening into the proximal trachea. The tube is then further advanced off the stylet, and the scope is removed by forward rotation of the proximal end back toward the patient's chest.

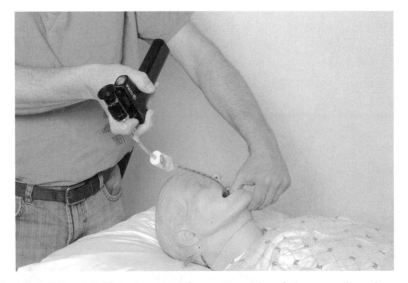

Figure 6–26. The Shikani SOS is inserted from the side of the mouth, advanced over the molars, and then rotated upright.

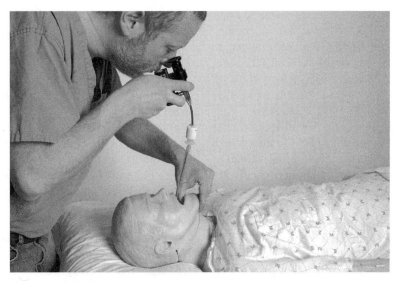

Figure 6–27. While maintaining a jaw lift, the user looks through the proximal eyepiece of the SOS in an attempt to view the glottic structures.

Fiberoptic Stylet Troubleshooting

- **Getting "lost."** It should be appreciated that navigation of any fiberoptic instrument through the airway is contingent on advancing the device through a patent airway lumen. While an awake patient will maintain airway patency, an obtunded or relaxed patient (as during an RSI) must have a patent lumen created by a laryngoscope blade, with a jaw thrust, or gentle tongue traction during the procedure. The stylet should *not* be blindly advanced if no lumen is appreciable. In the event that orientation is lost (often manifested by "pink-out"), the scope should be partially withdrawn until an anatomic landmark (e.g., uvula or epiglottis) can be reidentified and at that point, advancement can resume.
- **Fogging.** If fogging is encountered once the stylet is already in use, briefly holding the stylet tip against the patient's buccal mucosa will help clear the view.
- **Blood and secretions.** It should be understood that there is no integrated suction

mechanism with most of these instruments. Blood, secretions, and vomitus will make use of an indirect fiberoptic system difficult. For this reason, fiberoptic scope use should always be preceded by suctioning of the oropharynx. Also, as blood and secretions will pool posteriorly, the scope should be kept anterior in the airway during navigation toward the laryngeal inlet. The difficulty which blood and secretions can cause with the use of a fiberoptic scope points to the need for its early use, before the airway has been traumatized by multiple intubation attempts!

Fiberoptic Stylet Effectiveness

ROUTINE AND DIFFICULT AIRWAY MANAGEMENT

Shikani studied 120 patients, 74 of them children, including 7 patients with Cormack Grade 3 or 4 views. All patients in the series, including 5 awake patients, were successfully intubated with the scope, 88% on the first attempt. Five of the seven Grade 3 and 4 patients required concomitant direct laryngoscopy.[41] Bein et al.[42] studied use of the Bonfils fiberoptic stylet in 80 patients with predictors of difficult DL, comparing it to LMA Fastrach use. Thirty-nine of 40 patients randomized to the Bonfils were intubated on the first attempt, in contrast to a 70% first attempt success rate for the Fastrach. A second study looked at Bonfils use after failed DL. In 25 patients recruited following two failed DL attempts, 88% were successfully intubated with the Bonfils at the first attempt, and all but one (96%) by the second attempt.[43] Evans and coworkers compared the SOS to the bougie in a manikin study with a fixed Grade 3 view. In this model, the SOS resulted in faster intubation times than the bougie, with significantly fewer esophageal intubations.[44] A second manikin study, this one comparing the bougie with the Levitan FPS scope, showed the fiberoptic scope to be significantly more successful than the bougie in managing a simulated Grade 3B view,[45] but did not demonstrate a significant difference in intubation success in a simulated Grade 3A view. The latter finding has been confirmed in a subsequent human study using simulated Grade 3 views in elective surgical patients, in which the bougie was found to be equally effective to the Levitan FPS scope.[46] Finally, a recently published case series has documented successful use of the Bonfils in six patients in whom difficulty had been encountered in the prehsopital setting.[47]

SKILLS ACQUISITION

These devices are relatively easy to learn on manikins, as dealing with "pink out" is rarely an issue, and the upper airway lumen is widely patent. Skill transfer to the live setting is likely to be more challenging. One study looking at the learning curve of the Bonfils stylet suggested that proficiency was attained after 20–25 intubations.[48] Other studies with fiberoptic stylets have reported that most of the failed intubations occurred within the first 10 uses of the device.[41,49] The fact that the fiberoptic stylet can

be used as an adjunct to the core skill of direct laryngoscopy may contribute to an easier learning curve.

C-SPINE PRECAUTIONS

In a study comparing intubation using Macintosh blade direct laryngoscopy with the Bonfils stylet, Bullard laryngoscope, or LMA Fastrach, each of the Bonfils, Bullard, and Fastrach resulted in significantly less C-spine movement than Macintosh blade-facilitated intubation, although Bonfils and Fastrach intubations took significantly longer than those using the Macintosh and Bullard blades.[50] A second study, also using fluoroscopy to assess C-spine movement, found that Bonfils intubations caused significantly less extension of the upper C-spine than Macintosh laryngoscope-aided intubations.[51]

▶ VIDEOLARYNGOSCOPY

Displaying the view obtained at laryngoscopy on a video monitor has a number of advantages:

- Display of an enlarged, panoramic viewing field.[52]
- In those devices using integrated video technology on rigid blades, as the camera is located toward the distal end of the blade, an improved view may be obtained compared to direct laryngoscopy.
- Aids in teaching.
- Assisting personnel can see the results of their manipulations, for example, external laryngeal manipulation (ELM).
- The procedure can be digitally stored for documentation, teaching, or research purposes.
- The user is at a greater distance away from the patient's face, decreasing the chance of exposure to potentially infectious respiratory secretions and spray.

Video technology can be applied in two ways: (a) using an adapter, a video camera can be attached to the eyepiece of conventional fiberoptic devices such as the Shikani, Levitan FPS, Bullard, or flexible fiberoptic bronchoscopes, or (b) integrated video is used as the primary viewing mechanism (e.g., the Glidescope).

The Glidescope

Commercially introduced in 2002, the Glidescope® (GVL®) is a video laryngoscope which has become increasingly available in and out of the OR, as an alternative intubation device. The one-piece blade and handle is made of a durable medical-grade plastic. The blade has a vertical profile of 14.5 mm, a 60° bend midblade, and distally, houses a miniature video camera and light-emitting diode (LED) light source. The image obtained by the camera is projected by cable to a liquid-crystal display (LCD) color monitor. A heating element covering the camera provides effective antifogging after the device has been turned on for 10–30 seconds. The reusable blades are available in large (patients 30 kg and up), midsize

(10 kg and up), and small (1.5 kg and up) sizes, and can be sterilized. More recently introduced versions of the GVL include the **GVL Ranger**, which is a compact, battery-based unit, and the **GVL Cobalt**, which features a reusable internal video baton for placement within large or small-sized disposable blades.

The GVL is inserted orally in the midline. As the scope is advanced, the uvula, base of tongue and then epiglottis will be visualized on the screen, helping to retain orientation to the midline. Although the blade is designed to be placed above the epiglottis in the vallecula, in contrast to direct laryngoscopy, the blade tip need not be advanced completely into the glossoepiglottic fold: a more proximal tip location allows a wider field of view and more room for ETT manipulation (Fig. 6–28). A styletted ETT is inserted immediately on the right side of the blade and is navigated to the laryngeal inlet under indirect visualization on the LCD screen. An accompanying nonmalleable, reusable stylet has been made available by the manufacturer to facilitate tube passage (Fig. 6–29), or a regular malleable stylet can be used, angled at about 60°

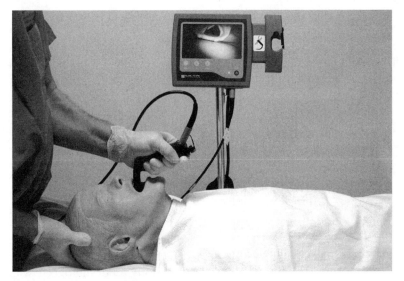

Figure 6–28. Glidescope video system use.

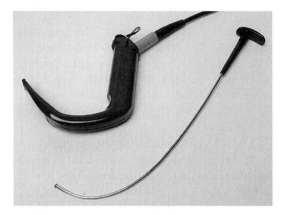

Figure 6–29. Dedicated rigid stylet (below) for use with the Glidescope.

just proximal to the cuff.[53,54] Once the tip of the ETT has been passed through the cords, the stylet should be withdrawn 2 inches (4 cm), whereupon the tube can be further advanced off the stylet down the trachea.[55]

There is a growing literature on the use of this device, primarily in the OR setting. It is clear that the GVL does provide good and often superior views of the glottic opening when compared with conventional laryngoscopy, including a high rate of conversion of Cormack Grade 3 (epiglottis only) views to Grade 2 or better.[53,54,56,57] However, somewhat longer intubation times have been reported with the GVL compared to DL, even in the setting of Grade 1 views by DL, possibly related to user inexperience with tube delivery.[54,57–59]

The GVL has been successfully used for awake intubations in adults.[60] C-spine motion during GVL use has been compared, using fluoroscopy, to that incurred with Macintosh blade DL. Motion with GVL use was less than that incurred by Macintosh laryngoscopy at only one (C2-5) of 4 neck levels studied.[37]

There are some recent reports of upper airway trauma during GVL use.[55,61,62] This suggests that especially in the patient with a smaller oral cavity, awareness of the ETT tip location must be maintained as it is advanced, ideally by direct vision of the ETT until it has passed the palatoglossal arch. Thereafter, the clinician's vision can be transferred to the screen and indirect, videoscopic ETT navigation can occur to and through the cords. Alternatively, some clinicians prefer to place the ETT into the patient's pharynx prior to insertion of the GVL blade.[55]

The Berci-Kaplan DCI Video Laryngoscope

The Berci-Kaplan DCI video laryngoscope (Karl Storz Endoscopy, Culver City, CA) is a hybrid of fiberoptic and video technology: an image-light bundle in a laryngoscope blade delivers an image to a video camera located in the handle of what otherwise looks like a regular direct laryngoscope. A cable attaches the device to a cart-based camera-control unit, and also delivers light from the remote light source. The image obtained is displayed on a video monitor. Macintosh # 3, Mac 4, adult- and pediatric-sized Miller, and Dörges blades are available for use with the system. This system offers the advantage of being a familiar intubation technique and may deliver a superior view of the laryngeal inlet compared to that obtained with direct laryngoscopy.[52]

The LMA CTrach

The LMA CTrach (LMA North America Inc, San Diego CA) is a version of the previously discussed LMA Fastrach™ which adds video-guidance capability (Fig. 6–30). Looking otherwise like the LMA Fastrach™, the CTrach mask contains fiberoptic bundles for light and image transmission, emerging at the distal end of the airway barrel. In addition, a removable viewing monitor (the CTrach Viewer) attaches to the CTrach handle by way of a magnetic latch connector. The battery-powered viewer is rechargeable, and provides controls for focusing and image adjustment. For use, the CTrach Viewer is detached, and the mask is deflated, lubricated posteriorly, and antifogged with application of an appropriate solution to the fiberoptic lenses. Mask insertion is identical to the technique used

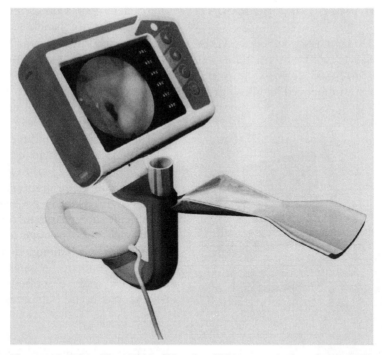

Figure 6–30. The LMA CTrach. (With permission from LMA North America).

for the LMA Fastrach™, with the head and neck in a neutral position. Once seated, the mask is inflated and the patient ventilated. The CTrach viewer is then turned on and attached to the magnetic latch connector on the mask, while firmly holding the CTrach handle. The mask is then manipulated as needed to attain a clear image of the glottic opening. For intubation, while lifting vertically on the CTrach handle (i.e., the Chandy maneuver, as described for LMA Fastrach™ intubation), the dedicated silicone-based ETT is advanced through the cords under indirect vision. The ETT cuff is inflated, and tube position confirmed. The viewer is then detached, whereupon the CTrach mask can be removed in identical fashion to the Fastrach, leaving the ETT in situ.

At the time of writing, early published clinical experience with the CTrach suggests a high rate of successful mask insertion and patient ventilation, as with the LMA-Fastrach™.[63,64] Although a view of the cords is not always easily

attained, even after manipulation.[63,64] a number of corrective maneuvers will help to attain or improve the view of the laryngeal inlet.[65–68] As with the LMA Fastrach™, the "up-down" (withdrawing the inflated mask 6 cm, then readvancing it) will often help release a down-folded epiglottis.[65,66,68] If only the posterior cartilages are visualized, withdrawing the mask 1-cm and lifting will improve the view.[65] The need for medial-lateral corrections of the mask can also be visualized on the screen.[66] Once a good view is attained, intubation usually succeeds, and even with poor visualization, successful intubation follows in some cases.[63–65] In published series, CTrach use has permitted visualization of the larynx and successful intubation in most patients presenting Grade 3 or worse views at direct laryngoscopy.[63, 64, 68] Other case reports and series have detailed successful CTrach intubation in very difficult situations,[68] even when the LMA Fastrach™ had failed.[69]

The McGrath Video Laryngoscope

The McGrath video laryngoscope Series 5 (LMA North America, San Diego, CA) is an additional example of a video-based device (Fig. 6–31). The scope features a rubberized handle with an attached 1.7-inch video screen. The screen tilts and rotates on the handle to optimize the viewing angle for the clinician. The blade is somewhat adjustable in length for different patients, and is designed for use with a single-use disposable plastic sleeve. The entire unit is portable, and operates using a single AA battery. As with the Glidescope, once the laryngeal inlet has been indirectly visualized, the clinician guides a styletted tube toward and through the cords. Early experience suggests easy McGrath blade insertion and a good view of the larynx, even in patients with predictors of difficult direct laryngoscopy.[70] As with the Glidescope, tube passage to and through the larynx can be challenging until the learning curve is ascended.[70] A similar intubation technique to that described above for the Glidescope should be successful.

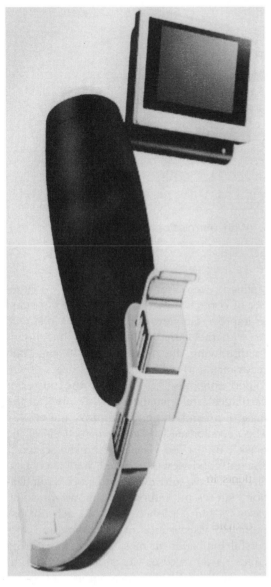

Figure 6–31. The McGrath Video laryngoscope Series 5.

▶ OTHER RIGID AND FLEXIBLE FIBEROPTIC AND OPTICAL INSTRUMENTS

Rigid Fiberoptic Devices

Other rigid fiberoptic scopes exist. Some have attained a small but loyal following, mainly in the OR setting, however due to expense or unfavorable learning curves, as a group, they are rarely used in out-of-OR settings. One such is the **Bullard laryngoscope** (Fig. 6–32), an L-shaped rigid fiberoptic laryngoscope. The Bullard has a blade enabling good tongue control, and a choice of two dedicated attached stylets to facilitate tube passage. With or without the attached stylet, tube passage can be difficult, however, and this fact has limited its popularity over the years. The Bullard has been shown to result in less cervical spine movement than that caused by Macintosh or Miller laryngoscopy,[71] although the clinical significance of this finding is unclear. Similar J- or L-shaped rigid fiberoptic scopes include the UpsherScope Ultra and the WuScope System.

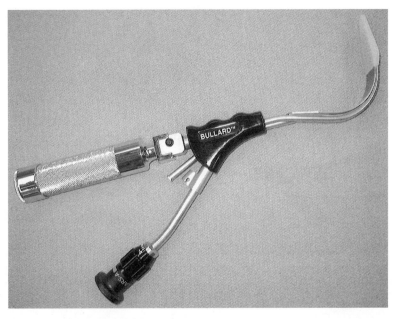

Figure 6–32. Bullard laryngoscope.

Rigid Optical Device: The Airtraq

The **Airtraq** optical laryngoscope (King Systems Corp., Noblesville, IN) is a single-use, L-shaped device which uses a series of mirrors to deliver an image of the laryngeal inlet to a proximal eyepiece (Fig. 6–33). Insertion of the device begins with the handle parallel to the patient's chest. As the blade is advanced into the oropharynx, it is rotated down and around the tongue, with the clinician looking through the eyepiece to visualize airway structures. The blade tip is placed into the vallecula and the cords centered in the viewfinder, whereupon the pre-loaded ETT is advanced into the trachea via a built-in tube delivery channel. The ETT is then separated from the delivery channel to the side, and while holding the tube in place, the scope is rotated back out of the patient. At the time of writing, the Airtraq was available in two sizes: "Regular," accommodating tube sizes 7.0–8.5 mm ID, and "Small Adult", appropriate for use with ETTs of size 6.0–7.5 mm ID.

Early manikin studies comparing the Airtraq to Macintosh direct laryngoscopy have shown a favorable learning curve for novice[72] and inexperienced[73] clinicians. With "difficult airway" simulator features activated, tracheal intubation has required less time and fewer attempts by experienced clinicians using the Airtraq, compared to Macintosh laryngoscopy.[74] In elective surgical patients with no predictors of difficult laryngoscopy, performance of the Airtraq was comparable to Macintosh DL.[75] With known difficult laryngoscopy, however, the Airtraq was successful in providing a view and enabling intubation in a series of 8 elective surgical patients in whom a Cormack Lehane Grade 4 laryngoscopy had been encountered.[76]

Flexible Fiberoptic and Video Devices

Flexible fiberoptic or video-based bronchoscopes have been the mainstay of difficult airway management in the OR. Most awake

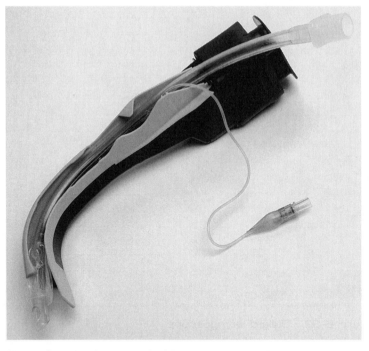

Figure 6–33. Airtraq optical laryngoscope (single-use).

intubations are performed with flexible fiberoptic bronchoscopes in this setting, although many of the other techniques and devices described in this and other chapters (including direct laryngoscopy) can also be used on the awake patient. Unfortunately, flexible fiberoptic- or videobronchoscopes are expensive to attain and maintain, and skills acquisition is also an issue, resulting in these instruments rarely being used for intubation by non-anesthesia clinicians. Having said this, flexible fiberoptic scopes can be used in various capacities, including nasopharyngoscopic upper airway assessment, or flexible fiberoptic guided intubation through the LMA Fastrach™ or AirQ extraglottic devices. With time, flexible fiberoptic intubation may become a more commonly used technique for awake intubation of the difficult airway patient in out-of-OR locations, by non-anesthesia personnel. For more details on the technique, the reader is referred to reviews[77] in other publications.

▶ PEDIATRIC ALTERNATIVE INTUBATION OPTIONS

For those departments or environments having care of pediatric patients in their mandate, when choosing equipment, consideration should be directed toward whether it is available in pediatric sizes. It must be emphasized that most children without congenital dysmorphisms can be successfully intubated with direct laryngoscopy and can almost always be easily bag-mask ventilated. However, in the event that difficulty is encountered with direct laryngoscopy, the following is a summary of the availability of pediatric versions of the devices discussed above:

- **LMA Fastrach™.** At the time of writing, the smallest reusable or disposable Fastrach available is the adult #3, appropriate for use in patients weighing 30–50 kg.

- **AirQ.** The smallest size is the 1.5, for use in patients weighing 10–20 kg.
- **Trachlight.** The Trachlight is available in two pediatric sizes (child and infant). Clinicians experienced with Trachlight use in children have commented that, while effective, the thin necks of the very young make it difficult to distinguish the glow of a tube correctly placed in the trachea from incorrect esophageal placement. This is particularly problematic in infants.
- **Fiberoptic Stylets.** The SOS is available in a pediatric size, 27 cm in length and accepting tubes down to 2.5 mm ID. One small case series has described its successful use in four children with various dysmorphisms.[78] The Bonfils Retromolar Intubation Endoscope in the pediatric/ small adult size will accept tube sizes from 4.0 to 5.5 mm ID, while the Brambrinck Intubation Endoscope (both marketed by Karl Storz) will accept a minimum tube size of 2.5 mm ID.
- **Video laryngoscopes.** The mid-size (minimum patient weight, 10 kg) and small (patient weight, 1.5 kg) Glidescope blades are appropriate for pediatric use. Pediatric and neonatal blades are available for use with the Berci-Kaplan DCI Video Laryngoscope.
- **Other devices.** The Bullard laryngoscope is available in child and neonatal blade sizes, while flexible fiberoptic bronchoscopes are available in an array of pediatric sizes, compatible with flexible fiberoptic intubation of even infants.

▶ SUMMARY

Many alternative intubation devices are available. They differ in their degree of history, published evidence of their effectiveness, cost, and whether they are blind techniques or allow indirect vision. Most are probably similar in their learning curve and success rates in difficult situations. Unfortunately, many clinical trials of these devices have been performed in comparison to conventional DL, leaving unanswered the question of how they compare to best look DL (i.e., using head lift, ELM, and adjuncts such as the bougie). However, case reports, case series, and studies of patients with actual difficult airways do suggest their utility in difficult situations (although often, in the hands of expert users). Certainly, moving on to an alternative intubation device after a best look laryngoscopy has failed is preferable to multiple futile attempts at direct laryngoscopic intubation. Which alternative intubation device or devices the clinician chooses to become familiar with will depend on individual or institutional preference. However, no matter which device, the clinician must make the effort to gain experience by using it in lower-acuity or routine situations until competence and confidence in its use are attained.

REFERENCES

1. Crosby ET, Cooper RM, Douglas MJ, et al. The unanticipated difficult airway with recommendations for management. *Can J Anaesth.* 1998;45(8):757–776.
2. Mort TC. Emergency tracheal intubation: complications associated with repeated laryngoscopic attempts. *Anesth Analg.* 2004;99(2):607–613, table of contents.
3. Hung OR, Pytka S, Morris I, Murphy M, Stewart RD. Lightwand intubation: II—Clinical trial of a new lightwand for tracheal intubation in patients with difficult airways. *Can J Anaesth.* 1995;42(9):826–830.
4. Brimacombe JR. Intubating LMA for airway intubation. *Laryngeal Mask Anesthesia: Principles and Practice.* Second ed. Philadelphia: Saunders; 2005:469–504.
5. Reardon RF, Martel M. The intubating laryngeal mask airway: suggestions for use in the emergency department. *Acad Emerg Med.* 2001;8(8):833–838.
6. Lu PP, Yang CH, Ho AC, Shyr MH. The intubating LMA: a comparison of insertion techniques with conventional tracheal tubes. *Can J Anaesth.* 2000;47(9):849–853.
7. Joo H, Rose K. Fastrach—a new intubating laryngeal mask airway: successful use in patients with difficult airways. *Can J Anaesth.* 1998;45(3):253–256.

8. Kihara S, Yaguchi Y, Brimacombe J, Watanabe S, Taguchi N, Hosoya N. Intubating laryngeal mask airway size selection: a randomized triple crossover study in paralyzed, anesthetized male and female adult patients. *Anesth Analg.* 2002;94(4):1023–1027.

9. Fan KH, Hung OR, Agro F. A comparative study of tracheal intubation using an intubating laryngeal mask (Fastrach) alone or together with a lightwand (Trachlight). *J Clin Anesth.* 2000;12(8):581–585.

10. Martel M, Reardon RF, Cochrane J. Initial experience of emergency physicians using the intubating laryngeal mask airway: a case series. *Acad Emerg Med.* 2001;8(8):815–822.

11. Rosenblatt WH, Murphy M. The intubating laryngeal mask: use of a new ventilating-intubating device in the emergency department. *Ann Emerg Med.* 1999;33(2):234–238.

12. Watson NC, Hokanson M, Maltby JR, Todesco JM. The intubating laryngeal mask airway in failed fibreoptic intubation. *Can J Anaesth.* 1999;46(4):376–378.

13. Ferson DZ, Rosenblatt WH, Johansen MJ, Osborn I, Ovassapian A. Use of the intubating LMA-Fastrach in 254 patients with difficult-to-manage airways. *Anesthesiology.* 2001;95(5):1175–1181.

14. Shung J, Avidan MS, Ing R, Klein DC, Pott L. Awake intubation of the difficult airway with the intubating laryngeal mask airway. *Anaesthesia.* 1998;53(7):645–649.

15. Frappier J, Guenoun T, Journois D, et al. Airway management using the intubating laryngeal mask airway for the morbidly obese patient. *Anesth Analg.* 2003;96(5):1510–1515.

16. Choyce A, Avidan MS, Shariff A, Del Aguila M, Radcliffe JJ, Chan T. A comparison of the intubating and standard laryngeal mask airways for airway management by inexperienced personnel. *Anaesthesia.* 2001;56(4):357–360.

17. Baskett PJ, Parr MJ, Nolan JP. The intubating laryngeal mask. Results of a multicentre trial with experience of 500 cases. *Anaesthesia.* 1998;53(12):1174–1179.

18. Agro F, Hung OR, Cataldo R, Carassiti M, Gherardi S. Lightwand intubation using the Trachlight: a brief review of current knowledge. *Can J Anaesth.* 2001; 48(6):592–599.

19. Hung OR, Stewart RD. Lightwand intubation: I—a new lightwand device. *Can J Anaesth.* 1995;42 (9):820–825.

20. Stewart RD, LaRosee A, Kaplan RM, Ilkhanipour K. Correct positioning of an endotracheal tube using a flexible lighted stylet. *Crit Care Med.* 1990; 18(1):97–99.

21. Locker GJ, Staudinger T, Knapp S, et al. Assessment of the proper depth of endotracheal tube placement with the Trachlight. *J Clin Anesth.* 1998;10(5):389–393.

22. Hung OR, Tibbet JS, Cheng R, Law JA. Proper preparation of the Trachlight and endotracheal tube to facilitate intubation. *Can J Anaesth.* 2006;53(1):107–108.

23. Hung OR, Pytka S, Morris I, et al. Clinical trial of a new lightwand device (Trachlight) to intubate the trachea. *Anesthesiology.* 1995;83(3):509–514.

24. Iwama H, Ohmori S, Kaneko T, Watanabe K. Ambient light requirements for successful intubation with the Trachlight in adults. *Anaesthesia.* 1997;52(8):801.

25. Hodgson RE, Gopalan PD, Burrows RC, Zuma K. Effect of cricoid pressure on the success of endotracheal intubation with a lightwand. *Anesthesiology.* 2001;94(2):259–262.

26. Masso E, Sabate S, Hinojosa M, Vila P, Canet J, Langeron O. Lightwand tracheal intubation with and without muscle relaxation. *Anesthesiology.* 2006;104(2):249–254.

27. Agro F, Brimacombe J, Carassiti M, Morelli A, Giampalmo M, Cataldo R. Use of a lighted stylet for intubation via the laryngeal mask airway. *Can J Anaesth.* 1998;45(6):556–560.

28. Agro F, Benumof JL, Carassiti M, Cataldo R, Gherardi S, Barzoi G. Efficacy of a combined technique using the Trachlight together with direct laryngoscopy under simulated difficult airway conditions in 350 anesthetized patients. *Can J Anaesth.* 2002;49(5):525–526.

29. Wada H, Nakamura K, Nishiike S, Seki S, Tsuchida H. [The combined use of laryngoscope and Trachlight: another option for endotracheal intubation in patients with large epiglottic cysts]. *Masui.* 2006;55(4):468–470.

30. Agro F, Brimacombe J, Marchionni L, Carassiti M, Cataldo R. Nasal intubation with the Trachlight. *Can J Anaesth.* 1999;46(9):907–908.

31. Favaro R, Tordiglione P, Di Lascio F, et al. Effective nasotracheal intubation using a modified transillumination technique. *Can J Anaesth.* 2002;49(1):91–95.

32. Margolis GS, Menegazzi J, Abdlehak M, Delbridge TR. The efficacy of a standard training program for

transillumination-guided endotracheal intubation. *Acad Emerg Med.* 1996;3(4):371–377.

33. Wik L, Naess AC, Steen PA. Intubation with laryngoscope versus transillumination performed by paramedic students on manikins and cadavers. *Resuscitation.* 1997;33(3):215–218.

34. Soh CR, Kong CF, Kong CS, Ip–Yam PC, Chin E, Goh MH. Tracheal intubation by novice staff: the direct vision laryngoscope or the lighted stylet (Trachlight)? *Emerg Med J.* 2002;19(4):292–294.

35. Yamamoto T, Aoyama K, Takenaka I, Kadoya T, Uehara H. [Light-guided tracheal intubation using a Trachlight: causes of difficulty and skill acquisition]. *Masui.* 1999;48(6):672–677.

36. Konishi A, Kikuchi K, Sasui M. [Cervival spine movement during light-guided orotracheal intubation with lightwand stylet (Trachlight)]. *Masui.* 1998;47(1):94–97.

37. Turkstra TP, Craen RA, Pelz DM, Gelb AW. Cervical spine motion: a fluoroscopic comparison during intubation with lighted stylet, GlideScope, and Macintosh laryngoscope. *Anesth Analg.* 2005;101(3):910–915.

38. Inoue Y, Koga K, Shigematsu A. A comparison of two tracheal intubation techniques with Trachlight and Fastrach in patients with cervical spine disorders. *Anesth Analg.* 2002;94(3):667–671.

39. Levitan RM. Design rationale and intended use of a short optical stylet for routine fiberoptic augmentation of emergency laryngoscopy. *Am J Emerg Med.* 2006;24(4):490–495.

40. Kovacs G, Law AJ, Petrie D. Awake fiberoptic intubation using an optical stylet in an anticipated difficult airway. *Ann Emerg Med.* 2007;49(1):81–83.

41. Shikani AH. New "seeing" stylet-scope and method for the management of the difficult airway. *Otolaryngol Head Neck Surg.* 1999;120(1):113–116.

42. Bein B, Worthmann F, Scholz J, et al. A comparison of the intubating laryngeal mask airway and the Bonfils intubation fibrescope in patients with predicted difficult airways. *Anaesthesia.* 2004;59(7):668–674.

43. Bein B, Yan M, Tonner PH, Scholz J, Steinfath M, Dorges V. Tracheal intubation using the Bonfils intubation fibrescope after failed direct laryngoscopy. *Anaesthesia.* 2004;59(12):1207–1209.

44. Evans A, Morris S, Petterson J, Hall JE. A comparison of the Seeing Optical Stylet and the gum elastic bougie in simulated difficult tracheal intubation: a manikin study. *Anaesthesia.* 2006;61(5):478–481.

45. Kovacs G, Law JA, McCrossin C. A comparison of a fiberoptic stylet and a bougie as adjuncts to direct laryngoscopy in a manikin simulated difficult airway. *Ann Emerg Med.* 2007 [E pub ahead of print].

46. Greenland KB, Liu G, Tan H, Edwards M, Irwin MG. Comparison of the Levitan FPS Scope and the single-use bougie for simulated difficult intubation in anaesthetised patients. *Anaesthesia.* 2007;62(5):509–515.

47. Byhahn C, Meininger D, Walcher F, Hofstetter C, Zwissler B. Prehospital emergency endotracheal intubation using the Bonfils intubation fiberscope. *Eur J Emerg Med.* 2007;14(1):43–46.

48. Halligan M, Charters P. Learning curve for the Bonfils intubation fibrescope. *British Journal of Anaesthesia.* 2003;90:826P.

49. Halligan M, Charters P. A clinical evaluation of the Bonfils Intubation Fibrescope. *Anaesthesia.* 2003;58(11):1087–1091.

50. Wahlen BM, Gercek E. Three-dimensional cervical spine movement during intubation using the Macintosh and Bullard laryngoscopes, the bonfils fibrescope and the intubating laryngeal mask airway. *Eur J Anaesthesiol.* 2004;21(11):907–913.

51. Rudolph C, Schneider JP, Wallenborn J, Schaffranietz L. Movement of the upper cervical spine during laryngoscopy: a comparison of the Bonfils intubation fibrescope and the Macintosh laryngoscope. *Anaesthesia.* 2005;60(7):668–672.

52. Kaplan MB, Ward D, Hagberg CA, Berci G, Hagiike M. Seeing is believing: the importance of video laryngoscopy in teaching and in managing the difficult airway. *Surg Endosc.* 2006;20 Suppl 2:S479–483.

53. Agro F, Barzoi G, Montecchia F. Tracheal intubation using a Macintosh laryngoscope or a GlideScope in 15 patients with cervical spine immobilization. *Br J Anaesth.* 2003;90(5):705–706.

54. Cooper RM, Pacey JA, Bishop MJ, McCluskey SA. Early clinical experience with a new videolaryngoscope (GlideScope) in 728 patients. *Can J Anaesth.* 2005;52(2):191–198.

55. Cooper RM. Complications associated with the use of the GlideScope videolaryngoscope. *Can J Anaesth.* 2007;54(1):54–57.

56. Hsiao WT, Lin YH, Wu HS, Chen CL. Does a new videolaryngoscope (glidescope) provide better glottic exposure? *Acta Anaesthesiol Taiwan.* 2005;43(3):147–151.

57. Sun DA, Warriner CB, Parsons DG, Klein R, Umedaly HS, Moult M. The GlideScope Video Laryngoscope: randomized clinical trial in 200 patients. *Br J Anaesth*. 2005;94(3):381–384.

58. Rai MR, Dering A, Verghese C. The Glidescope system: a clinical assessment of performance. *Anaesthesia*. 2005;60(1):60–64.

59. Cooper RM. The GlideScope videolaryngoscope. *Anaesthesia*. 2005;60(10):1042.

60. Doyle DJ. Awake intubation using the GlideScope video laryngoscope: initial experience in four cases. *Can J Anaesth*. 2004;51(5):520–521.

61. Malik AM, Frogel JK. Anterior tonsillar pillar perforation during GlideScope video laryngoscopy. *Anesth Analg*. 2007;104(6):1610–1611; discussion 1611.

62. Hsu WT, Hsu SC, Lee YL, Huang JS, Chen CL. Penetrating injury of the soft palate during GlideScope intubation. *Anesth Analg*. 2007;104(6): 1609–1610; discussion 1611.

63. Timmermann A, Russo S, Graf BM. Evaluation of the CTrach—an intubating LMA with integrated fibreoptic system. *Br J Anaesth*. 2006;96(4): 516–521.

64. Liu EH, Goy RW, Chen FG. The LMA CTrach, a new laryngeal mask airway for endotracheal intubation under vision: evaluation in 100 patients. *Br J Anaesth*. 2006;96(3):396–400.

65. Liu EH, Goy RW, Chen FG. An evaluation of poor LMA CTrach views with a fibreoptic laryngoscope and the effectiveness of corrective measures. *Br J Anaesth*. 2006;97(6):878–882.

66. Dhonneur G, Ndoko SK, Yavchitz A, et al. Tracheal intubation of morbidly obese patients: LMA CTrach vs direct laryngoscopy. *Br J Anaesth*. 2006;97(5): 742–745.

67. Timmermann A, Russo S, Natge U, Heuer J, Graf BM. [LMA CTrachtrade mark : initial experiences in patients with difficult-to-manage airways.]. *Anaesthesist*. 2006;55(5):528–534.

68. Goldman AJ, Rosenblatt WH. The LMA CTrach in airway resuscitation: six case reports. *Anaesthesia*. 2006;61(10):975–977.

69. Goldman AJ, Rosenblatt WH. Use of the fibreoptic intubating LMA-CTrach in two patients with difficult airways. *Anaesthesia*. 2006;61(6): 601–603.

70. Shippey B, Ray D, McKeown D. Case series: the McGrath videolaryngoscope—an initial clinical evaluation. *Can J Anaesth*. 2007;54(4):307–313.

71. Watts AD, Gelb AW, Bach DB, Pelz DM. Comparison of the Bullard and Macintosh laryngoscopes for endotracheal intubation of patients with a potential cervical spine injury. *Anesthesiology*. 1997;87(6):1335–1342.

72. Maharaj CH, Costello JF, Higgins BD, Harte BH, Laffey JG. Learning and performance of tracheal intubation by novice personnel: a comparison of the Airtraq and Macintosh laryngoscope. *Anaesthesia*. 2006;61(7):671–677.

73. Maharaj CH, Ni Chonghaile M, Higgins BD, Harte BH, Laffey JG. Tracheal intubation by inexperienced medical residents using the Airtraq and Macintosh laryngoscopes—a manikin study. *Am J Emerg Med*. 2006;24(7):769–774.

74. Maharaj CH, Higgins BD, Harte BH, Laffey JG. Evaluation of intubation using the Airtraq or Macintosh laryngoscope by anaesthetists in easy and simulated difficult laryngoscopy—a manikin study. *Anaesthesia*. 2006;61(5):469–477.

75. Maharaj CH, O'Croinin D, Curley G, Harte BH, Laffey JG. A comparison of tracheal intubation using the Airtraq or the Macintosh laryngoscope in routine airway management: a randomised, controlled clinical trial. *Anaesthesia*. 2006;61(11): 1093–1099.

76. Maharaj CH, Costello JF, McDonnell JG, Harte BH, Laffey JG. The Airtraq as a rescue airway device following failed direct laryngoscopy: a case series. *Anaesthesia*. 2007;62(6):598–601.

77. Morris IR. Fibreoptic intubation. *Can J Anaesth*. 1994;41(10):996–1007; discussion 1007–1008.

78. Shukry M, Hanson RD, Koveleskie JR, Ramadhyani U. Management of the difficult pediatric airway with Shikani Optical Stylet. *Paediatr Anaesth*. 2005;15(4):342–345.

CHAPTER 7

Rescue Oxygenation

▶ KEY POINTS

- Failed oxygenation may be defined as the inability to tracheally intubate the patient in conjunction with failure to maintain oxygen saturation above 90% with bag mask ventilation.
- Failed oxygenation implies the immediate need to proceed with cricothyrotomy, although a brief attempt at extraglottic device (EGD) placement should occur first.
- By successfully enabling rescue oxygenation, EGD use will often preclude the need for a cricothyrotomy
- Widespread clinical experience and a significant body of literature support the use of EGDs such as the Laryngeal Mask Airway or Combitube as a primary and rescue airway.
- The LMA Fastrach™ is an effective rescue EGD that also provides a means of facilitating blind endotracheal intubation.
- Extraglottic devices will not necessarily work if obstructing pathology exists at or below the cords.
- As an alternative to an open surgical cricothyrotomy, kits are available containing cuffed cannulae for percutaneous, needle-guided insertion.

▶ INTRODUCTION TO RESCUE OXYGENATION

Following a failed intubation attempt using direct laryngoscopy or an alternative intubating technique, ease of bag mask ventilation (BMV) should be assessed, and the patient reoxygenated as needed. As discussed in more detail in Chap. 12, as long as oxygenation with BMV is non-problematic, additional attempts at tracheal intubation can then be made. However, total attempts at intubation should be limited in this setting, as patient morbidity and mortality climbs with three or more attempts.[1] After three attempts at intubation, unless a more experienced clinician has arrived or additional equipment is obtained, oxygenation should revert to BMV or may proceed with the placement of an **extraglottic device (EGD)** while plans are made for definitive care. In the more ominous situation where tracheal intubation has failed and the patient can't be oxygenated with BMV, the so-called "can't intubate/can't oxygenate" scenario, preparations should be made to rapidly proceed with a **cricothyrotomy**. However, even in this scenario, a quick trial of EGD placement is usually warranted before proceeding with the cricothyrotomy, as reoxygenation of the patient often results. Indeed, since their introduction, EGDs have enabled rescue oxygenation in many failed airway situations, returning the patient to a "you have time" scenario whereby cricothyrotomy can be avoided. Additional expertise or equipment can then be obtained for successful oral or nasal intubation, or if tracheostomy is elected, it can be performed under more controlled conditions.

Extraglottic devices (alternatively termed *supra*glottic devices), well-known examples of which include the **Laryngeal Mask Airway** (LMA; LMA North America Inc, San Diego, CA) and the **Esophageal-Tracheal Combitube** (ETC; Tyco-Kendall-Sheridan, Mansfield, MA) are so-named as they enable ventilation from outside (i.e., above) the cords. Unlike bag mask ventilation, however, these devices sit distal to where a relaxed soft palate and tongue may fall back to obstruct the airway, and as such are more likely to result in successful patient oxygenation and ventilation. Equally, their extraglottic location also represents a potential limitation to EGD effectiveness, when obstructing pathology is present at or below the cords. Thus, while widespread availability and use of EGDs may have diminished the need for cricothyrotomy, any clinician with airway management responsibilities should still be prepared to rapidly perform a cricothyrotomy to access the airway below the cords.

This chapter will describe equipment and techniques for rescue oxygenation using EGDs and cricothyrotomy. More information on decision-making about when to use these techniques appears in Chap. 12.

▶ THE LARYNGEAL MASK AIRWAY (LMA)

Available for clinical use since the late 1980s, the LMA has an established place as a device to provide a hands-free airway in routine operating room (OR) cases. It has also been successfully used on many occasions in airway emergencies, both in and out of the OR. It is reasonably easy to insert, even by unskilled personnel,[2–4] and most versions require no additional tools for placement. Now available in a number of reusable and disposable formats, the LMA consists of a plastic airway tube attached distally to a cuffed, inflatable mask. When properly seated in the pharynx, the inflated cuff forms a seal around the laryngeal inlet, enabling ventilation from immediately above the cords, while bypassing more proximal sources of obstruction.

Relative contraindications to LMA use include a high risk of passive regurgitation of gastric contents; the need for high airway ventilation pressures, and pathology that would prevent, or be aggravated by its insertion.[5] However, none of these conditions preclude an attempt at LMA use as a rescue device in an emergency, failed oxygenation situation.

LMA Devices: Description

LMA Classic™ and Unique
The original LMA was introduced in 1988 and has now been used well over 100 million times. It remains in widespread use in its reusable format, the LMA Classic™ (Fig. 7–1), and a more recently introduced disposable version, the LMA Unique. Both versions are latex-free and consist of a large-bore airway tube with proximal standard 15-mm connector, and a bowl-shaped distal cuff which is inflated via a valve on an inflation line. With the opening of its lumen facing the laryngeal inlet, the mask conforms to the shape of the pharynx. Both the LMA Classic™ and Unique are available in a full range of sizes, from neonatal to large adult.

LMA ProSeal
The LMA ProSeal (Fig. 7–2) was introduced in 2000. This version of the LMA includes a drain tube, which originates from an orifice in the distal tip of the mask cuff and travels proximally alongside the airway lumen. The drain tube is designed to accept a catheter which can be used for suctioning esophageal contents.

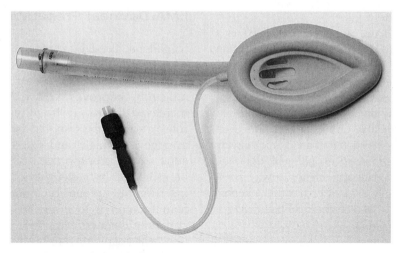

Figure 7-1.   The LMA Classic.

The cuff of the LMA ProSeal has also undergone modifications, including the addition of a posterior component (only in the adult sizes) to better conform to the shape of the pharynx. These cuff modifications allow for an airway seal pressure up to 10 cm H_2O higher than that of the LMA Classic™.[5] A built-in proximal bite block has also been added. With its improved seal and provision for gastric tube placement, the ProSeal offers more protection of the airway against aspiration of gastric contents, and allows ventilation at higher airway pressures, perhaps making it a better choice than the LMA Classic™ or Unique for use in emergencies.

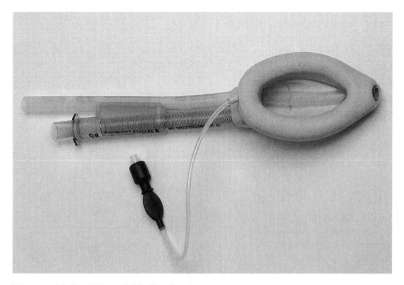

Figure 7-2.   The LMA ProSeal.

LMA Supreme

The single-use LMA Supreme (Fig. 7–3) is a recent addition to the LMA family. It features an L-shaped airway tube, a modified cuff to enable ventilation at higher airway pressures, a second lumen for esophageal drainage, and a proximal bite block. At the time of writing, no published literature was available on this device. However, designed for easy insertion (L-shaped tube), airway protection (presence of esophageal drainage lumen), and ventilation at higher airway pressures (cuff design), this device has the potential to become a good choice of single-use EGD for the emergency patient.

LMA Fastrach™ and CTrach

The L-shaped LMA Fastrach™ and its similarly shaped video-based sibling, the LMA CTrach, were designed to enable blind or video-aided intubation, respectively. However, both are also effective as rescue oxygenation and ventilation devices, with a high first attempt insertion and successful ventilation rate. The LMA Fastrach™ has been shown to have an oropharyngeal leak pressure 5–10 cm H_2O higher than the LMA Classic™.[5] As they were designed to also facilitate intubation, these devices have been discussed in more detail in Chap. 6.

LMA Devices: Preparation for Use

In general, the largest-sized LMA compatible with insertion should be selected. Studies in adults indicate that the use of larger sizes significantly improves seal efficacy with no increased insertion difficulty.[5] As a general rule, a size 5 mask should be chosen for an average adult male, and size 4 for an average adult female. Appropriate pediatric sizing can be estimated by patient weight. The classic™ insertion technique recommended by the manufacturer is to insert the mask with the cuff fully deflated (Fig. 7–4). For cuff deflation, while aspirating air via a syringe attached to the inflation line, the mask should be pressed down against a flat surface, as this will help maintain the appropriate cuff shape. Prior to insertion, the posterior surface of the mask should be lubricated with a water-soluble lubricant. The LMA ProSeal is supplied with an L-shaped insertion tool: if this is used, the distal end of the tool should be introduced into the strap at the junction of cuff and tube. The airway and drain tubes are then bent around its convex surface, and proximally, the airway tube is snapped into a matching slot[5] (Fig. 7–5).

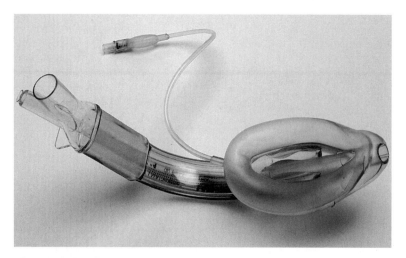

Figure 7–3. The LMA Supreme.

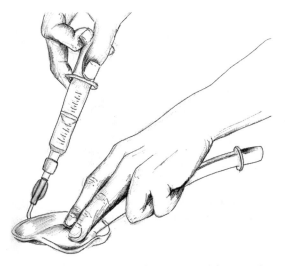

Figure 7–4. The LMA is prepared for use by fully deflating the cuff of air while pressing the mask against a flat surface.

LMA Devices: Insertion Techniques

LMA Classic™ and Unique
To ease LMA placement, the head should be extended, when not contraindicated. Through an opened mouth, the mask is inserted midline, with the operator's forefinger at the junction of the tube with the inflatable cuff. Once the tip of the inserting forefinger has passed the upper teeth, pushing cephalad on the mask with this digit (Figs. 7–6 to 7–8) during further advancement will encourage the LMA to take on the curve of the hard palate, increasing the ease of negotiating the turn down into the pharynx. The LMA is then advanced gently until resistance is encountered. Once placed, the LMA cuff is inflated using the recommended cuff volume printed on the side of the LMA barrel, or simply using the cuff volume formula "(LMA size–1) × 10." Note that some authorities prefer to initially inflate the cuff with only 2/3 of this recommended volume, with additional inflation used only to overcome a poor seal.[5] However, for use in emergency, failed airway situations, the full recommended volume should be used primarily. The proximal connector of the LMA is attached to a manual resuscitator, and ventilation attempted: appropriate chest rise and bag compliance with positive pressure ventilation suggest correct placement.

Many modified insertion techniques have been suggested for the LMA Classic™, reflecting the fact that placement does not always succeed on the first attempt. One study found similar

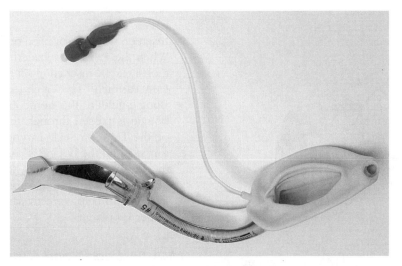

Figure 7–5. An L-shaped insertion tool can be used to facilitate correct placement of the LMA ProSeal.

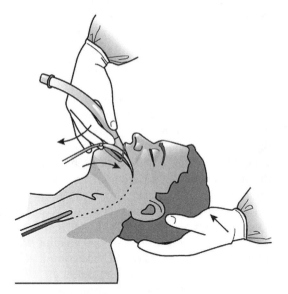

Figure 7-6. LMA Classic insertion begins by inserting the mask tip behind the upper teeth (With permission, LMA North America).

success rates when placing the single-use LMA Unique with or without intraoral finger use.[6] In general, however, the manufacturer's recommended technique for the LMA Classic™ and Unique is the most reliable and should be used for the initial insertion attempt.

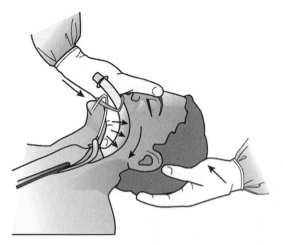

Figure 7-7. As the LMA is advanced, the index finger pushes the mask cephalad against the hard palate (With permission, LMA North America).

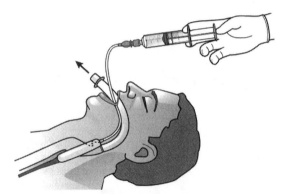

Figure 7-8. Once in place, the LMA cuff is inflated (With permission, LMA North America).

LMA Supreme

The LMA Supreme can be inserted without intra-oral finger use. Held at its proximal end, while applying a jaw lift, it is simply rotated into the patient, down and around the tongue, following the curve of the hard palate.

LMA ProSeal

A few insertion techniques have been described for the LMA ProSeal:

- Mask insertion with intraoral finger use, identical to that described above for the LMA Classic™;
- Insertion with the supplied rigid insertion tool. When the ProSeal is loaded on the insertion tool, it can be inserted in similar fashion to the LMA Fastrach™ or CTrach (see next section);
- Bougie-guided: the non-coudé-tip end of a bougie is passed through the drainage tube of the LMA ProSeal. Laryngoscopy is performed, and the bougie is passed deliberately into the upper esophagus. The bougie then acts as a guide during subsequent ProSeal insertion, to help correctly situate its tip in the upper esophagus

LMA Fastrach™ and CTrach

Both these devices, as well as the ProSeal when using the rigid insertion tool, can be inserted while holding the external guiding handle. A jaw lift is performed, the mask tip is inserted behind the upper teeth, whereupon the mask is rotated down into the pharynx, following and maintaining pressure against the palate.

Cricoid pressure impedes successful placement of an LMA,[5] and should be at least transiently released during LMA placement. After the LMA is correctly situated, cricoid pressure can be reapplied, but should only be maintained if it does not impede ventilation.

LMA Devices: Troubleshooting

Difficulty is occasionally encountered in negotiating the turn into the pharynx, particularly with attempted LMA Classic™ placement. The following strategies can be used in response:

- *Lateral approach:* Advancing the LMA from the side of the oral cavity, aiming toward the midline, sometimes results in successful passage into the pharynx;
- *Cuff partially inflated:* Partially inflating the cuff may result in a softer leading edge to the advancing LMA, potentially helping navigation "around the corner" into the pharynx;[5]
- *Laryngoscope-aided:* If difficulty is still encountered, use of the direct laryngoscope to control soft tissues enables the LMA to be directly placed into the pharynx.

LMA Devices: Clinical Effectiveness

Routine and Difficult Airway Management

Data for the LMA Classic™ derived largely from an OR population, using the standard insertion technique, suggests first-attempt and overall success rates of 87% and 98%, respectively. In the difficult airway population, ease of LMA insertion is independent of both Mallampati and Cormack-Lehane scoring.[5] Both the LMA Classic™ and LMA Fastrach™ have high success rates in achieving ventilation in patients with predicted and unanticipated difficult airways, including patients who could not be intubated, or could not be intubated or ventilated.[5] In this latter

scenario, one analysis of 21 case reports[5] and a descriptive study of 17 cases[7] reported success in establishing ventilation using the LMA in 92% and 94% of cases, respectively. Similar efficacy of LMA devices in the difficult airway has been reported in the pediatric population.[5]

Skills Acquisition

Good success rates have been achieved by novices with LMA placement in human patients after appropriate manikin training.[6] However, as common sense would suggest, there is evidence that with more experience, success rates increase.[5]

C-spine Precautions

In a study of various airway devices using a cadaver with a posteriorly destabilized C3 vertebra, LMA Classic™ insertion and LMA Fastrach™ insertion with subsequent intubation resulted in movement comparable to both laryngoscopic intubation and facemask ventilation.[8] LMA insertion would also be expected to be more difficult in situations where head extension is contraindicated. Some movement of the intact upper C-spine has been shown with LMA Fastrach™ insertion and intubation[8,9] although this is of uncertain clinical significance and does not preclude use of this or other EGD for rescue oxygenation, if other techniques have failed.

▶ THE ESOPHAGEAL-TRACHEAL COMBITUBE (ETC)

The Combitube (Fig. 7–9) is another EGD with an extensive history of use, primarily in the prehospital resuscitation setting. It has also been used in-hospital as a rescue ventilation device, both in and out of the OR. As with the LMA, it is easily used by inexperienced personnel. Its strength lies in the ability to achieve patient ventilation irrespective of its location: esophagus or trachea. The Combitube may be placed blindly or using a laryngoscope for soft tissue control. With blind placement, esophageal placement of the Combitube will occur in over 90% of cases.[5]

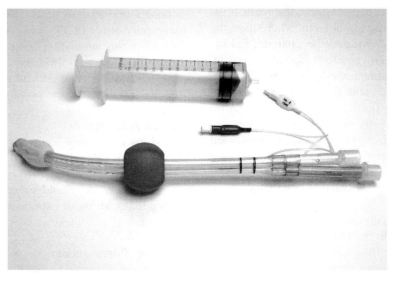

Figure 7–9. The Esophageal-Tracheal Combitube (ETC).

The ETC is available in two sizes, the Combitube (41 French) and the Combitube SA (37 French). Manufacturer recommendations are for use of the larger Combitube in patients over 5 ft (152 cm), although a number of authors have observed that the smaller Combitube SA works well in patients from 4–6 ft (122–183 cm) in height.[10,11] At the time of writing, there was no pediatric version.

As with other blind techniques, Combitube use may be relatively contraindicated in the presence of airway pathology. Reports of esophageal perforation with its use exist,[12, 13] possibly in the context of an excessive volume of air having been injected into the distal, esophageal cuff. Finally, it is important to recognize that as with the LMA, the Combitube ventilates from an extraglottic position when located in the esophagus, so will not necessarily work if obstructing pathology exists at or below the cords.

Combitube Description

Designed for blind insertion, the Combitube consists of a double-lumened tube, with a distal and more proximal cuff. With the more likely esophageal placement, the distal cuff seals the upper esophagus, and the more proximal and larger pharyngeal cuff seals the oro- and nasopharynx. Applied ventilation through the blind-ending esophageal lumen (labeled No. 1 and blue in color) exits through multiple fenestrations between the inflated distal and proximal cuffs and travels through the cords into the trachea (Fig. 7–10). With tracheal placement, ventilation would occur distally, through the other lumen (labeled No. 2, Fig. 7–11) as with a regular endotracheal tube.

When situated in the esophagus, the inflated distal cuff helps protect the hypopharynx from gastric contents,[11] and the open tracheal lumen can be suctioned for liquid matter. Equally, the more proximal pharyngeal cuff also provides reasonable protection from tracheal soiling by oral cavity contents (e.g., blood).[14] Oropharyngeal leak pressure is 25–40 cm H_2O.

Combitube Preparation for Use

The device is removed from its packaging and both cuffs are checked, then fully deflated. Some clinicians elect to bend the Combitube anteriorly to 90° or more for a few seconds prior to insertion, (the "Lipp maneuver") to augment

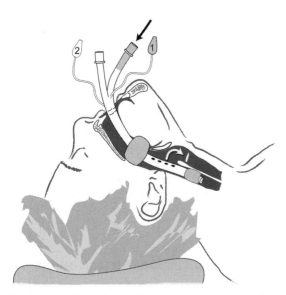

Figure 7–10. Ventilation pathway when the Combitube is located in the esophagus, through lumen No. 1.

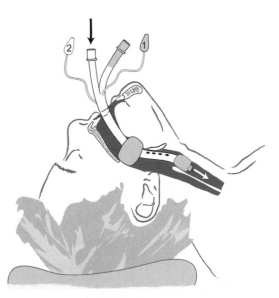

Figure 7–11. Ventilation is through lumen No. 2 when the Combitube is located in the trachea.

the curve and help it to better conform to the shape of the oropharyngeal curve.

Combitube Insertion

The Combitube is ideally inserted in conjunction with direct laryngoscopy (Fig. 7–12), to help control the tongue and improve the angle of insertion. However, for blind placement, slight head extension and a jaw lift will help (Fig. 7–13). The Combitube is advanced gently through the mouth in a curved, downward motion. Once in the posterior pharynx, further advancement should ideally be with the distal end of the device parallel to the patient's anterior chest wall, and not angled further posteriorly. Once inserted, two transverse lines appearing proximally on the Combitube should be adjacent to the upper teeth or alveolar ridges. During emergency use, once placed, the two cuffs are inflated: first the proximal (pharyngeal) occluding cuff (Combitube SA 85 mL; Combitube 100 mL) using the blue pilot balloon (labeled "No. 1"). The distal (esophageal) cuff is then inflated (Combitube SA 5–12 mL; Combitube 5–15 mL) using the

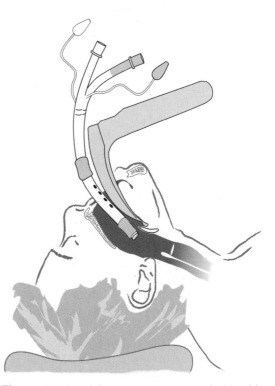

Figure 7–12. A laryngoscope may help with Combitube placement.

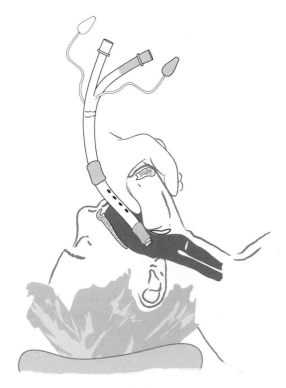

Figures 7-13. A jaw lift and head extension are performed to aid blind Combitube insertion.

white pilot balloon (labeled "No. 2"). Particularly for the distal cuff, overinflation should be avoided, as esophageal rupture can otherwise occur.[12] Once a seal has been achieved and the correct lumen identified, many clinicians remove air from the proximal cuff until the "minimum leak" volume is found, to help avoid danger of mucosal damage.

Ventilation through the Combitube should first be attempted through the blue lumen, labeled "No. 1", which will allow ventilation from an esophageal location. End-tidal CO_2 detection will help confirm the correct lumen, as will the clinical signs of chest rise, breath sounds with positive pressure, and manual resuscitator bag compliance. If this is judged not to be the correct lumen, ventilation should be attempted through the other, clear lumen (labeled "No. 2"). This will be the correct lumen on the rare occasion that tracheal placement has occurred. In this

case, the Combitube will act as a regular ETT, and the proximal cuff can be deflated.

Combitube Troubleshooting

If suboptimal ventilation is obtained through both lumens, most often the Combitube is located too far distally, and the pharyngeal cuff is occluding the laryngeal inlet. In this situation, the Combitube should be pulled back in small (1 cm) increments, up to a total of 3 cm, until ventilation succeeds through the blue, esophageal lumen.

Combitube Clinical Effectiveness

ROUTINE AND DIFFICULT AIRWAY MANAGEMENT
Published success rates for Combitube insertion and ventilation are 97–99% for in-hospital populations.[5] Slightly higher success rates in the surgical population occur with laryngoscope-guided placement. In the prehospital setting, rescue ventilation with the Combitube following failed laryngoscopic intubation has been reported to be successful in 75–100% of cases.[15–18]

C-SPINE PRECAUTIONS
Combitube insertion has been shown to have a lower success rate in patients wearing a rigid cervical collar[19] although most failures could be corrected using adjunctive laryngoscopy. However, once placed, the presence of a C-collar does not impede ventilation through a Combitube.[20] In a cadaver model with a destabilized C3 segment, Combitube insertion caused movement comparable to oral intubation with direct laryngoscopy, and exceeded that caused by LMA Fastrach™ intubation or LMA Classic™ placement.[8]

▶ NEWER EXTRAGLOTTIC DEVICES

In recent years, numerous new extraglottic devices have been introduced. Many, but not all, are single-use items. Some have more accompanying narrative in the literature than others, however early experience looks promising for many in terms of ease of insertion and effectiveness. As many hospitals are trending toward the use of disposable equipment, the clinician should be prepared to be presented with an unfamiliar device from time to time!

The disposable **Portex Soft-Seal laryngeal mask** (Smiths Medical, Inc., St. Paul, MN) is similar in shape to the LMA Unique, but with a blunter distal cuff, a deeper bowl, wider airway tube, and no mask aperture bars.[21] Compared to the LMA Unique or Classic™, the Soft-Seal has similar reported insertion success rates, oropharyngeal leak pressure,[22,23] and ease of ventilation.[24] The Soft-Seal (Fig. 7–14) is available in adult and pediatric sizes.

Ambu (Ambu Inc., Glen Burnie, MD) also markets an extraglottic airway in both reusable (the **Aura40**) and disposable (the **AuraOnce**) formats (Fig. 7–15). It differs from the LMA Classic™/Unique and Portex Soft-Seal in having a premolded L-shaped airway tube proximal to the distal cuff. The cuff is manufactured from a soft material and has a reinforced tip to resist bending during insertion. For insertion, the cuff is deflated, and, holding the device proximally, the tip is inserted behind the upper teeth. Following the hard and soft palate, it is then rotated down into the pharynx. The Aura extraglottic airways are available in adult and pediatric (Table 7–1) sizes. Early data suggests a good first attempt success rate, and an oropharyngeal leak pressure of 18–25 cm H_2O.[24,25]

The King **Laryngeal Tube** (LT; King Systems Corporation, Noblesville, IN, Fig. 7–16) consists of an airway tube with two cuffs: one distal, to seal the esophagus, and one proximal midway up the tube, to seal the oro- and nasopharynx. Between the two cuffs are multiple ventilation apertures. As with the Combitube, ventilation emerges from these apertures, between the proximal pharyngeal and distal esophageal cuffs. Unlike the Combitube, inflation of both cuffs occurs through a single pilot line. The LT is available in adult and pediatric sizes, in reusable (LT) and disposable (LT-D) versions. A disposable version with a separate gastric drainage channel (LTS-D) is also available. Insertion is begun with the head and neck in the 'sniffing' position, with concomitant jaw lift. The lubricated LT is inserted through the mouth and advanced behind the base of

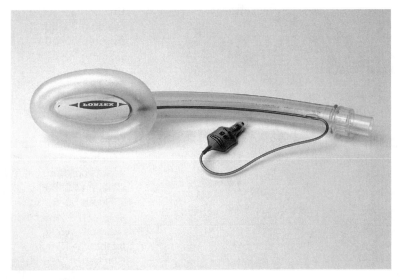

Figure 7–14. The Portex Soft Seal laryngeal.

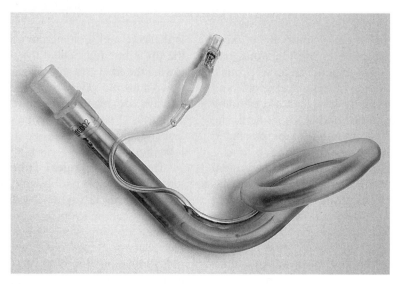

Figure 7–15. The Ambu AuraOnce.

▶ **TABLE 7–1** SAMPLE PEDIATRIC OPTIONS OF EXTRAGLOTTIC DEVICE (EGD)

Device	Mask Size(s)	Patient Size Guidelines
LMA Classic™ and LMA Unique	1	Neonates/infants up to 5 kg
	11/2	Infants 5–10 kg
	2	Infants/children 10–20 kg
	21/2	Children 20–30 kg
	3	Children 30–50 kg
LMA ProSeal	11/2	Infants 5–10 kg
	2	Children 10–20 kg
	21/2	Children 20–30 kg
	3	Children 30–50 kg
LMA Fastrach™	3	Children 30–50 kg
AirQ	1.5	Children 10–20 kg
	2.5	Children 20–50 kg
Ambu Aura40 and AuraOnce	1	<5 kg
	11/2	5–10 kg
	2	10–20 kg
	21/2	20–30 kg
	3	30–50 kg
Portex Soft-Seal Laryngeal Mask	1	Neonates/infants up to 5 kg
	1.5	Infants 5–10 kg
	2	Infants/children10–20 kg
	2.5	Children 20–30 kg
	3	Children 30–50 kg
Combitube SA		4–6 ft, 122–186 cm in height
King LT, LT-D, and LTS-D	0	Newborn, <5 kg
	1	Infants, 5–12 kg
	2	Children, 12–25 kg
	3	Small adult, 122–155 cm

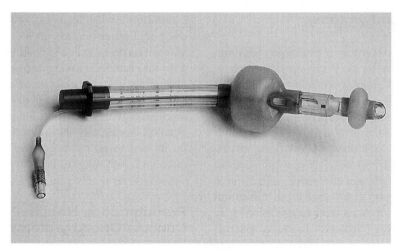

Figure 7–16. The King LTS-D.

the tongue. It is advanced until (a) resistance is encountered, or (b) the connector base is aligned with teeth or gums. The cuffs are then inflated (Size 3–45 to 60 mL; size 4–60 to 80 mL; size 5–70 to 90 mL). A self-inflating manual resuscitator is attached, and if necessary, the LT can be slowly withdrawn until easy ventilation is achieved. Studies of ease and success of insertion have been favorable, with a quoted success rate of 97%–100%.[26] Comparison studies with the LMA Classic™ have generally shown equivalent efficacy.[26]

Other EGDs continue to be introduced, for example, the cuffed **Cobra Perilaryngeal Airway** (Engineered Medical Systems Inc, Indianapolis, IN) and the cuffless **SLIPA (**Slipa Medical Ltd, London, UK) and **I-gel** (Intersurgical Ltd., Wokingham, UK) airways. Indeed, it is probably safe to say that each passing year will see additional devices come to market. While some may have a price advantage over more traditional extraglottic devices, it must be said that the burden of proof lies on the new devices to have their safety and efficacy demonstrated before their routine use can be espoused over EGDs with a long history of safe use. In addition, using an EGD that is in common use in an institution's operating rooms increases the opportunity for obtaining experience in the nonemergency setting.

▶ CRICOTHYROTOMY

Rarely, access to the airway below the vocal cords will be necessary as the primary approach to obtaining an airway. More commonly, cricothyrotomy follows the failure of attempts to secure the airway from above the cords, coupled with an inability to oxygenate the patient by bag-mask ventilation or EGD: the **failed oxygenation** *(can't intubate, can't oxygenate)* situation. In most cases, emergency access is obtained through the cricothyroid membrane, as this location is generally easy to locate by external palpation, and may be less vascular than more distal locations. Needle; percutaneous needle-guided cannula, and open surgical cricothyrotomy have been used, with varying success.

All clinicians with airway management responsibilities must be prepared with the will, the knowledge, and the equipment to perform a cricothyrotomy in a can't intubate/can't oxygenate situation.

Needle Cricothyrotomy

Needle cricothyrotomy is a technique with significant limitations to its effectiveness and safety, and at least in the adult population, is falling out of favor. Most often performed with a large-bore intravenous or similar purpose-made catheter, ventilation and oxygenation is attempted either via intermittent application of low-flow oxygen (at 15 L/min) or by jet ventilation at pressures of 45–50 lb/in^2.[27] However, bench and animal research suggests that ventilation (although admittedly less important than oxygenation) may be ineffectual with low-flow oxygen via this route, particularly in the face of complete proximal airway obstruction.[27] Conversely, use of jet ventilation, while more effective in achieving good ventilation, has a substantial risk of barotrauma. In addition, jet ventilators are not commonly available in out-of-OR settings. For these and other reasons, including a lack of airway protection against aspiration of gastric contents and catheter kinking or dislodgement, many authorities now consider needle cricothyrotomy to be the least desirable option for infraglottic rescue oxygenation in the adult patient.[27, 28] More detailed description of adult techniques will thus be limited to percutaneous needle-guided cannula and open surgical cricothyrotomy.

Percutaneous Needle-Guided Cannula Cricothyrotomy

Commercial kits are now available containing equipment for needle-guided placement of a wide-bore cuffed cannula via the cricothyroid membrane (Fig. 7–17). Many of these kits originally

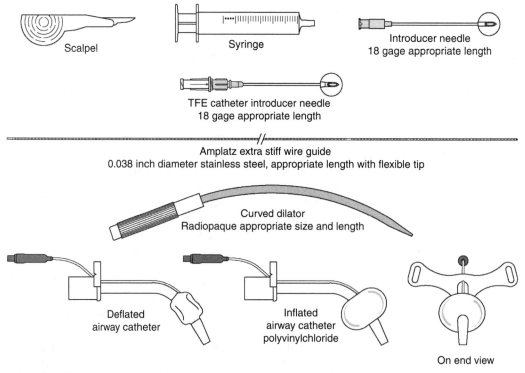

Scalpel

Syringe

Introducer needle
18 gage appropriate length

TFE catheter introducer needle
18 gage appropriate length

Amplatz extra stiff wire guide
0.038 inch diameter stainless steel, appropriate length with flexible tip

Curved dilator
Radiopaque appropriate size and length

Deflated
airway catheter

Inflated
airway catheter
polyvinylchloride

On end view

Set consists of items shown above and cloth tracheostomy tape strip for fixation of airway catheter.

Figure 7–17. Contents of the Melker Emergency Cricothyrotomy Catheter Set. (Cook Critical Care, Bloomington, IN)

contained uncuffed cannulae of varying caliber, introducing the possibility of resultant inadequate ventilation.[29] The preferred cuffed cannula allows the airway to be secured and protected against aspiration of gastric contents and permits adequate ventilation in the face of decreased pulmonary compliance, even with an airway patent from above. Examples of such kits are the **Melker Emergency Cricothyrotomy Catheter Set** (Cook Medical, Inc., Bloomington, IN) and the **PCK–Portex® Cricothyroidotomy Kit** (PCK, Smiths Medical Inc., St. Paul, MN). The Melker uses a familiar Seldinger over-the-wire placement technique, while the PCK uses Veress needle technology to indicate successful airway access.

Needle-Guided Cricothyrotomy Technique: Melker

The patient is ideally placed with the head and neck in the extended position, to help with anatomy identification and access. The cricothyroid membrane is palpated and the area is prepped. In an obese neck where landmark identification is difficult, a small midline vertical incision can be made to better identify the membrane, and indeed, some espouse routine placement of a small vertical skin nick over the cricothyroid membrane prior to needle insertion. A catheter/introducer needle attached to a syringe is advanced through the cricothyroid membrane in a caudad direction, with continuous aspiration (Fig. 7–18). Tracheal entry will be suggested by free aspiration of air into the syringe. The catheter is then advanced off the introducer needle into the trachea, and the needle is removed (Fig. 7–19). Through the catheter, a wire is advanced several centimeters into the trachea. Note that the supplied wire has a stiff and a supple end: the nontraumatic supple end should be advanced into the patient. The catheter is removed, leaving only the wire in the trachea (Fig. 7–20). If not already done, a small vertical incision is now made with a scalpel blade in the skin alongside the entry point of the wire (Fig. 7–21). Subsequently, the dilator/cannula assembly is "railroaded" over the wire into the trachea. Note that during this process, the outer cannula must be held tightly onto the inner dilator (Fig. 7–22), as the dilator will otherwise back away from the cannula, causing difficulty in passage of the blunt end of the cannula. Once the cannula is seated in the trachea, the dilator and wire are removed together. The cuff is inflated with 8–10 mL of air (Fig. 7–23), and the cannula's connector is attached directly to a manual resuscitator device. False passage can occur, so usual objective means of confirming endotracheal placement must be sought, with CO_2 monitoring as the gold standard.

The cuffed Melker cricothyrotomy cannula has an inner diameter (ID) of 5.5 mm. Use of the older uncuffed Melker cannulae, particularly in the patient with decreased lung or chest wall compliance, may result in applied positive pressure preferentially exiting the mouth and nose. The obvious solution is exclusive use of the cuffed version, however faced with the foregoing situation, squeezing the nostrils, holding the mouth firmly closed during ventilation, or packing the hypopharynx with moist gauze have all been described as temporizing solutions,[29] together with rapid conversion to open cricothyrotomy or formal tracheostomy. Both latter options permit a cuffed tube to be placed.

Mastering the Melker can easily be done in a manikin-type setting. The learning curve flattens after five insertions in manikins, with no further accuracy or shortening of placement time (about 40 seconds) attained after this.[30] Effectiveness of skills transfer from a manikin to the human in an emergency setting is unknown.

Needle-Guided Cricothyrotomy Technique: PCK

The PCK device is packaged assembled, with a Veress needle and ensleeved dilator placed through the cuffed 6-mm ID cannula. For use, after identification of the cricothyroid membrane, the manufacturer recommends making a 2-cm horizontal incision through the overlying skin. The cricothyroid membrane is reidentified

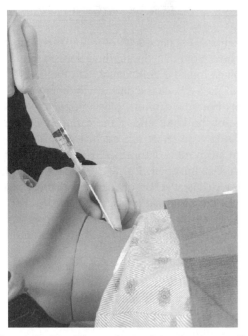

Figure 7–18. The catheter introducer needle/syringe assembly is advanced through the cricothyroid membrane. Tracheal access is indicated by free aspiration of air.

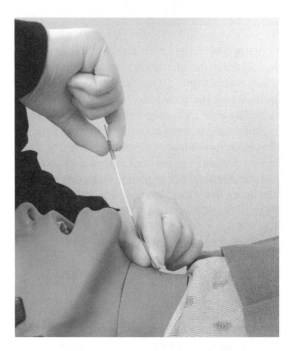

Figure 7–20. The pliable end of the supplied wire is passed through the catheter into the trachea, after which the catheter is removed over the wire.

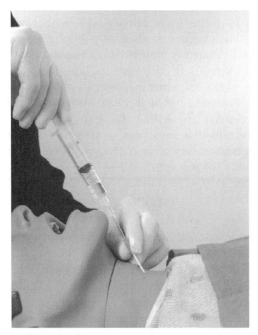

Figure 7–19. Once tracheal access is achieved, the catheter is advanced off the needle into the trachea.

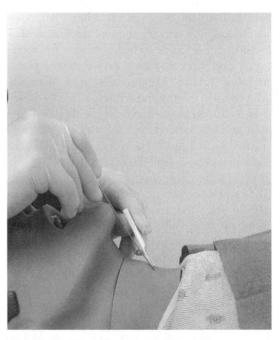

Figure 7–21. If not already done, a small incision is made along the wire through the cricothyroid membrane.

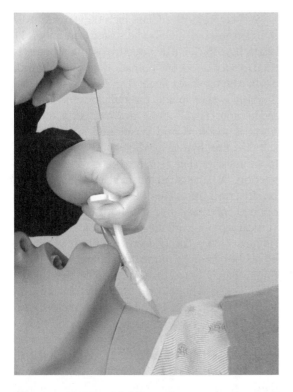

Figure 7-22. Holding the cannula and curved dilator together, the assembly is passed caudad over the wire, through the cricothyroid membrane.

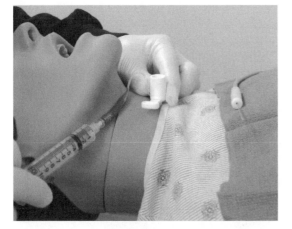

Figure 7-23. The cuff is inflated, and cannula position in the trachea is confirmed with the usual objective criteria.

by palpation in the wound. From an initial position above and perpendicular to the cricothyroid membrane, the needle tip of the cannula/dilator/needle assembly is advanced posteriorly through the cricothyroid membrane. As long as the needle tip remains in contact with tissue, a red indicator will be visible in the needle hub (Fig. 7–24). Once the red indicator flag disappears, indicating tracheal entry, the assembly is carefully advanced further until contact with the posterior aspect of the cricoid ring is signaled by reappearance of the indicator. At that point, the assembly is angled caudad and advanced 1–2 cm. The needle is then removed, and the outer cannula is advanced off the dilator. Once the cannula is fully advanced, the dilator is removed, the cuff is inflated, and positioning is verified in the usual fashion.

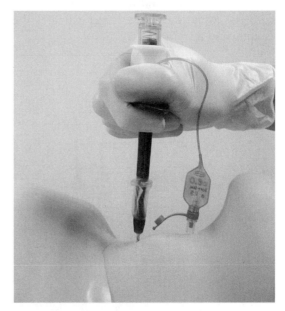

Figure 7-24. The PCK needle cricothyrotomy device. As long as the needle tip remains in contact with tissue, a red indicator will be visible in the needle hub. With entry into the free lumen of the trachea, the red indicator disappears.

► OPEN (SURGICAL) CRICOTHYROTOMY

For those familiar with the anatomy and skilled in the procedure, an open cricothyrotomy offers the benefit of placement of a cuffed endotracheal or tracheostomy tube. It can be done quickly, with only a few instruments (Fig. 7–25). A tray with the needed sterilized surgical equipment should be available and stored with other airway equipment. Commercially available kits containing equipment for both percutaneous needle-guided and open surgical approaches are now in the market.[31]

In the classical open surgical approach, the clinician stands beside the patient, face to face, at the level of the shoulders. The patient's head and neck should be extended. To proceed, the fingers of the clinician's nondominant hand are placed on the thyroid cartilage. The long finger and thumb of this hand remain on the thyroid cartilage, while the index finger palpates the cricothyroid membrane (Fig. 7–26)

A 3-cm vertical midline incision is made over the cricothyroid membrane, using a number 11 blade (Fig. 7–27). The cricothyroid membrane is then reidentified by palpation in the wound, again with the index finger (Fig. 7–28). A transverse incision is then made through the cricothyroid membrane (Fig. 7–29). Once incised, a tracheal hook is inserted and positioned superiorly to stabilize the thyroid cartilage, and is handed off to an assistant (Fig. 7–30), who provides upward traction. A Trousseau tracheal dilator can then be inserted into the incision with its arms opened inferiorly and superiorly to enlarge the vertical opening in the cricothyroid membrane (Figure 7–31). The chosen cannula (e.g., Shiley #4 trachesostomy cannula or #6.0 mm ID ETT) is then placed between the arms of the dilator (Fig. 7–32), whereupon the dilator/cannula (or ETT) complex is rotated counterclockwise 90° down and into the trachea, all in one movement (Fig. 7–33). The Trousseau dilator is then removed, and the cannula or ETT cuff is inflated. An ETT can now be connected directly to a standard manual resuscitator device and intratracheal

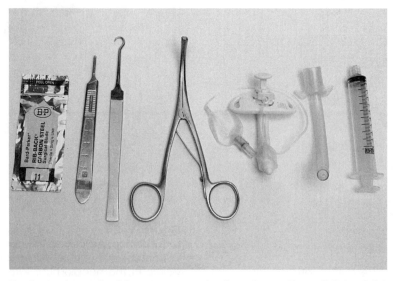

Figure 7–25. Equipment required for an open cricothyrotomy. From left to right: a scalpel handle, # 11 blade, tracheal hook, Trousseau dilator, #4 Shiley tracheostomy tube, 10-cc syringe.

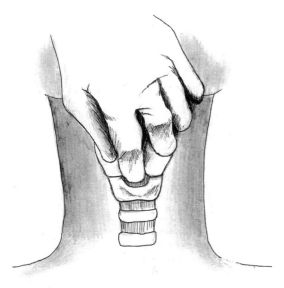

Figure 7–26. With thumb and long finger stabilizing the thyroid cartilage, the index finger palpates the cricothyroid membrane.

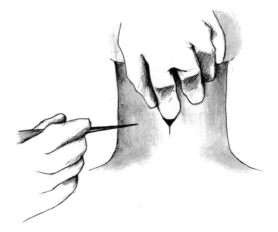

Figure 7–28. The index finger re-palpates the cricothyroid membrane within the wound.

position confirmed in the usual fashion. A Shiley tracheostomy tube will have to have its inner dilator removed and replaced with the inner cannula. Once tracheal placement has been confirmed, the tracheal hook is removed, and the cannula or ETT is secured.

Early complications of cricothyrotomy include bleeding, incorrect or unsuccessful tube placement, cricoid cartilage fracture, obstruction and subcutaneous emphysema. Rarely, laryngeal, esophageal, or mediastinal injury can occur. Pneumothorax, pneumomediastinum, and aspiration are also infrequent complications. After the situation has stabilized, a cricothyrotomy should be replaced either by intubation from above, or by conversion to a formal tracheostomy. This will help minimize

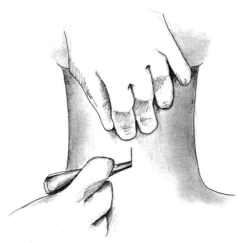

Figure 7–27. A 3-cm vertical incision is made over the cricothyroid membrane.

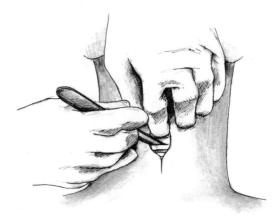

Figure 7–29. A horizontal incision is then made in the cricothyroid membrane.

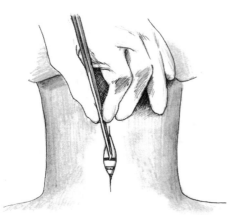

Figure 7–30. A tracheal hook picks up and stabilizes the inferior border of the thyroid cartilage, and is passed off to an assistant.

vocal cord morbidity or the occurrence of subglottic stenosis at the level of the cricoid ring.

▶ PEDIATRIC OPTIONS FOR RESCUE OXYGENATION

At the outset, it must be said that a failed oxygenation situation is very unusual in the pediatric population, due in no small measure to the fact that this population is almost always easy to bagmask ventilate. However, as in the adult, if intu-

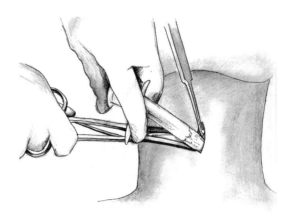

Figure 7–32. A #4 tracheostomy tube is placed between the arms of the Trousseau dilator, into the cricothyrotomy opening.

bation has failed and difficulty is encountered in maintaining oxygen saturation with BMV, rescue oxygenation can be achieved with both extraglottic devices as well as via transtracheal access.

Extraglottic Device Use in the Pediatric Patient

Most of the extraglottic devices on the market are available in pediatric sizes. Some are available in a full array of sizes while others are

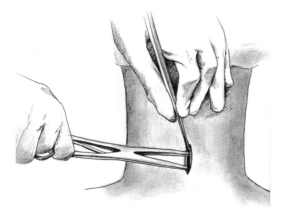

Figure 7–31. A Trousseau dilator is placed in the cricothyrotomy, and is used to enlarge the opening, vertically.

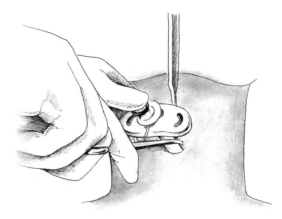

Figure 7–33. The Trousseau dilator and tube are rotated 90° counter-clockwise, and the cannula is concurrently advanced down the trachea.

suitable for use only in larger children (Table 7-1). As with adults, case reports attest to successful ventilation achieved by EGD use after BMV had failed.[5]

Pediatric Cricothyrotomy

Cricothyrotomy is not performed in children under the age of eight. In this age group, there is no developed space between the cricoid ring and the thyroid cartilage. In addition, significant narrowing occurs at the level of the cricoid ring, which could impede cannula passage in an emergency. Thirdly, as the cricoid ring is necessary to help maintain patency of an otherwise substantially membranous trachea, its fracture during attempted cricothyrotomy could jeopardize subsequent airway patency. For these reasons, if trans-tracheal access is required in an emergency in the patient under 8, it should be obtained below the cricoid ring.

In keeping with the rare nature of the event, there is very little literature on emergency cricothyrotomy or tracheotomy in children. Most clinicians would avoid an open surgical technique in a pediatric emergency owing to poor landmarks and the vascularity of the area. Two other options exist:

- **Needle cricothyrotomy or tracheotomy** with ventilation through an attached pediatric-sized manual resuscitator. A large-bore IV catheter can be used to access the trachea, and is connected to the manual resuscitator in one of two ways: (a) insertion of the connector of a 3.0 mm ID ETT into the IV catheter hub or (b) attaching the barrel of a 3 cc syringe, then pushing the connector of a 7.0 mm ID ETT into the end of the syringe barrel (Figure 7–34). Both options then permit attachment of a manual resuscitator via the 15-mm ETT connector. Manual ventilation ensues with 100% oxygen. The chest must be observed for deflation between ventilations, to avoid the risk of barotrauma.
- A **pediatric cricothyrotomy** kit (e.g., the Pedia-Trake Pediatric Emergency Cricothyro-

tomy Kit, Smiths Medical, St. Paul MN) is available with uncuffed cannulae in sizes of 3, 4, and 5 mm ID.

▶ PREDICTING DIFFICULT RESCUE OXYGENATION

As is the case with predictors of difficult bag-mask ventilation and difficult laryngoscopic intubation, the clinician should evaluate whether rescue oxygenation via EGD or cricothyrotomy is predicted to succeed. This is of particular importance when a rapid-sequence intubation (RSI) is contemplated in

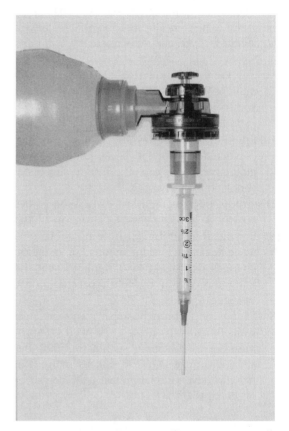

Figure 7–34. Needle cricothyrotomy set-up using a large-bore IV, the barrel of a 3-cc syringe attached to the connector of a 7.0 ETT. The assembly is attached to a BVM device.

the uncooperative patient with predictors of difficult bag mask ventilation as well as difficult laryngoscopy (see Chap. 11).

Predictors of Difficult Extraglottic Device Use

Simply expressed, EGD use can fail due to an inability to place the device into or through the mouth; or even if it has been advanced through the oral cavity, it can't be seated in front of the laryngeal inlet. Thirdly, even if seated well in front of the laryngeal inlet, adequate ventilation through the EGD may fail owing to obstructing pathology at or below the glottis, or poor lung compliance.

Alternatively, the mnemonic **"MOODS"** may be useful to help recall predictors of difficulty in achieving EGD rescue ventilation:

Mouth **O**pening limitation. Mouth opening may be functionally impaired by trismus and a clenched jaw, or anatomically by TMJ pathology.
Obstruction at or below the glottic opening. Glottic edema, foreign body, tumor, or subglottic conditions can all preclude successful ventilation via an EGD.
Distortion, displacement, or disruption of the airway. Displacement or distortion of the laryngeal inlet by pathology such as a neck hematoma, blunt trauma, or radiation changes may make it difficult to seat the EGD directly in the path of the glottic opening.
Stiff lungs (e.g., bronchospasm) and/or chest wall. Bronchospasm or chest wall compromise due to conditions such as morbid obesity may cause EGDs to fail, as many (but not all) have oropharyngeal leak pressures of 25 cm H_2O or less.

Predictors of Difficult Cricothyrotomy

The default course of action in a failed oxygenation scenario is cricothyrotomy. As with EGD use, assessment of the patient for predictors of difficult cricothyrotomy is important, particularly if difficulty with laryngoscopy as well as BMV is predicted. Difficulty can occur if there are impediments to identifying the location of the cricothyroid membrane, or even if its location is evident, if problems are anticipated in accessing the trachea through it. The mnemonic **"DART"** can help recall these predictors.

Distortion of the anatomy from trauma, expanding neck hematoma, infection, or other pathology.
Access problems from obesity or extreme neck flexion (e.g., ankylosing spondylitis).
Radiation therapy to the neck area in the past.
Tumors.

If RSI is being contemplated in an uncooperative patient with predictors of difficult laryngoscopy and difficult bag-mask ventilation, before proceeding, the clinician should locate the cricothyroid membrane by palpation. Some situations will mandate a formal "double setup", whereby RSI is undertaken only once the cricothyroid membrane has already been marked and prepped, and equipment and personnel are available for immediate cricothyrotomy should failed oxygenation ensue.

▶ SUMMARY

With application of a consistent approach to difficult bag-mask ventilation and difficult laryngoscopy, failed intubation or failed oxygenation scenarios will be only infrequently encountered. However, when the need arises, extraglottic device use has transformed the airway management landscape away from the old "can't intubate—cut the neck" directive. That being said, every clinician with a practice mandate that includes airway management should be familiar with indications for, and knowledge of how to rapidly perform a cricothyrotomy.

REFERENCES

1. Mort TC. Emergency tracheal intubation: complications associated with repeated laryngoscopic attempts. *Anesth Analg*. 2004;99(2):607–613, table of contents.

2. Davies PR, Tighe SQ, Greenslade GL, Evans GH. Laryngeal mask airway and tracheal tube insertion by unskilled personnel. *Lancet*. 1990;336(8721):977–979.

3. Levitan RM, Ochroch EA, Stuart S, Hollander JE. Use of the intubating laryngeal mask airway by medical and nonmedical personnel. *Am J Emerg Med*. 2000;18(1):12–16.

4. Yardy N, Hancox D, Strang T. A comparison of two airway aids for emergency use by unskilled personnel. The Combitube and laryngeal mask. *Anaesthesia*. 1999;54(2):181–183.

5. Brimacombe JR. *Laryngeal Mask Anesthesia Principles and Practice*. 2nd ed. Philadelphia: Saunders; 2005.

6. Brimacombe J, Keller C. Insertion of the LMA-Unique with and without digital intraoral manipulation by inexperienced personnel after manikin-only training. *J Emerg Med*. 2004;26(1):1–5.

7. Parmet JL, Colonna-Romano P, Horrow JC, Miller F, Gonzales J, Rosenberg H. The laryngeal mask airway reliably provides rescue ventilation in cases of unanticipated difficult tracheal intubation along with difficult mask ventilation. *Anesth Analg*. 1998;87(3):661–665.

8. Brimacombe J, Keller C, Kunzel KH, Gaber O, Boehler M, Puhringer F. Cervical spine motion during airway management: a cinefluoroscopic study of the posteriorly destabilized third cervical vertebrae in human cadavers. *Anesth Analg*. 2000;91(5):1274–1278.

9. Keller C, Brimacombe J, Keller K. Pressures exerted against the cervical vertebrae by the standard and intubating laryngeal mask airways: a randomized, controlled, cross-over study in fresh cadavers. *Anesth Analg*. 1999;89(5):1296–1300.

10. Levitan RM, Frass M. The Combitube as rescue device: recommended use of the small adult size for all patients six feet tall or shorter. *Ann Emerg Med*. 2004;44(1):92; author reply 92–93.

11. Urtubia RM, Aguila CM, Cumsille MA. Combitube: a study for proper use. *Anesth Analg*. 2000;90(4):958–962.

12. Vezina D, Lessard MR, Bussieres J, Topping C, Trepanier CA. Complications associated with the use of the Esophageal-Tracheal Combitube. *Can J Anaesth*. 1998;45(1):76–80.

13. Klein H, Williamson M, Sue-Ling HM, Vucevic M, Quinn AC. Esophageal rupture associated with the use of the Combitube. *Anesth Analg*. 1997;85(4):937–939.

14. Mercer MH. An assessment of protection of the airway from aspiration of oropharyngeal contents using the Combitube airway. *Resuscitation*. 2001;51(2):135–138.

15. Davis DP, Valentine C, Ochs M, Vilke GM, Hoyt DB. The Combitube as a salvage airway device for paramedic rapid sequence intubation. *Ann Emerg Med*. 2003;42(5):697–704.

16. Calkins TR, Miller K, Langdorf MI. Success and complication rates with prehospital placement of an esophageal-tracheal combitube as a rescue airway. *Prehospital Disaster Med*. 2006;21(2 Suppl 2):97–100.

17. Staudinger T, Brugger S, Roggla M, et al. [Comparison of the Combitube with the endotracheal tube in cardiopulmonary resuscitation in the prehospital phase]. *Wien Klin Wochenschr*. 1994;106(13):412–415.

18. Blostein PA, Koestner AJ, Hoak S. Failed rapid sequence intubation in trauma patients: esophageal tracheal combitube is a useful adjunct. *J Trauma*. 1998;44(3):534–537.

19. Mercer MH, Gabbott DA. Insertion of the Combitube airway with the cervical spine immobilised in a rigid cervical collar. *Anaesthesia*. 1998;53(10):971–974.

20. Mercer MH, Gabbott DA. The influence of neck position on ventilation using the Combitube airway. *Anaesthesia*. 1998;53(2):146–150.

21. Brimacombe J, von Goedecke A, Keller C, Brimacombe L, Brimacombe M. The laryngeal mask airway Unique versus the Soft Seal laryngeal mask: a randomized, crossover study in paralyzed, anesthetized patients. *Anesth Analg*. 2004;99(5):1560–1563; table of contents.

22. Hanning SJ, McCulloch TJ, Orr B, Anderson SP. A comparison of the oropharyngeal leak pressure between the reusable Classic laryngeal mask airway and the single-use Soft Seal laryngeal mask airway. *Anaesth Intensive Care*. 2006;34(2):237–239.

23. Francksen H, Bein B, Cavus E, et al. Comparison of LMA Unique, Ambu laryngeal mask and Soft Seal laryngeal mask during routine surgical procedures. *Eur J Anaesthesiol*. 2006:1–7.

24. Tan MG, Chin ER, Kong CS, Chan YH, Ip-Yam PC. Comparison of the re-usable LMA Classic and two single-use laryngeal masks (LMA Unique and Soft-Seal) in airway management by novice personnel. *Anaesth Intensive Care.* 2005;33(6):739–743.

25. Sudhir G, Redfern D, Hall JE, Wilkes AR, Cann C. A comparison of the disposable Ambu AuraOnce(trade mark) Laryngeal Mask with the reusable LMA Classic(trade mark) laryngeal mask airway. *Anaesthesia.* 2007;62(7):719–722.

26. Asai T, Shingu K. The laryngeal tube. *Br J Anaesth.* 2005;95(6):729–736.

27. Scrase I, Woollard M. Needle vs surgical cricothyroidotomy: a short cut to effective ventilation. *Anaesthesia.* 2006;61(10):962–974.

28. Frerk C, Frampton C. Cricothyroidotomy; time for change. *Anaesthesia.* 2006;61(10):921–923.

29. Sulaiman L, Tighe SQ, Nelson RA. Surgical vs wire-guided cricothyroidotomy: a randomised crossover study of cuffed and uncuffed tracheal tube insertion. *Anaesthesia.* 2006;61(6): 565–570.

30. Wong DT, Prabhu AJ, Coloma M, Imasogie N, Chung FF. What is the minimum training required for successful cricothyroidotomy?: a study in mannequins. *Anesthesiology.* 2003;98(2):349–353.

31. Melker JS, Gabrielli A. Melker cricothyrotomy kit: an alternative to the surgical technique. *Ann Otol Rhinol Laryngol.* 2005;114(7):525–528.

CHAPTER 8

How to do Awake Tracheal Intubations—Oral and Nasal

▶ KEY POINTS

- If a difficult airway is considered likely and clinically significant, an "awake" approach should be considered, if patient cooperation permits.
- An awake approach describes an intubation technique facilitated by upper airway anesthesia applied topically or with nerve blocks, with or without light doses of sedation.
- Although commonly used, "deep sedation" should never be counted upon to "relax" or alleviate clenched teeth, nor should it be used to compensate for poor topical airway anesthesia.
- In general, awake intubation should proceed by the route with which the clinician has the most comfort and the greatest experience.
- Local anesthetics can be topically applied in ointment, jelly, nebulized or atomized forms through mouth or nose. Nerve blocks and transtracheal injection are also options.
- If blood pressure permits, an awake intubation can be performed in the semisitting or sitting position.
- 'Precision' laryngoscopy, whereby the operator carefully guides a laryngoscope blade into the mouth using the digits of

the right hand, will aid in performing awake direct laryngoscopy.
- Acute-care clinicians should be as competent in performing an awake intubation as they are in performing a rapid-sequence intubation.

▶ GENERAL CONSIDERATIONS FOR THE AWAKE TRACHEAL INTUBATION

Generally, tracheal intubations are performed in one of three ways:

- Using rapid-sequence intubation (RSI)
- With an "awake" technique, following application of topical airway anesthesia
- Facilitated by deep sedation, but without pharmacologic paralysis

The occasional patient will require a primary surgical airway. Advantages and disadvantages of each route appear in Table 8–1 and are discussed further in Chap. 11.

The American Society of Anesthesiologists' (ASA) difficult airway algorithm is predicated upon the clinician first assessing the "likelihood and clinical impact" of encountering difficulty.[1] If a difficult airway is considered likely and clinically significant, the algorithm suggests an awake approach. An awake approach to the airway generally describes an intubation technique facilitated by upper airway anesthesia applied topically or with nerve blocks, in combination with light (e.g., anxiolytic) doses of sedation. "Awake" in the context of emergency airway management is perhaps a misnomer, as the patient requiring emergency tracheal intubation often has an impaired level of consciousness (LOC). However, "awake intubation", even in the patient with a depressed LOC, is distinct from traditional procedural sedation, where the patient's LOC might be *intentionally* altered in an attempt to overcome resistance to laryngoscopy. This latter technique of using deep sedation without paralysis, although still commonly practiced, has none of the benefits of either awake or rapid sequence (RSI) approaches to tracheal intubation: indeed, the use of deep sedation is referred to by some as "tiger" country in airway management.[2]

Currently, RSI is both the most common primary and secondary rescue approach used to facilitate tracheal intubation in emergency departments (EDs) in North America.[3] The literature supports the use of RSI in the hands of trained and experienced emergency physicians (EPs).[4] The decision to use RSI follows an assessment of the likelihood of encountering difficulty during the process. In face of predicted difficulty, awake intubation becomes an attractive alternative that may provide a wider margin of safety in many instances. Unfortunately, skillful awake tracheal intubation receives little attention in the emergency medicine (EM) literature or practice. This may relate to a combination of lack of perceived need, patient cooperation issues, or deficits in awake intubation skills teaching and experience.

As with RSI, acute-care clinicians should be competent and experienced in performing an awake intubation. This chapter will review the awake intubation process using either the oral or nasal route.

The Advantages of Awake Tracheal Intubation

As reviewed in Table 8–1, in a conscious patient, an awake tracheal intubation delivers the following advantages:

- The patient continues to breathe spontaneously.
- The patient continues to maintain a patent airway.
- The patient continues to protect the airway against aspiration of gastric contents.
- Light (or omitted) doses of sedative/hypnotic agent will generally not present the same risk of hypotension as those used for RSI.

Patient Cooperation and Awake Tracheal Intubation

A degree of patient cooperation is required for an awake intubation. This may exclude a significant proportion of patients requiring emergency tracheal intubation. Indeed, the cooperation issue is one which has made the use of RSI so widespread in EDs. Patient cooperation figures prominently in the decision-making process on how to proceed with tracheal intubation (Fig. 11–3, Chap. 11). However, a blanket dismissal of a patient's ability to cooperate with an awake intubation is also not appropriate: patients will and can cooperate more often than commonly perceived. The "actively" uncooperative, physically agitated patient will often not be rendered cooperative by any means. However, other patients can be described as "passively" uncooperative (e.g., the patient in respiratory failure), and will often permit airway topicalization and awake instrumentation. Patients in the early stages of upper airway obstruction are usually mentating normally and are ideal candidates for an awake approach, as discussed below.

▶ **TABLE 8-1** COMPARISON OF DIFFERENT METHODS OF PROCEEDING WITH TRACHEAL INTUBATION

Intubation Method	Advantages	Disadvantages

Awake intubation	• Patient continues to:
	  ○ Breathe spontaneously
	  ○ Maintain
	  ○ Protect
	  . . .his or her airway.
	  "No bridges burned".
	• Avoids adverse effects of RSI medications.
	• Avoids risk of hypoxemia during transition from spontaneous respirations to taking over positive pressure ventilation.
		• Clinician perception of patient discomfort.
		• Requires an element of patient cooperation.
		• As with RSI, requires training in indications, performing airway anesthesia and direct laryngoscopic or indirect fiber/videoscopic techniques.

Deep sedation	• Perception of a sense of security:
	  "I haven't burned any bridges by giving a muscle relaxant. . ."
	• May help control an uncooperative patient.
	• Perception of a more humane procedure.
		• Often gives a **false** sense of security.
		• Retains many of the downsides of RSI while not delivering the upside of facilitated conditions.
		• Undesirable reflexes intact:
		  ○ gag/vomiting
		  ○ laryngospasm
		• No guarantee that deep sedative doses will leave the patient breathing spontaneously or maintaining an airway.
		• Airway protection ablated in a full stomach patient, often with no applied cricoid pressure.
		• Deep sedative doses of medication can still hemo-dynamically "crash" the patient.
		• Scientific literature clearly documents less optimal intubating conditions using only deep sedation.[35-37]

(*Continued*)

Intubation Method	Advantages	Disadvantages
RSI	• Skeletal muscle relaxation facilitates conditions for direct laryngoscopy. • Application of cricoid pressure may decrease risk of aspiration. • Not dependent on patient cooperation. • Drugs may help control undesirable physiologic responses, for example, ICP, HR. • High success rates in experienced hands.[4]	• Induction drugs may cause profound drop in blood pressure, for example, in shock states. • Not all physicians are adequately trained in or comfortable using RSI. • "Rescue RSI" not appropriate for all uncooperative patients, for example, those with obstructing airway pathology. • Succinylcholine will not always wear off in time to have patient resume spontaneous ventilation before life-threatening hypoxemia occurs in "can't intubate, can't oxygenate" situations. • Fear of "what if I can't intubate or ventilate?" • Requires intimate knowledge of all drugs and contraindications to technique. • Requires requisite surgical skills and equipment.
Awake tracheotomy or cricothyrotomy	• In the patient presenting with obstructing airway pathology, less risk of losing the airway during application of topical airway anesthesia or attempted tube passage from above.	

When and Why to do an Awake Tracheal Intubation

There are three broad reasons to consider an awake tracheal intubation in emergencies:

A. **Predicted difficult airway.** An awake intubation should be considered primarily if a question exists about whether the clinician can easily take over what the patient is presently doing for him- or herself. Especially if difficulty is predicted in both intubating the patient and maintaining oxygenation with either bag-mask or a rescue oxygenation technique, then awake intubation should be considered. A classic scenario would include the patient with obstructing pathologic changes in the airway.

B. **Predicted exaggerated hypotensive response to induction medications used for RSI.** Some patients present with significant hemodynamic instability and concern may exist over the effects of RSI induction agents on the blood pressure. While careful choice of induction agent and dose, together with a fluid bolus, will often enable safe conduct of an RSI in this situation, an awake intubation is a second option to help maintain blood pressure during tracheal intubation.

C. **RSI not needed: the arrested, critically ill, or intrinsically sedated patient:** Many patients requiring intubation in emergencies have a markedly decreased LOC as part of their presenting condition. Such patients may be arrested, critically ill, or intrinsically sedated by their presenting condition, such as hypercarbia due to respiratory failure. While not truly "awake" or overtly cooperative, these patients will often not resist a primary laryngoscopy. This indication is particularly relevant in the profoundly hypotensive or arrested patient. In contrast, the unconscious head-injured patient is still best intubated with RSI.

Oral or Nasal Route?

In general, awake tracheal intubation should proceed by the route with which the clinician has the most comfort and the greatest experience. For most, this will mean an oral approach. Blind nasotracheal intubation (BNTI) may be considered an option when the patient's mouth opening is restricted and RSI is contraindicated. However, BNTI has relative contraindications in certain trauma patients, more complications, and a lower success rate than RSI.[4] With either route (oral or nasal), attempts should be made to topically anesthetize the airway.

Tools for Awake Tracheal Intubation

Almost any intubating device can be used for an awake intubation. Most awake intubations in the operating room (OR) are performed using a flexible fiberoptic bronchoscope. However, **direct laryngoscopy**, a familiar technique, can also be used and realistically would be used for most awake intubations in the emergency, out-of-OR setting. Other tools used for awake intubations include video-based and rigid or semi-rigid fiberoptic scopes.[5] A description of fiberoptic stylet use in the awake patient appears in Chap. 6.

▶ TOPICAL AIRWAY ANESTHESIA

The very presence of so many different published techniques of applying topical airway anesthesia bears witness to the fact that there is probably no one *best* agent or technique. Local anesthetics can be topically applied in ointment, jelly, nebulized and atomized forms through the mouth or nose. Nerve blocks and transtracheal injection of local anesthetic are also options.

Review of Airway Innervation

The glossopharyngeal nerve innervates the posterior third of the tongue down to and including the vallecula, as well as the soft palate and palatoglossal folds (Fig. 3–10, Chap. 3). A "gag" response will be elicited if the laryngoscope blade touches or applies pressure to sensitive structures innervated by this nerve. These structures can be blocked with topically applied local anesthetics. The inferior aspect of the epiglottis and the larynx above the cords are supplied by the internal branch of the superior laryngeal nerve (SLN). Touch or pressure to these structures without anesthesia can stimulate reflex glottic closure. The SLN can also be blocked topically by application of local anesthetic in the region of the piriform recesses, located on either side of the laryngeal inlet. Alternatively, it can be blocked by injecting a small volume of local anesthetic (e.g., 2 mL of lidocaine 2%) in the proximity of the nerve as it pierces the thyrohyoid membrane near the lateral edges of the hyoid bone. Below the cords, sensation is provided by the recurrent laryngeal branch of the vagus nerve. Tracheal anesthesia can be attained with inhalation or application of atomized local anesthetic, or a transcricothyroid membrane injection of local anesthetic.

Topical Airway Anesthesia for Orotracheal Intubation

Adequate anesthesia for awake oral intubation using direct laryngoscopy can be achieved with anesthetic agents applied mainly to the distribution of the glossopharyngeal nerve (Fig. 3–10, Chap. 3). Lidocaine can be used as a sole agent: once applied to the mucosa, it will have maximal effect in 2–5 minutes, and will act for about 20 minutes. Lidocaine ointment (in a 5% concentration) or jelly (2% concentration) (Fig. 8–1) is applied with a tongue depressor from the front to back of the tongue, targeting especially the posterior third. The ointment, if used, is quite thick and must be applied slowly, allowing it to "melt" on the tongue surface (Fig. 8–2). The 2% jelly is easier to apply and will usually be adequate. The very cooperative

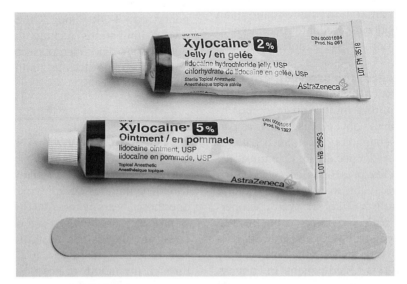

Figure 8–1. Lidocaine ointment (in a 5% concentration) or jelly (2% concentration) may be applied with a tongue depressor.

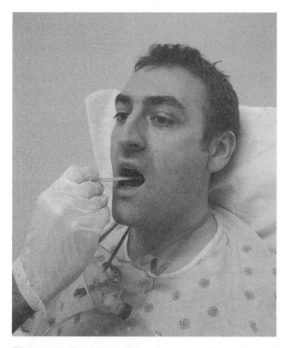

Figure 8–2. Lidocaine ointment once placed on a tongue depressor is applied to the posterior third of the tongue.

patient can also be coached to "gargle and swish" liquid 4% lidocaine. Thereafter, other sensitive areas, including the soft palate, posterior pharynx, tonsillar pillars and hypopharynx should be targeted, using a "spray as you go" technique (Fig. 8–3). Lidocaine endotracheal spray (in a 10% concentration = 10 mg/spray; not currently available in the USA) can be used, or 4% lidocaine administered by an atomizing device. Atomizers include the venerable DeVilbiss atomizer (Fig. 8–4) and the newer Mucosal Atomization Devices (e.g., MADgic®, [Wolfe Tory Medical Inc., Salt Lake City, UT], Fig. 8–5).

Although the above regimen will generally allow for awake direct laryngoscopy, if time permits, additional doses of local anesthetic can be applied to progressively deeper structures (e.g., the laryngeal inlet). Gradually deeper insertion of the laryngoscope blade will help expose the epiglottis, and then glottic opening for additional sprays of anesthetic agent (Fig. 8–6). Oxygen can be readministered as required in between doses.

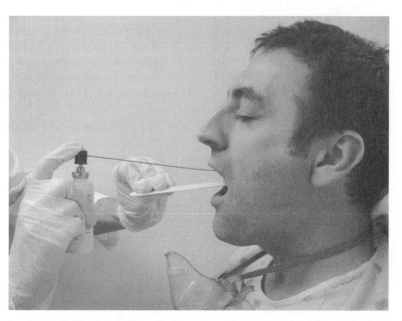

Figure 8–3. The soft palate, posterior pharynx, tonsillar pillars, and hypopharynx should be targeted, using a "spray as you go" technique.

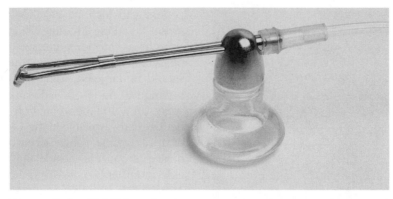

Figure 8–4. DeVilbiss atomizer.

Alternatively, 4 mL of 4% lidocaine with or without neosynephrine 0.5% (1 mL) can be nebulized and delivered either by mask or a mouth piece (Fig. 8–7). This technique requires some time (10–15 minutes) and a degree of patient cooperation.

However applied, care should be taken to ensure that the maximum recommended dose of lidocaine (5–7 mg/kg) is not exceeded.

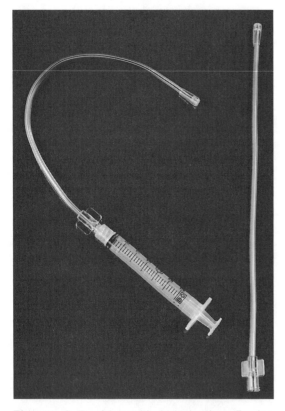

Figure 8–5. Mucosal Atomization Device (MADgic®, courtesy of Wolfe Tory Medical Inc., Salt Lake City, UT).

Topical Airway Anesthesia for Nasotracheal Intubation

A. Vasoconstriction of the nasal mucosa can be achieved with phenylephrine 0.5% or oxymetazoline drops. Compared with cocaine for the prevention of epistaxis, studies suggest that phenylephrine and oxymetazoline are no less effective (although other studies have failed to show any advantage over saline).[6–9]

B. The nares can be anesthetized by applying 2% lidocaine jelly to, and inserting a nasopharyngeal airway, or using a cotton pledget soaked with 2% lidocaine with epinephrine. Alternatively, one of the previously mentioned atomizing devices (e.g., DeVilbiss or MAD® Nasal) can be used.

C. The pharynx is anesthetized with lidocaine spray, as described in the above section on "oral" anesthesia.

D. Lidocaine can be simultaneously delivered to oral and nasal cavities by nebulizer mask. Although an easy modality to use, results are usually not as good as those obtained with more focused application of local anesthetic.

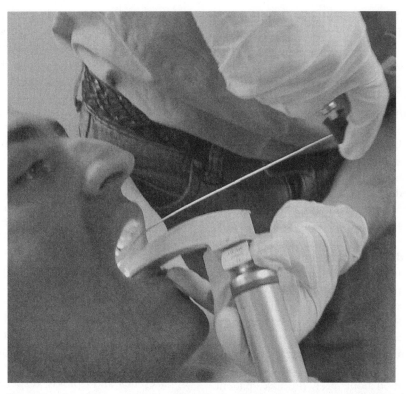

Figure 8–6. Deeper structures may be targeted with topical airway anesthesia during the awake laryngoscopy.

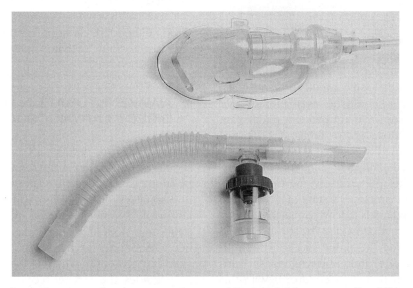

Figure 8–7. A mask or mouth-piece may be used to administer aerosolized lidocaine.

▶ SEDATION FOR THE AWAKE INTUBATION

Light sedation is the intended state for awake intubation. It represents a depth of sedation characterized by anxiolysis, and possibly decreased pain perception, yet the patient is readily rousable with verbal or at most, light physical stimulation. The patient is able to maintain protective airway reflexes and a patent airway, and should be at no risk of becoming apneic. **No sedation** is also an option, and may be most appropriate for the patient presenting with a tenuous airway due to obstructing airway pathology.

Deep sedation represents a state of unconsciousness which may impair the patient's respiratory drive and ability to protect the airway. Deep sedation can be an unintended complication of light sedation. Consequences of unintended deep sedation include vomiting and aspiration with airway instrumentation, laryngospasm, and apnea. It should also be recognized that sedation alone rarely produces patient cooperation in the actively combative patient. Although commonly used, deep sedation should never be counted upon to relax or alleviate clenched teeth, nor should it be used to compensate for poor topical airway anesthesia.

Sedation Pearls

A. **Titrate to effect.** Individuals respond differently to the same medication dosages. Small doses should be used initially, for example, in a 70-kg patient: midazolam 0.25–1 mg/dose and/or fentanyl 25–50 μg/dose, repeated as needed. Other agents to consider would include haloperidol (2–5 mg/dose) or ketamine (20–40 mg/dose). This latter agent produces a state of dissociative amnesia and tends to leave protective airway reflexes intact. However, by sensitizing the upper airway, ketamine has the theoretical potential to induce laryngospasm (primarily seen in young children). With this

potential, and its tendency to increase secretions, some clinicians have suggested that ketamine may not be an ideal sedative agent for awake intubation. Other sedative agents with potential application to awake intubation include remifentanil and dexmedetomidine (Chap. 13).

B. **Age differences.** The elderly require less drug to achieve sedation, while children in general require comparatively more (in mg/kg).

C. **Physiological differences.** The patient with high sympathetic tone (frequently the case in the emergency intubation population) is highly sensitive to low doses of sedative agents.

D. **Pathological differences.** The neurologically impaired patient, for example, has lower requirements.

E. **Reversal agents.** Although more often required in nonairway procedural sedation, reversal agents (Flumazenil and Naloxone) should be readily available for benzodiazepines and opioids, respectively.

Note that the mainstay of the awake intubation is topical airway anesthesia. Sedatives, anxiolytics, or narcotics should be used only as needed. An awake intubation should be just that! Additional sedation can be administered, if needed, as soon as the patient has been successfully intubated and tube position is confirmed.

▶ AWAKE INTUBATION USING DIRECT LARYNGOSCOPY

If blood pressure permits, an awake intubation should be performed in the semisitting or sitting position. This will be mandatory for the patient in respiratory distress, who will be very reluctant to lie supine. If needed, the clinician can stand on a stool or a chair. Once the patient has been prepared, laryngoscopy begins. "Precision" laryngoscopy, whereby the operator carefully guides the laryngoscope blade into the mouth using the digits of the right hand (Fig. 8–8), will aid in keeping the blade in the lumen of the oral cavity, avoiding contact with sensitive mucosa until absolutely necessary. As the blade reaches the back of the oral cavity, gentle tongue compression will begin, aiming to visualize the epiglottis. The patient can experience some "pressure" at this stage. Once the epiglottis is seen, the blade is positioned, centered, in the vallecula (Fig. 8–9). At this point, the patient should be warned that transient discomfort will be felt during the increased pressure caused by the laryngoscope "lift" needed to expose the cords (Figure 8–10). Once seen, the clinician

should maintain visual contact with the cords, while having a coached assistant place the endotracheal tube (ETT) in his or her hand in the correct orientation. Expeditious intubation should then occur while the cords are abducted during patient inspiration. If the cords are transiently adducted, the clinician should pause with the ETT poised at the cords until abduction occurs. As used in the accompanying figures, curved blade (Macintosh) laryngoscopy is recommended for awake laryngoscopy, as a direct lift of the SLN-innervated undersurface of the epiglottis could otherwise stimulate reflex glottic closure.

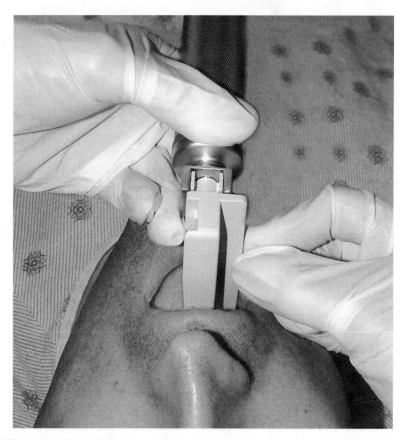

Figure 8–8. "Precision" laryngoscopy, whereby the operator carefully guides the laryngoscope blade into the mouth using the digits of the right hand.

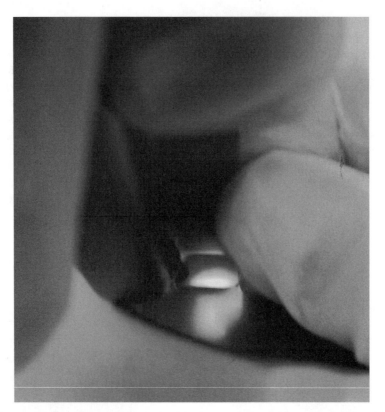

Figure 8–9. Once the epiglottis is seen, the blade can be positioned, centered in the vallecula.

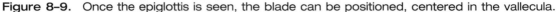

▶ AWAKE ORAL INTUBATION—A GENERIC APPROACH

A. **Preoxygenation** with a nonrebreathing face mask or manual resuscitator should occur for 2–5 minutes (as time permits). Supplemental oxygen should be continued, as possible, during the application of topical airway anesthesia.

B. **Preparation** of monitors, oxygen, BVM device, suction, ETTs, stylet, laryngoscope and blades, drugs, alternative intubation options and rescue devices should be complete. Note that **psychological preparation** should be performed with the mentating patient: the patient should be told the rationale for the procedure and what to expect, with reassurance. The patient's cooperation should be elicited (if possible) with mouth opening, tongue protrusion, and avoidance of struggling against the laryngoscope blade.

C. **Topical airway anesthesia** should be applied, as described above. Sedation can be titrated to effect, recognizing the need for ongoing patient cooperation.

D. **Awake direct laryngoscopy** is performed, as described above. Unpleasant as this may sound, it is often well tolerated.

E. **The tube location is confirmed.** Once intubated, the ETT cuff is inflated. Often, the patient will cough, and expiratory flow can be felt and heard issuing from the proximal tube. The patient should not be able to vocalize. However, objective confirmation of placement with an ETCO$_2$ detector should still be sought. The patient should be reassured that the procedure has been successfully completed, that he won't be able to talk.

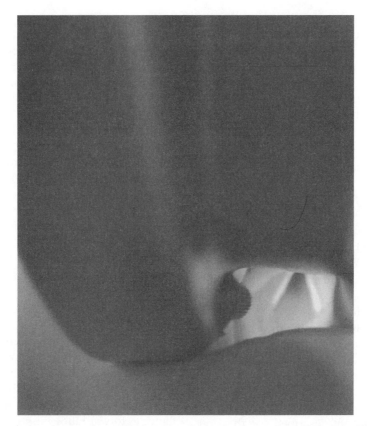

Figure 8–10. Once the blade is positioned in the vallecula, an appropriate lift will expose the cords.

F. **Additional analgesia and sedation** should be introduced, as blood pressure permits. Vital signs should be rechecked.

▶ BLIND NASOTRACHEAL INTUBATION (BNTI)

BNTI Introduction

BNTI has become increasingly rare in contemporary practice. This is appropriate, as it can be technically challenging, has a higher complication rate, and compared to RSI, is less frequently successful.[4] However, it is also a technique that "occasionally, in cases where laryngoscopy is difficult, [may permit] a nasal tube [to] enter the trachea blindly with remarkable ease."[10] As is

implied in its name, BNTI is performed without direct visualization of the laryngeal inlet, in a spontaneously breathing patient. Guided by breath sounds, a regular endotracheal tube is placed through the nose and advanced into the trachea. Corrective maneuvers, if needed, are suggested by clinical signs. BNTI may be an option to consider in a patient with predictors of significant difficulty when RSI is relatively contraindicated and/or cooperation with an awake oral intubation may not be expected.

All contraindications to BNTI (including apnea) are relative, and include upper airway foreign bodies, bleeding diathesis (including heparinized, warfarinized, or recently thrombolyzed patients), or obstructing airway pathology. Midface and/or basal skull fracture[11] has historically been included as a relative contraindication to BNTI, based on a small number of case reports of accidental intracranial passage of nasogastric[12-15] or nasotracheal tubes.[16-18] However, other published reports have failed to demonstrate adverse outcomes following nasal intubation in this same population in the prehospital,[19,20] ED,[19] or OR settings.[19,21]

BNTI Technique

As with any other technique, all needed equipment should be assembled. An uncut ETT one full size smaller than would normally be used for orotracheal intubation should be selected, for example, 6.5–7.0-mm internal diameter (ID) for a female or 7.0–7.5-mm ID for a male. Both nostrils should be medicated with local anesthetic with or without a vasoconstrictor, as detailed earlier in this chapter. A nasopharyngeal airway covered in lidocaine jelly or ointment can help with application of the anesthetic while also assessing the nasal passage for patency. An attempt should also be made to apply local anesthetic to the pharynx (if feasible) in a manner similar to that previously described for the oral approach.

The head and neck should be placed in the "sniffing" position.[10] The well-lubricated tube should be placed in the right nostril (if the option exists), with the bevel facing the septum. This tube orientation keeps the leading edge of the ETT's bevel away from the vascular Kiesselbach's plexus on the nasal septum. Other clinicians advocate preferentially using the most patent nostril. The tube should be directed inferiorly, along the floor of the nasal passage, to stay within the major nasal airway, beneath the inferior turbinate. This will also direct the tube away from the thin bone of the more superiorly located cribriform plate.[22] A gentle twisting motion during tube advancement will help avoid obstruction.

There will be some resistance in the posterior nasopharynx (as is the case when inserting a nasogastric tube). Gentle pressure and a twisting

motion (e.g., 90° to the left) should allow passage. As the ETT is advanced, fogging will be seen and breath sounds should be heard from the end of the tube. The ETT is further advanced, with the clinician's ear near the proximal end of the ETT, monitoring breath sounds. Maximal breath sounds will be heard when the ETT is at the glottic opening. The ETT should then be quickly advanced through the cords during inspiration, when the cords are maximally abducted. The cuff is inflated, and tube position confirmed in the usual objective fashion. The ETT should be sited at approximately 28 cm at the nares in males and 26 cm in females.

BNTI Troubleshooting

Due to the intrinsic shape of the ETT and the path traveled as it is advanced through the nasopharynx, the tube is often perfectly directed up toward the larynx. However, one of four malpositions can occur.[23] Diagnosis of a malposition should be possible by evaluating (a) breath sounds through the tube; (b) resistance to forward tube passage; and (c) palpation or observation of tube impingement in the anterior neck. Corrective maneuvers include directing the tube more anteriorly (by extending the head) or posteriorly (by lifting then flexing the head); or by directing it laterally (by twisting the tube to left or right), as needed. Diagnostic features of, and corrective maneuvers needed for the four BNTI malpositions appear in Table 8–2.

Continued difficulty in spite of these corrective maneuvers can occasionally be addressed by some of the suggestions in the next section, useful in the patient requiring C-spine precautions.

Performing BNTI with C-Spine Precautions

For BNTI in the patient requiring manual in-line neck stabilization, head extension is not an option if additional anterior direction of the tube

▶ **TABLE 8–2** BLIND NASAL INTUBATION: DIAGNOSING AND CORRECTING MALPOSITIONS

Malposition	Breath Sounds	Resistance to Forward Passage	Neck Palpation	Corrective Maneuver
(None: Correct location)	Present	None	Nothing palpable	None needed
Caught up on adducted cords, anterior commissure, or cricoid	Present	Present	Nothing palpable	Flex head slightly (for anterior commissure hang-up), rotate tube slightly, and readvance
Caught up in vallecula	Muffled or absent	Present	Tube tip in midline of neck	Withdraw, flex head slightly, do jaw lift and readvance
Piriform sinus	Muffled or absent	Present	Tube tip felt in lateral neck	Withdraw slightly, rotate tube in contralateral direction, readvance
Esophagus	Absent	None	Nothing palpable	Withdraw tube until breath sounds heard, extend head, readvance tube

is needed. The following three maneuvers can be used as alternatives:

A. Backward pressure can be applied to the thyroid cartilage (akin to external laryngeal manipulation (ELM) performed to improve the view at direct laryngoscopy), to "bring the larynx to the tube".
B. If available, an Endotrol® tube[24–26] (Mallinckrodt Inc., St. Louis, MO) can be used. This tube has a directable tip, controlled by a small loop near its proximal end (Fig. 8–11). By pulling on the loop, the ETT tip is flexed, causing it to move anteriorly.
C. With the tube sitting in the oropharynx, inflation of the ETT cuff with 10–15 mL of air will elevate the ETT tip up and toward the laryngeal inlet. The tube is then advanced until resistance is encountered, with loud breath sounds. The cuff is deflated to allow tube passage through the cords, and is reinflated once tracheal intubation has been successfully completed.[27, 28] This

maneuver can also be used with Trachlight guidance, using the device with its inner stylet removed.

Although the "sniffing" position has long been thought to be the ideal position for BNTI,[10] the neutral position with cuff inflation appears to result in similar success rates.[29]

BNTI Complications

In addition to failure to intubate, complications of BNTI may include epistaxis and bacteremia. Epistaxis severe enough to interfere with intubation or require posterior nasal packing is unusual, occurring in less than 2.5% of cases.[8,30,31] Moderate bleeding, usually described as blood visible in, or enough to suction from the posterior pharynx, occurs more often, in up to 14% of cases.[8,9,30,31] This latter degree of bleeding would be unlikely to interfere with intubation attempts, however.

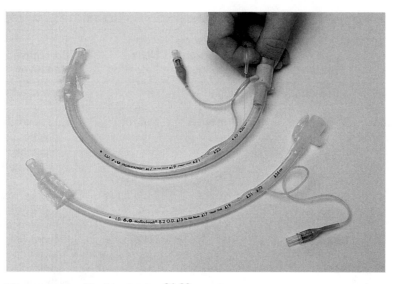

Figure 8–11. Endotrol tube [24–26] (Mallinckrodt Inc., St. Louis, MO).

Bacteremia occurred with nasotracheal intubation[32] in 5.5% of patients in one OR series. Retropharyngeal perforation, with a risk of submucosal false passage, has been described.[30] As previously mentioned, intracranial endotracheal tube passage has also been reported.[16–18]

BNTI Effectiveness

ROUTINE AND DIFFICULT AIRWAY MANAGEMENT

In the hands of seasoned clinicians, BNTI success rates of up to 92% have been reported in both routine and difficult airway situations.[11,30,31] Other series have reported first attempt success rates of 55%–61% in the hands of novices "within a reasonable time frame."[11,33] Both overall and first-attempt success rates are lower than those reported using other techniques.[4,33]

C-SPINE PRECAUTIONS

Historically, BNTI was advocated as the method of choice for intubation of the patient with a suspected C-spine injury. In fact, neither neurologic outcome nor C-spine movement with BNTI in this population has been shown to differ from that resulting from oral intubation by direct laryngoscopy.[34] Currently, known or suspected C-spine injury is not by itself considered an indication for nasotracheal intubation, blind or otherwise.

▶ SUMMARY

Compared with RSI, awake intubation may be perceived as a more technically challenging procedure. In contrast to RSI, an element of patient cooperation is needed to successfully manage a patient's airway using an awake approach. Awake intubation is a necessary skill and should not become a vanishing art. Success is linked not only to patient selection but also to the deliberate acquisition and maintenance of awake intubation skills. Clinicians should be as competent and comfortable in performing an awake tracheal intubation as they are in performing an RSI.

REFERENCES

1. Practice guidelines for management of the difficult airway: an updated report by the American Society of Anesthesiologists Task Force on Management of the Difficult Airway. *Anesthesiology.* 2003;98(5): 1269–1277.

2. Donati F. Tracheal intubation: unconsciousness, analgesia and muscle relaxation. *Can J Anaesth.* 2003;50(2):99–103.

3. Sagarin MJ, Barton ED, Chng YM, et al. Airway management by US and Canadian emergency medicine residents: a multicenter analysis of more than 6,000 endotracheal intubation attempts. *Ann Emerg Med.* 2005;46(4):328–336.

4. Kovacs G, Law JA, Ross J, et al. Acute airway management in the emergency department by non-anesthesiologists. *Can J Anaesth.* 2004;51(2): 174–180.

5. Kovacs G, Law JA, Petrie D. Awake fiberoptic intubation using an optical stylet in an anticipated difficult airway. *Ann Emerg Med.* 2007;49(1):81–83.

6. Gross JB, Hartigan ML, Schaffer DW. A suitable substitute for 4% cocaine before blind nasotracheal intubation: 3% lidocaine-0.25% phenylephrine nasal spray. *Anesth Analg.* 1984;63(10):915–918.

7. Latorre F, Otter W, Kleemann PP, et al. Cocaine or phenylephrine/lignocaine for nasal fibreoptic intubation? *European Journal of Anaesthesiology.* 1996;13:577–581.

8. Katz RI, Hovagim AR, Finkelstein HS, et al. A comparison of cocaine, lidocaine with epinephrine, and oxymetazoline for prevention of epistaxis on nasotracheal intubation. *J Clin Anesth.* 1990;2(1):16–20.

9. Rector FT, DeNuccio DJ, Alden MA. A comparison of cocaine, oxymetazoline, and saline for nasotracheal intubation. *Aana J.* 1987;55(1):49–54.

10. Magill IW, Macintosh R, Hewer CL, et al. Lest we forget. A historic meeting of the Section of Anaesthetics of Royal Society of Medicine on 6 Decemeber 1974. Divynyl ether. *Anaesthesia.* 1975;30(5): 630–632.

11. Iserson KV. Blind nasotracheal intubation. *Ann Emerg Med.* 1981;10(9):468–471.

12. Fremstad JD, Martin SH. Lethal complication from insertion of nasogastric tube after severe basilar skull fracture. *J Trauma.* 1978;18(12): 820–822.

13. Fletcher SA, Henderson LT, Miner ME, et al. The successful surgical removal of intracranial nasogastric tubes. *J Trauma.* 1987;27(8): 948–952.

14. Gregory JA, Turner PT, Reynolds AF. A complication of nasogastric intubation: intracranial penetration. *J Trauma.* 1978;18(12):823–824.

15. Bouzarth WF. Intracranial nasogastric tube insertion. *J Trauma.* 1978;18(12):818–819.

16. Horellou MF, Mathe D, Feiss P. A hazard of naso-tracheal intubation. *Anaesthesia.* 1978;33(1): 73–74.

17. Cameron D, Lupton BA. Inadvertent brain penetration during neonatal nasotracheal intubation. *Arch Dis Child.* 1993;69(1 Spec No):79–80.

18. Marlow TJ, Goltra DD, Jr., Schabel SI. Intracranial placement of a nasotracheal tube after facial fracture: a rare complication. *J Emerg Med.* 1997;15(2): 187–191.

19. Rosen CL, Wolfe RE, Chew SE, et al. Blind nasotracheal intubation in the presence of facial trauma. *J Emerg Med.* 1997;15(2): 141–145.

20. Rhee KJ, Muntz CB, Donald PJ, et al. Does nasotracheal intubation increase complications in patients with skull base fractures? *Ann Emerg Med.* 1993;22(7):1145–1147.

21. Bahr W, Stoll P. Nasal intubation in the presence of frontobasal fractures: a retrospective study. *J Oral Maxillofac Surg.* 1992;50(5):445–447.

22. Goodisson DW, Shaw GM, Snape L. Intracranial intubation in patients with maxillofacial injuries associated with base of skull fractures? *J Trauma.* 2001;50(2):363–366.

23. Jacoby J. Nasal endotracheal intubation by an external visual technic. *Anesth Analg.* 1970;49(5): 731–739.

24. Asai T. Endotrol tube for blind nasotracheal intubation. *Anaesthesia.* 1996;51(5):507.

25. Hooker EA, Hagan S, Coleman R, et al. Directional-tip endotracheal tubes for blind nasotracheal intubation. *Acad Emerg Med.* 1996;3(6):586–589.

26. O'Connor R E, Megargel RE, Schnyder ME, et al. Paramedic success rate for blind nasotracheal intubation is improved with the use of an endotracheal tube with directional tip control. *Ann Emerg Med.* 2000;36(4):328–332.

27. van Elstraete AC, Pennant JH, Gajraj NM, et al. Tracheal tube cuff inflation as an aid to blind nasotracheal intubation. *Br J Anaesth.* 1993;70(6): 691–693.

28. Gorback MS. Inflation of the endotracheal tube cuff as an aid to blind nasal endotracheal intubation. *Anesth Analg.* 1987;66(9):916–917.

29. Chung YT, Sun MS, Wu HS. Blind nasotracheal intubation is facilitated by neutral head position and endotracheal tube cuff inflation in spontaneously

breathing patients. *Can J Anaesth*. 2003;50(5): 511–513.

30. Tintinalli JE, Claffey J. Complications of nasotracheal intubation. *Ann Emerg Med*. 1981;10(3): 142–144.

31. Danzl DF, Thomas DM. Nasotracheal intubations in the emergency department. *Crit Care Med*. 1980;8(11):677–682.

32. Dinner M, Tjeuw M, Artusio JF, Jr. Bacteremia as a complication of nasotracheal intubation. *Anesth Analg*. 1987;66(5):460–462.

33. Roppolo LP, Vilke GM, Chan TC, et al. Nasotracheal intubation in the emergency department, revisited. *J Emerg Med*. 1999;17(5):791–799.

34. Crosby ET. Airway management in adults after cervical spine trauma. *Anesthesiology*. 2006;104(6): 1293–1318.

35. Lieutaud T, Billard V, Khalaf H, et al. Muscle relaxation and increasing doses of propofol improve intubating conditions. *Can J Anaesth*. 2003;50(2): 121–126.

36. Erhan E, Ugur G, Gunusen I, et al. Propofol—not thiopental or etomidate—with remifentanil provides adequate intubating conditions in the absence of neuromuscular blockade. *Can J Anaesth*. 2003;50(2):108–115.

37. Collins L, Prentice J, Vaghadia H. Tracheal intubation of outpatients with and without muscle relaxants. *Can J Anaesth*. 2000;47(5):427–432.

CHAPTER 9

Rapid Sequence Intubation—Why and How to do it

▶ KEY POINTS

- For clinicians with the requisite skills, rapid-sequence intubation should become the method of choice for tracheal intubation in emergencies, unless contraindicated.
- The emergency medicine literature suggests high success rates and low morbidity with the use of RSI in experienced hands.
- "Successful" tracheal intubation does not by itself necessarily represent a successful outcome.
- The evidence favoring pretreatment medications is not compelling. Emphasis should instead be placed on preventing hypoxia and hypotension.
- If rapid oxygen desaturation occurs (or is likely to occur) with onset of apnea during an RSI, gentle bag-mask ventilation can and should be performed while awaiting onset of the muscle relaxant.
- Cricoid pressure has the potential to impair the view at laryngoscopy, cause difficulty with bag-mask ventilation (BMV) and impair extraglottic device (EGD) placement.
- Laryngoscopy and intubation should proceed only once the muscle relaxant has taken effect.

▶ INTRODUCTION TO RAPID-SEQUENCE INTUBATION (RSI)

Historically, the term "RSI" has referred to Rapid Sequence *Induction* (of anesthesia), used to minimize the risk of aspiration in surgical patients felt to have a "full stomach." In emergency medicine the term RSI refers to Rapid Sequence *Intubation* (RSI). The difference in semantics refers to a different end-point: in the operating room (OR), patients are intubated to provide anesthesia, while in the emergency department (ED), patients are anesthetized to facilitate tracheal intubation.[1]

Rapid sequence *induction* was originally described in the anesthesia literature as a method of airway management undertaken to minimize the risk of aspiration in parturients undergoing emergency Caesarean section.[2] Despite initial controversy, RSI has now also become part of everyday emergency medicine (EM) practice. RSI in emergency care involves the use of a combination of specific pharmacologic agents to obtain optimal conditions for tracheal intubation.

RSI use has been shown to increase the likelihood of successful tracheal intubation and decrease complications when compared to other methods, in most settings.[3] However, these results assume trained and experienced clinicians who have learned the process and are familiar with the drugs used.

Unless contraindicated, RSI should be strongly considered for emergency intubations. *Relative* contraindications to RSI include the following:

A. **Inadequate prerequisite clinician factors:** The clinician performing RSI must have the necessary knowledge and skills. Needed airway equipment and trained help must also be available.

B. **Anticipated difficult airway:** RSI should be avoided if difficult tracheal intubation is predicted, especially if bag-mask ventilation (BMV) may also be problematic. In this situation, an "awake" intubation should be considered, if the patient can cooperate. In particular, the patient presenting with obstructing airway pathology should rarely be intubated using RSI.

C. **Unnecessary:** RSI may not be needed in situations where "facilitation" is not needed, for example, in the arrested patient.

In most cases, RSI will facilitate emergency intubations. However, the decision to proceed with RSI should follow an airway assessment, and in the face of predictors of significant difficulty, should only proceed if lack of patient cooperation precludes an awake attempt. In addition, if RSI is undertaken in the patient with predictors of difficulty, rescue oxygenation techniques such as extraglottic device use or cricothyrotomy must be predicted to succeed. As discussed in more detail in Chap. 11, the benefit of proceeding with RSI in the face of difficulty should outweigh the risk of encountering a failed airway situation. It is also important to appreciate that RSI is only one way to facilitate tracheal intubation, and that intubation in turn is only one facet of airway management.

▶ RSI IN EMERGENCIES: WHY USE IT?

RSI is being used increasingly in emergency departments and selected other settings. As an example of its broader dissemination, Advanced Trauma Life Support (ATLS) now supports the use of RSI to facilitate airway management in trauma patients.[4] As a means of securing the airway, RSI holds the following advantages, reproduced here from Table 8–1:

- RSI is not dependent on patient cooperation and, with appropriate preparation, can usually be expeditiously performed.
- Skeletal muscle relaxation facilitates conditions for direct laryngoscopy and intubation.
- Application of cricoid pressure may decrease the risk of aspiration.
- Drugs used during RSI may help control undesirable physiologic responses to laryngoscopy and intubation such as gagging, or increases in intracranial pressure (ICP), heart rate, or blood pressure.
- RSI has a high success rate in experienced hands.

However, much as RSI will most often facilitate intubation, it is just as important to appreciate when it may **not** be the technique of first choice. Used in the wrong patient (e.g., the patient presenting with obstructing airway pathology), adverse effects can include a failed airway, "can't intubate, can't oxygenate" situation. Morbidity can also occur with use of an incorrect choice or dosage of induction medication. The practicing clinician adopting RSI use must therefore make the effort to attain the needed cognitive and psychomotor airway skills. A number of established educational programs exist to help attain and augment these skills. Additional experience in the use of RSI medications can often be obtained in hospital ORs.

▶ RSI IN EMERGENCIES: WHAT IS THE CURRENT STATE OF EVIDENCE?

Many reports have described various institutions' experiences with RSI in the ED.[5–10] Despite the growing evidence to support its use, RSI is still not routinely practiced in many hospital EDs, particularly outside teaching centers. There also remains a resistance to RSI use in emergency settings outside the ED. Various perceptions have been cited for this and might include:

- "Administration of paralytics outside of an OR is dangerous."
- "Nonanesthesiologists have no role giving anesthetic drugs."
- "RSI is unnecessary."
- "What if I can't see the cords after the patient is paralyzed?"
- "Midazolam or propofol are safer because the patient maintains spontaneous ventilation."

In the 1970s and into the early 1980s, orotracheal intubation was performed chiefly in patients in cardiopulmonary arrest, while the nasotracheal route was used in spontaneously breathing patients requiring intubation. Anesthesiologists were commonly summoned to the ED to aid in airway management. Over subsequent years, more data began to appear describing RSI use in the ED.[3] Gradually, RSI began to be claimed by EM as a method of airway management within their domain of practice. By the late 1990s, over 95% of U.S. emergency medicine teaching programs reported routine use of neuromuscular blocking agents to facilitate intubation.[11] In 1997, 15 years after the first published use of succinylcholine in the ED, the American College of Emergency Physicians (ACEP) made a Policy Statement on RSI, which included the following statements:

- "Physicians performing RSI should possess training, knowledge, and experience in the techniques and pharmacologic agents used to perform RSI.
- "Neuromuscular blocking agents and appropriate sedative and induction agents should be immediately available in the ED and accessible to all physicians who perform RSI in the ED.
- "Quality review and patient monitoring should be addressed when policies about RSI are developed in the ED."[12]

Data from prospective, randomized controlled trials comparing RSI to other approaches for tracheal intubation in the ED is not available. However, available data does support the use of RSI by emergency physicians as both an effective and safe method to facilitate intubation.[5–10]

On the other hand, the use of deep sedation alone to facilitate tracheal intubation remains very common outside the OR. This practice continues despite growing literature consistently demonstrating that even with potent combinations of sedatives and narcotic (without paralytics) in the hands of experienced clinicians, optimal intubating conditions occur in less than 50% of cases.[3,13–16] Most of these studies were done in elective surgical, physiologically normal patients. The acutely ill emergency patient would likely respond quite differently, with such large doses of sedatives and narcotics creating a more dangerous combination of apnea, hypotension and suboptimal intubating conditions.

Most of the EM literature on RSI originates from relatively large volume centers and in that setting, success rates approaching 100% are reported. Although this data is important, it tends to minimize the concept of airway management as a process. Ten to twenty percent of ED RSIs require more than one attempt at tracheal intubation.[3,5–10] With each attempt there is an increasing potential for complications.[17] The exact nature and rate of complications from emergency intubation are inconsistently reported in the literature. Thus, the true incidence of process-related adverse events such as hypotension and hypoxia related to emergency airway management is not clear. "Successful" tracheal intubation does not necessarily represent a successful outcome by itself, if, for example, significant hypoxia has occurred during the process. RSI is simply one tool to aid successful airway management, along with good planning, preparation, and a timely response to both anticipated and unanticipated clinical events. Throughout the process, it is important to maintain a "bigger picture" perspective and ensure patient oxygenation is maintained, for example, with BMV between attempts.

▶ RSI: DEFINITION AND THE PROCESS

Rapid sequence intubation is a process that involves pharmacologically inducing unconsciousness and paralyzing the patient in a manner that facilitates tracheal intubation, while minimizing the risk of aspiration using application of cricoid pressure. "Rapid-sequence" refers to the fact that the induction agent and the neuromuscular blocker are given in quick succession, and are not titrated to effect. In addition, "rapid" can refer to the fact that one is taking the patient from a conscious state (with the airway protected by the patient) to the placement of a tube in the trachea with the cuff inflated (when the airway is again protected, this time by the ETT cuff) with as little intervening time as possible.

The following discussion assumes that a decision has been made to undertake an RSI, and presents the process from that point to postintubation.

▶ RSI: HOW TO DO IT

The RSI process involves several steps:

A. Preparation.
B. Preoxygenation.
C. Fluid preloading and pretreatment.
D. Induction and pharmacologic paralysis.
E. Application of cricoid pressure.
F. Intubation and confirmation of tube placement.
G. Postintubation management.

Preparation

This involves preparation of the patient and equipment, as discussed in Chap. 5. To review, the following elements are important in preparing for RSI:

Personnel: Airway management is not a one-person job. At least one assistant, and ideally two, are needed to help, guided by specific directions. The assistants should be briefed about the location of the cricoid cartilage and need for cricoid pressure. If difficulty is anticipated, this should be communicated to the team, together with the planned response to difficult laryngoscopy, recognizing that more than one attempt at laryngoscopy may be required.

Equipment: Needed equipment should be assembled. The previously presented mnemonic **STOP "I" "C" BARS** (Chap. 5) can serve as a reminder of the basics needed for routine and potentially difficult tracheal intubations. Suction should be running and immediately available.

Medications. All medications needed for pretreatment (if used), induction, and neuromuscular blockade should be drawn up *and labeled*. Rescue vasopressor agents such as ephedrine or phenylephrine for bolus injection should be drawn up and available to manage postintubation hypotension.

Positioning. The patient and clinician should be **optimally positioned** for the situation.

Preoxygenation

Administration of 100% oxygen for 3–5 minutes in a normal healthy adult will result in "nitrogen washout" and the establishment of an oxygen reservoir using the functional residual capacity (FRC). A similar effect can be achieved by having the patient take 4–8 deep (vital capacity) breaths of 100% oxygen over a one minute period.[18] Preoxygenation will prolong the time available for tracheal intubation before oxygen desaturation occurs. FRC is compromised in situations such as obesity and advanced stages of pregnancy. In addition, in critically ill patients and children, oxygen consumption is increased, leading to more rapid desaturation. Time to desaturation may be delayed in some of these patients by preoxygenating them in the "head-up" position.[19]

In the spontaneously breathing patient, preoxygenation is best performed by tightly applying the mask of a manual resuscitator to the face. Classic teaching of RSI usually includes avoidance of positive pressure ventilation with the manual resuscitator during preoxygenation to avoid insufflating the stomach. However, if the patient's spontaneous ventilation is inadequate and/or the patient's oxygen saturation does not improve with passive oxygen delivery, then assisted BMV is appropriate to preoxygenate the patient. Assisted BMV during preoxygenation may also be appropriate in the patient in whom a difficult airway is suspected. In this situation, briefly attempting BMV before proceeding with RSI helps to test (a) appropriate mask fit and (b) effective delivery of positive pressure ventilation before committing to paralyzing the patient.

Fluid Loading and Pretreatment

The pretreatment step involves the use of medications to prevent adverse physiologic effects resulting from laryngoscopy, or the use of succinylcholine. Historically, the term "pretreatment" has referred to the use of lidocaine, fentanyl, a defasciculation agent or atropine (in children) given at least 3 minutes prior to induction. However, as discussed in more detail in Chap. 13, no outcome data firmly supports the use of these agents, although their administration probably does not cause harm. On the other hand, hypotension and hypoxia are still relatively common adverse events during emergency tracheal intubation using RSI.[4,20,21] For these reasons **the only two routinely mandatory interventions required in the pretreatment phase of an RSI are the administration of 100% oxygen to prevent desaturation and a fluid bolus of 10–20 mL/kg, in an attempt to minimize postintubation hypotension.**

Induction and Pharmacologic Paralysis

In this step, a potent sedative-hypnotic (e.g., propofol, etomidate, or thiopental) or other agent such as the dissociative amnestic ketamine is given with the goal of inducing unconsciousness. This should be done with the correct dose of an agent with rapid onset and with a side effect profile that minimizes exacerbating the patient's underlying condition. Dosing of induction agents is based on the patient's weight and is adjusted down (or up) in consideration of the following factors:

- **Age:** Dosing is adjusted upward for the pediatric patient, and downward for the older patient.
- **Volume status:** Dosage should be adjusted downward in the hypovolemic patient. In the profoundly hypovolemic and hypotensive patient, induction agents, even in small doses, may be poorly tolerated.
- **Patient co-morbidities:** The patient with a depressed level of consciousness may need less induction agent, as is the case for a patient in a cardiogenic or other shock state.

Administration of an induction agent is followed in rapid sequence by a muscle relaxant. Succinylcholine or rocuronium are most often used (see Table 9–1), and both take time to onset. Many clinicians make the mistake of trying to intubate before complete paralysis has occurred or become too hurried after the onset of apnea despite stable oxygen saturation. Succinylcholine usually takes 45 seconds to act fully, and rocuronium (in a dose of 1.0 mg/kg) closer to 1 minute. The mandible should open easily. In the adequately preoxygenated patient, there is no need to bag the patient. However, if rapid oxygen desaturation occurs (or is likely to occur) with onset of apnea, gentle BMV can and should be undertaken, with continued application of cricoid pressure to prevent gastric insufflation.

▶ **TABLE 9–1** ADVANTAGES OF SUCCINYLCHOLINE AND ROCURONIUM FOR RSI

The Debate: Succinylcholine or Rocuronium for intubation? Clinicians are divided on which neuromuscular blocker to use for RSI in emergencies. Advantages of each are presented below:

Favoring the use of Succinylcholine	Favoring the use of Rocuronium
• Rapid onset and favorable intubating conditions.	• Longer duration of action of rocuronium allows orderly transition from Plan A to Plan B or C if difficulty is encountered.
• Perception of rapid offset: patient resumes spontaneous ventilation in a failed airway situation.	• In a failed oxygenation situation, *both succinylcholine and rocuronium* may take sufficiently long to wear off that irreversible hypoxic brain damage may have occurred before spontaneous ventilation resumes.
• Rocuronium has slightly longer onset time, especially if underdosed.	• Rocuronium has a favorable side effect profile compared to succinylcholine, especially for use in the patient where no history is available.
• Many clinicians are more familiar with succinylcholine.	• [A separate agent for the rapid reversal of rocuronium is on the horizon].

Application of Cricoid Pressure

Immediately before RSI begins, the assistant should locate and apply light pressure (10 Newtons [N]) on the cricoid cartilage. As the patient becomes unconscious during RSI, cricoid pressure (the Sellick maneuver) is increased to 30N* (3 kg).[23] Posterior pressure is applied on the cricoid with the thumb, index, and long fingers. The cricoid cartilage is a complete ring, so applied backward pressure should secondarily occlude the esophagus, while not occluding the airway. This pressure theoretically prevents passive regurgitation of gastric contents and also prevents gastric insufflation in the unconscious patient should BMV be undertaken. It is important to not apply full cricoid pressure in awake patients, and to release it

if the patient vomits. Cricoid pressure should continue until the ETT has been placed, the cuff inflated, and objective confirmation of its correct location has occurred.

Note that much as cricoid pressure may be considered standard of care for RSI in the full stomach patient, the published evidence supporting its use as an effective preventative measure is scant. Certainly, vigorous cricoid pressure has the potential to impair the view at laryngoscopy,[24–26] cause obstruction to BMV,[27–30] and impair extraglottic device (EGD) placement.[23] These risks should be balanced against the perceived benefits of cricoid pressure during RSI. Certainly, if substantial difficulty is encountered with BMV or laryngoscopy during RSI, cricoid pressure should be transiently released to determine if it is causing or contributing to difficulty. By the same token, as the distal tip of most EGDs sits in the upper esophagus, cricoid pressure should also be at least temporarily released during their placement.

---

*30N of applied force can be simulated using a 20 mL syringe. The plunger is withdrawn to the 20 mL mark, and its distal (Luer-lok) end occluded. The force needed to then depress the plunger from the 20 mL mark to 10 mL will approximate 30N.[22]

Intubation and Confirmation of Tube Placement

After onset of the muscle relaxant, laryngoscopy and intubation should be performed. "Best look" laryngoscopy should always be undertaken, as described in Chap. 5. An assistant should hand the clinician the ETT in the correct orientation, so that the cords are continuously visualized once seen. Laryngoscopy and intubation should take less than 30–45 seconds in most patients.

Postintubation Management

After tube placement, the cuff should be inflated *immediately* to minimize the period of time with an unprotected airway. If used, the stylet should be removed, if not already done. Cricoid pressure is released only after tracheal location of the ETT has been confirmed. The chest is auscultated for equality of breath sounds, and the tube is secured. A postinduction set of vital signs should be obtained early, with particular reference to the blood pressure.

In the event of inadvertent esophageal intubation, cricoid pressure should be maintained throughout the reintubation process, unless it was thought to be contributing to difficulty.

The ETT should be well secured and consideration given to postintubation sedation.

▶ PEDIATRIC RSI DIFFERENCES

Once again, it is important to emphasize that similarities of basic concepts in pediatric airway management outweigh the differences from those used in the adult. Armed with these basic concepts, and the help of a Broselow tape, the clinician should be able to successfully manage the pediatric airway. The following differences are important age-related considerations in RSI.

A. If using succinylcholine, a dose of 2 mg/kg should be used. Although atropine pretreatment has historically been used in children less than 6 years of age, its use as a prophylactic measure to prevent secondary bradydysrhythmias has been challenged in the literature.[31–34]

B. Apnea time after succinylcholine administration will be considerably less in the young child due to a higher volume of drug distribution and shorter redistribution times.

C. Basal oxygen consumption in children is twice that of adults, so that rapid oxygen desaturation should be anticipated.

SAMPLE RSIs

Table 9–2 contains sample timelines of an RSI performed in an adult and a pediatric patient.

SUMMARY

Successful RSI is all about planning. Patient assessment allows determination of whether RSI can safely be undertaken. Medications must be prepared, helpers briefed and equipment readied for what may be a routine or difficult intubation. Most often, RSI results in expeditious and safe tube placement. However, the clinician must recognize that applied cricoid pressure can create difficulty with laryngoscopy, BMV and EGD placement: if difficulty is encountered with these maneuvers, cricoid pressure should be transiently released. Postintubation care should initially emphasize confirmation of tube placement and reassessment of blood pressure.

▶ **TABLE 9-2** SAMPLE RSIs

Sample RSIs in an Adult and Pediatric Patient	
Adult: 75 kg, Systolic BP 140/	**Pediatric:** 20 kg, Systolic BP 100/
Time 0	
Pretreat with fluid bolus. Preoxygenate while preparing. Plan for difficulty. Position the patient.	Pretreat with fluid bolus (10–20 mL/kg). If used, atropine 0.02 mg/kg (minimum 0.1 mg). Preoxygenate while preparing. Plan for difficulty. Position the patient.
Time 3 minutes	
Pharmacologic induction: choice of. . . • Propofol 150 mg • Thiopental 250 mg • Ketamine 120 mg • Etomidate 20 mg	Pharmacologic induction: choice of. . . • Ketamine 1–2 mg/kg • Propofol 2–3 mg/kg • Thiopental 3–7 mg/kg • Etomidate 0.3 mg/kg
followed immediately by. . .	
Muscle relaxation: • Succinylcholine 120 mg or. . . • Rocuronium 80 mg	Muscle relaxation: • Succinylcholine 2 mg/kg • Rocuronium 1 mg/kg
• Doses must be adjusted according to weight, hemodynamics, level of consciousness and age. • *Cricoid pressure applied when patient rendered unconscious*	
Time 3 minutes 45 seconds	
Perform laryngoscopy and tracheal intubation, then post intubation care: • Objective confirmation of endotracheal location. • Release cricoid pressure. • Reassess blood pressure. • Secure ETT and consider ongoing sedation requirements.	

REFERENCES

1. Dronen S. Rapid–sequence intubation: a safe but ill-defined procedure. *Acad Emerg Med.* 1999;6(1):1–2.
2. Stept WJ, Safar P. Rapid induction-intubation for prevention of gastric-content aspiration. *Anesth Analg.* 1970;49(4):633–636.
3. Kovacs G, Law JA, Ross J, et al. Acute airway management in the emergency department by non-anesthesiologists. *Can J Anaesth.* 2004;51(2): 174–180.
4. *Advanced Trauma Life Support for physicians*: American College of Surgeons Committee on Trauma. Chicago; 2004.
5. Simpson J, Munro PT, Graham CA. Rapid sequence intubation in the emergency department: 5 year trends. *Emerg Med J.* 2006;23(1):54–56.
6. Sagarin MJ, Barton ED, Chng YM, et al. Airway management by US and Canadian emergency medicine residents: a multicenter analysis of more than 6,000 endotracheal intubation attempts. *Ann Emerg Med.* 2005;46(4):328–336.
7. Graham CA, Beard D, Henry JM, et al. Rapid sequence intubation of trauma patients in Scotland. *J Trauma.* 2004;56(5):1123–1126.
8. Levitan RM, Rosenblatt B, Meiner EM, et al. Alternating day emergency medicine and anesthesia resident responsibility for management of the trauma airway: a study of laryngoscopy performance

and intubation success. *Ann Emerg Med.* 2004;43(1):48–53.

9. Bushra JS, McNeil B, Wald DA, et al. A comparison of trauma intubations managed by anesthesiologists and emergency physicians. *Acad Emerg Med.* 2004;11(1):66–70.

10. Sakles JC, Laurin EG, Rantapaa AA, et al. Airway management in the emergency department: a one–year study of 610 tracheal intubations. *Ann Emerg Med.* 1998;31(3):325–332.

11. Ma OJ, Bentley B, 2nd, Debehnke DJ. Airway management practices in emergency medicine residencies. *Am J Emerg Med.* 1995;13(5):501–504.

12. Rapid-sequence intubation. American College of Emergency Physicians. *Ann Emerg Med.* 1997;29(4):573.

13. Collins L, Prentice J, Vaghadia H. Tracheal intubation of outpatients with and without muscle relaxants. *Can J Anaesth.* 2000;47(5):427–432.

14. Lieutaud T, Billard V, Khalaf H, et al. Muscle relaxation and increasing doses of propofol improve intubating conditions. *Can J Anaesth.* 2003;50(2):121–126.

15. Erhan E, Ugur G, Gunusen I, et al. Propofol—not thiopental or etomidate—with remifentanil provides adequate intubating conditions in the absence of neuromuscular blockade. *Can J Anaesth.* 2003;50(2):108–115.

16. Naguib M, Samarkandi A, Riad W, et al. Optimal dose of succinylcholine revisited. *Anesthesiology.* 2003;99(5):1045–1049.

17. Mort TC. Emergency tracheal intubation: complications associated with repeated laryngoscopic attempts. *Anesth Analg.* 2004;99(2):607–613, table of contents.

18. Baraka AS, Taha SK, Aouad MT, et al. Preoxygenation: comparison of maximal breathing and tidal volume breathing techniques. *Anesthesiology.* 1999;91(3):612–616.

19. Dixon BJ, Dixon JB, Carden JR, et al. Preoxygenation is more effective in the 25 degrees head-up position than in the supine position in severely obese patients: a randomized controlled study. *Anesthesiology.* 2005;102(6):1110–1115; discussion 1115A.

20. Dunford JV, Davis DP, Ochs M, et al. Incidence of transient hypoxia and pulse rate reactivity during paramedic rapid sequence intubation. *Ann Emerg Med.* 2003;42(6):721–728.

21. Mort TC. Preoxygenation in critically ill patients requiring emergency tracheal intubation. *Crit Care Med.* 2005;33(11):2672–2675.

22. Wilson NP. No pressure! Just feel the force. *Anaesthesia.* 2003;58(11):1135–1136.

23. Brimacombe JR, Berry AM. Cricoid pressure. *Can J Anaesth.* 1997;44(4):414–425.

24. Levitan RM, Kinkle WC, Levin WJ, et al. Laryngeal view during laryngoscopy: a randomized trial comparing cricoid pressure, backward-upward-rightward pressure, and bimanual laryngoscopy. *Ann Emerg Med.* 2006;47(6):548–555.

25. Snider DD, Clarke D, Finucane BT. The "BURP" maneuver worsens the glottic view when applied in combination with cricoid pressure. *Can J Anaesth.* 2005;52(1):100–104.

26. Haslam N, Parker L, Duggan JE. Effect of cricoid pressure on the view at laryngoscopy. *Anaesthesia.* 2005;60(1):41–47.

27. Hocking G, Roberts FL, Thew ME. Airway obstruction with cricoid pressure and lateral tilt. *Anaesthesia.* 2001;56(9):825–828.

28. Hartsilver EL, Vanner RG. Airway obstruction with cricoid pressure. *Anaesthesia.* 2000;55(3):208–211.

29. Mac GPJH, Ball DR. The effect of cricoid pressure on the cricoid cartilage and vocal cords: an endoscopic study in anaesthetised patients. *Anaesthesia.* 2000;55(3):263–268.

30. Butler J, Sen A. Best evidence topic report. Cricoid pressure in emergency rapid sequence induction. *Emerg Med J.* 2005;22(11):815–816.

31. Rothrock SG, Pagane J. Pediatric rapid sequence intubation incidence of reflex bradycardia and effects of pretreatment with atropine. *Pediatr Emerg Care.* 2005;21(9):637–638.

32. Fleming B, McCollough M, Henderson HO. Myth: Atropine should be administered before succinylcholine for neonatal and pediatric intubation. *Can J Emerg Med.* 2005;7(2):114–117.

33. McAuliffe G, Bissonnette B, Boutin C. Should the routine use of atropine before succinylcholine in children be reconsidered? *Can J Anaesth.* 1995;42(8):724–729.

34. Fastle RK, Roback MG. Pediatric rapid sequence intubation: incidence of reflex bradycardia and effects of pretreatment with atropine. *Pediatr Emerg Care.* 2004;20(10):651–655.

CHAPTER 10

Postintubation Management

▶ KEY POINTS

- In the well preoxygenated patient, oxygen desaturation can be a relatively late event following an esophageal intubation.
- The heat of the moment leads even experienced clinicians to occasionally advance the tube too far once they've seen it go through the cords.
- Hypotension is common immediately postintubation, particularly if rapid-sequence intubation (RSI) was employed. However, full fluid resuscitation is frequently not possible prior to an emergency intubation.
- Preexisting hypovolemia will make hypotension more likely with institution of positive pressure ventilation.
- Postintubation sedation should begin before the patient "awakens" from the RSI.
- If a patient receiving positive pressure ventilation is at risk for pneumothorax (e.g., rib fractures, significant pulmonary contusion), serious consideration should be given to placement of a chest tube prior to transport.
- Accidental extubation can occur during patient transfer. As difficult as it may have been to intubate the patient in the emergency department (ED), it will be much more difficult in the confined space of an ambulance or helicopter.

▶ THE IMMEDIATE POSTINTUBATION PERIOD

Once the endotracheal tube (ETT) has been placed and its correct tracheal location confirmed, everyone's relief is palpable. However, despite the fact that the most stressful part of the resuscitation is completed, significant airway management concerns remain. This chapter reviews issues which should be addressed following tracheal intubation.

Confirmation of Endotracheal Tube Placement

After intubation, the immediate priority is to confirm the correct tracheal location of the ETT. As discussed in more detail in Chapter 5, objective means of confirmation of tracheal intubation should include visualization of the ETT passing between the cords, *as well as* end-tidal CO_2 ($ETCO_2$) detection or use of an esophageal detector device. The clinician must appreciate the advantages and limitations of these methods. In the well preoxygenated patient of normal body habitus, oxygen desaturation can be a relatively late event following an esophageal intubation.[1]

ETT Depth

After confirming tracheal placement of the ETT, the tube's tip should be confirmed to be above the carina. Endobronchial intubation is all too common in the operating room (OR), intensive care unit (ICU), and emergency department (ED).[2,3] The heat of the moment leads even experienced clinicians to occasionally advance the tube too far once they've seen it go through the cords! As inattention by an assistant can also allow distal migration of the tube during preparations for it being secured to the patient, the intubating clinician should ensure its fixation before moving on to other aspects of patient care. Endobronchial intubation has potentially serious side effects, including hypoxia, barotrauma, and even direct trauma to the lower airway.[3] The ETT should be visually inspected to confirm its depth (20–22 cm at the teeth in adults) using the numeric markings printed on its outer surface. Endobronchial intubation is avoided in the younger pediatric patient by aligning the distal transverse marking on uncuffed ETTs with the vocal cords. Auscultation (which should *not* be relied upon as a sole method of confirming ETT placement) should always be performed following intubation and unequal breath sounds explained. While the most frequent cause of unilaterally diminished air entry will be an endobronchial intubation, pneumothorax or hemothorax must also be considered, particularly in the trauma patient. A chest x-ray will help identify such pathology, in addition to confirming that the ETT tip is above the carina. After any changes in the patient's position, auscultation should again be performed to confirm the ETT's location above the carina.

Securing the ETT

Following confirmation of appropriate ETT positioning, the tube must be secured to the patient. This can be done in a number of different ways:

- Adhesive tape is often used in the elective surgical setting, but is suboptimal for most emergency patients. Perspiration, blood, vomitus, and other body liquids may interfere with tape adherence.

- Cotton twill tape is a cheap and effective method of securing the ETT. Care must be taken to ensure that the encircling tape is not too tight, particularly in the head-injured patient. A small piece of waterproof tape placed over the twill where it contacts the ETT will help prevent accidental tube advancement.

- Several single-use commercial ETT clamp-like devices are effective and safe.[4] These products sometimes also double as a bite block.

Initiation of Positive Pressure Ventilation

Following tracheal intubation, manual ventilation should be initiated to evaluate lung compliance. Indeed, in many cases, a ventilator may not be immediately available. However, while manually ventilating the patient, it is essential to **ensure that the patient is not being inadvertently hyperventilated**. This is particularly important in the asthmatic or chronic obstructive pulmonary disease (COPD) patient, as it can lead to hypotension and/or barotrauma through breath stacking and "auto-PEEP." Accidental hyperventilation is also undesirable in the head-injured patient without appropriate indications. Most self-inflating manual resuscitators contain a volume of 1600 mL. Completely compressing the bag during manual ventilation with both hands will therefore deliver an excessive tidal volume. A more appropriate volume of closer to 700 mL will be delivered if the clinician simply touches the thumb and opposing finger together through the bag with one hand while bagging.

The initial Fio_2 should be set high (100%) and subsequently weaned downward by titration to pulse oximetry or arterial blood-gas monitoring.

Note that shortly after tracheal intubation and initiation of positive pressure ventilation, the ETT may require suctioning. Proper bronchial toilet at this time will help reduce airway resistance during subsequent mechanical ventilation, and in the spontaneously breathing patient, it can decrease the work of breathing.

Blood Pressure Recheck

The patient's **blood pressure** should be checked immediately after intubation and frequently (i.e., every 1–3 minutes) for the first 15 minutes postintubation or until hemodynamics have stabilized. This is a vital component of airway management and is frequently overlooked in emergencies. Hypotension is common following tracheal intubation, particularly if RSI was employed.[5,6] Several mechanisms have been described,[7] including the following:

- Direct negative inotropic and vasodilating effects of RSI induction agents.
- The effect of positive pressure ventilation on impeding venous return to the heart, particularly in the volume depleted patient.
- In the patient with respiratory distress or critical illness, as the work of breathing is lessened by tracheal intubation and institution of mechanical ventilation, the accompanying catecholamine excess is alleviated.
- Pneumothorax is a consideration, particularly in the trauma patient with rib fractures or the asthmatic/COPD patient. In the patient with a pneumothorax, onset of positive pressure can lead to a tension pneumothorax with cardiovascular collapse.

Treatment of Postintubation Hypotension

Careful assessment and replenishment of any volume deficit and appropriate induction drug dosing will help minimize postintubation hypotension. However, full fluid resuscitation is frequently not possible prior to an emergency intubation. In addition, drug dosing always involves some degree of approximation. Even in the hands of a seasoned clinician, patients requiring urgent tracheal intubation frequently experience transient hypotension.

This hypotension is generally limited to 10–15 minutes and most often does not result in any significant sequellae. However, in certain patients, most notably those with head injuries, the effects of even transient hypotension can be devastating.[8] Patients with stenotic vascular lesions such as severe carotid artery disease, coronary artery (particularly severe left main) disease, and aortic valvular stenosis also tend to tolerate hypotension poorly.[7] In addition, the patient in advanced stages of pregnancy, or any patient already significantly hypotensive can ill afford a further drop in blood pressure.

Management of postintubation hypotension is best initiated with fluid administration. A crystalloid bolus of 10–20 mL/kg will help prevent or treat such hypotension. In addition, bolus doses of short-acting vasopressors such as ephedrine 5–10 mg IV or phenylephrine 40–100 µg IV (in the adult patient) may be given. Both agents generally have a duration of action of 5–10 minutes, and they may be repeated two to three times if needed. **They both require diluting before use.** More prolonged hypotension is often the result of the underlying disease process requiring tracheal intubation and should be treated as such.

Postintubation Hypertension

Although hypotension is more common, hypertension (often with tachycardia) may be observed following tracheal intubation. This response is generally self-limited and usually of little consequence. However, treatment is indicated in patients with aneurysmal disease and significant coronary artery disease. If a paralytic agent had been used to facilitate intubation, hypertension and tachycardia could signal patient awareness while paralyzed, indicating the need for more sedative/hypnotic agent.

Postintubation hypertension is best treated initially with additional doses of induction agent (with the exception of ketamine, which could exacerbate the situation). Commonly used benzodiazepines or opioids, either alone or in combination, can also be used (e.g., midazolam 1–2 mg or fentanyl 50–100 μg, in the adult patient). A beta blocker such as metoprolol can be used effectively to control tachycardia. Esmolol, an ultrashort acting beta blocking agent, may be used as an alternative to metoprolol in doses of 0.5–1 mg/kg.

It goes without saying that hemodynamic alterations can only be treated if they are observed. All patients being intubated should ideally have continuous electrocardiographic (ECG), pulse oximetry and noninvasive blood pressure (NIBP) or arterial line monitoring.

▶ POSTINTUBATION SEDATION AND PARALYSIS

Tracheal intubation in emergencies is often challenging and rarely defines a management endpoint. Most drugs used to facilitate intubation are short acting. When needed, postintubation sedation should begin before the patient 'awakens' from the RSI. The choice of sedative will depend on:

- Clinician comfort and familiarity with sedative agents.
- Patient hemodynamics.
- Anticipated natural history of the underlying illness.
- Time and transport issues.

Examples of choices for postintubation sedation include:

- Midazolam: 0.025–0.05 mg/kg IV q 30–60 min (e.g., 2–5 mg in a 70-kg patient).
- Propofol: 25–100 μg/kg/min (10–40 mL/h in a 70-kg patient) by infusion. A 0.2–0.6 mg/kg bolus may be necessary initially.

These sedative agents have no analgesic properties. Concomitant administration of a narcotic is often necessary. Both sedative and analgesic agents need to be titrated to effect with appropriate adjustment of drug doses and/or dosing intervals. Be aware, however, that the combined use of narcotic and benzodiazepine can lead to hypotension. Examples of narcotic analgesics include:

- Fentanyl: 0.5–2.0 μg/kg q 20–30 min *prn* (e.g., 50–100 μg in a 70-kg patient)
- Morphine: 0.025–0.1 mg/kg q 20–30 min *prn* (e.g., 2–5 mg in a 70-kg patient)

In most circumstances, initial control of the patient after tracheal intubation can be obtained without the use of muscle relaxants. However, occasionally ongoing muscle relaxation may be required to help manage ventilation or prevent accidental extubation with transfers or as a result of uncontrolled patient movement. As long as the clinician has clinically and objectively confirmed ETT location, the use of maintenance neuromuscular blockade is rarely a problem. Postintubation paralysis can be obtained and maintained with the following:

- Rocuronium: 0.6 mg/kg load, then 0.1–0.2 mg/kg q 20–30 min *prn* (e.g., 50 mg load followed by 10–20 mg q 30 min *prn* in a 70-kg patient)
- Vecuronium: 0.1 mg/kg load, then 0.01 mg q 30–45 min *prn* (e.g., 7 mg load followed by 1 mg q 30–45 min *prn* in a 70-kg patient)

Note that **muscle relaxants have no sedative or amnestic properties.** If muscle relaxants are deemed necessary after intubation, or if rocuronium was used for intubation (with its duration of 30 minutes or more), it is essential to co-administer some form of sedative/amnestic medication. Unfortunately, in the paralyzed patient there is no way to be assured of an adequate level of sedation. Although blood pressure and heart rate are crude indicators of a patient's level of awareness, they must be used together with knowledge of dosages and expected durations of the administered sedatives. On this latter point, it should be noted that patients who are critically ill and/or in shock have lower sedative/hypnotic requirements. In this population, a small dose should be given initially, with subsequent doses titrated to effect, while monitoring blood pressure.

▶ THE VENTILATED PATIENT

A detailed discussion of mechanical ventilation is beyond the scope of this monograph. In emergency airway management, the priority is always to ensure oxygenation and maintain perfusion: this does not generally necessitate knowledge of complex ventilation strategies. **Respiratory therapists are an important resource for problem-solving ventilator issues**. A brief overview of modes of ventilation follows.

Assist Control (AC)

Following RSI, most patients will require assist control (AC) ventilation. With AC, the ventilator does most of the work. To initiate AC, a basic strategy is to simply set the tidal volume and rate (i.e., the minute ventilation). Typical initial settings would be a tidal volume of 8–10 cc/kg with a rate of 10 breaths per minute. As the muscle relaxant wears off and the patient initiates an additional breath, he will get the prescribed tidal volume at a respiratory rate he dictates. However, with no spontaneous breathing, the minimum prescribed volume and rate are maintained. This mode of ventilation is designed to give the patient a complete rest from the work of breathing. As such, ideally, the patient should not be initiating any spontaneous breaths.

Airway pressures should be monitored in the ventilated patient. In patients with normal lungs, the peak airway pressure should be less than 25 cm H_2O with the foregoing settings. Common causes of increased airway pressures

include stiff lungs (e.g., asthma, COPD, congestive heart failure, lung contusion, aspiration, anaphylaxis, or pulmonary embolus); or extra-parenchymal issues causing decreased compliance (e.g., pneumo- or hemothorax, obesity or distended stomach/abdomen). Problems with the ventilator circuit or ETT, including endobronchial intubation, ETT kinking, or mucus plugging, should be ruled out. Coughing or bucking on the tube ("fighting the vent") may also result in high airway pressures. Coughing may be an indication that the ETT has migrated distally and is touching the carina. Peak pressures exceeding 35 cm H_2O increase the risk of barotrauma.

Adjustment of tidal volume, respiratory rate, and flow rate may be required to reduce peak airway pressure. By varying flow rates, the inspiration:expiration time (I:E ratio) may also be manipulated in an attempt to lower airway pressures. The I:E ratio is usually set at 1:2, although the expiratory time may need to be increased in air trapping situations such as severe asthma. Decreasing the respiratory rate will also allow more time for expiration and may help lower airway pressures. Most patients can tolerate an increase in CO_2 ("permissive hypercapnia") secondary to decreased minute ventilation, so that the limiting factor in adjusting ventilator parameters will be primarily that needed to maintain oxygenation. Bear in mind, however, that there are some situations in which CO_2 management is in fact critical, as in the patient with increased intracranial pressure (ICP) and signs of herniation. Finally, occasionally it will be necessary to ventilate with peak airway pressures over 35 cm H_2O to maintain acceptable gas exchange. In these situations, one should be prepared to urgently manage barotrauma by decompression, if required.

Assisted Ventilation

Assisted ventilation requires the patient to have some respiratory drive. There are many assisted ventilation methodologies. Some forms provide a set amount of positive pressure (e.g., pressure support ventilation) when the ventilator senses an inspiratory effort by the patient, while others ensure a minimum number of breaths per minute. Assisted ventilation is commonly used in the ICU, particularly for weaning patients. It is generally better tolerated, with a lower occurrence of fighting the ventilator. Such modes of ventilation can also be used to gradually increase the patient's work of breathing over time.

Pressure support ventilation (PSV) is one of the simplest forms of assisted ventilation and in the patient with good respiratory drive and normal or near-normal lungs, can be used to simply help the patient overcome the resistance of breathing through an ETT. PSV of 5–10 cm H_2O is usually sufficient for this purpose. As an example, PSV would be a good ventilatory mode for the patient intubated strictly for airway protection, but who is breathing adequately. PSV could also be used for the patient intubated to overcome airway obstruction at or above the level of the glottis. Higher levels of pressure support can be used, in certain circumstances, to help the spontaneously breathing patient maintain adequate tidal volumes. Other types of assist mode ventilation may be appropriate if the clinician in charge is knowledgeable in their use.

Positive End—Expiratory Pressure (PEEP)

Positive end–expiratory pressure (PEEP) is a strategy used to improve oxygenation by alveolar recruitment and increasing functional residual capacity (FRC). It has complex physiologic implications, including the potential to lower blood pressure through its adverse effect on venous return to the heart.[7] This relates to the amount of applied PEEP and is not usually a significant problem under 10 cm H_2O pressure unless the patient is hypovolemic. Higher levels of PEEP (i.e., 10–20 cm H_2O) will cause adverse

hemodynamic effects more consistently and may also increase risk of barotrauma.[9] PEEP may also impair cerebral venous drainage and should be used with caution in the head-injured patient, as it may interfere with cerebral perfusion pressure by both increasing ICP and lowering arterial blood pressure.

PEEP may help reduce atelectasis and, in this respect, most patients benefit from its application at a low level (e.g., 5 cm H_2O). PEEP is particularly useful in patients with pulmonary edema, and the morbidly obese. Relative contraindications to PEEP include marked hypotension or hypovolemia; airway pressures in excess of 35 cm H_2O; uncorrected intrathoracic pathology (pneumo- or hemothorax); and increased ICP.

Titration of PaO$_2$ and PaCO$_2$

The goal of ventilation is to maintain oxygenation and to eliminate CO_2. Oxygenation can be approximated with pulse oximetry but this is only accurate over a small range of values. Due to the shape of the oxygen-hemoglobin dissociation curve, the patient's oxygenation status (PaO_2) can actually deteriorate considerably before being reflected by the oxygen saturation (SaO_2): the patient being ventilated with an FiO_2 of 1.0 may deteriorate from a PaO_2 of 400 mm Hg to a PaO_2 of 100 mm Hg with an unchanged SaO_2 of 100%. In some patients it may be difficult or impossible to obtain an SaO_2 reading at all due to hypothermia, hypotension, or peripheral vascular disease. In this situation, FiO_2 will have to be titrated to PaO_2 readings obtained from arterial blood gases.

CO_2 elimination is the other half of the ventilation equation and is particularly important in the patient with increased ICP. The colorometric devices used to confirm successful ETT placement do not allow ongoing quantitative measurement of CO_2. Some clinical settings may have capnographic monitoring which will measure and continuously display $ETCO_2$. The relationship between $ETCO_2$ and $PaCO_2$ (typically the $ETCO_2$ is 5 mm Hg lower than actual $PaCO_2$) generally remains constant in the paralyzed, mechanically ventilated patient without significant lung pathology, as long as hemodynamic and ventilatory parameters remain unchanged.[10,11] In the manually ventilated patient or with a rapidly changing respiratory rate, this relationship is too volatile to be accurate. In the stable patient, $ETCO_2$ and SaO_2 can be used to monitor gas exchange, although blood gases should be repeated if there are major changes in hemodynamics or ventilation parameters. Although it is becoming more commonly available, continuous $ETCO_2$ monitoring is still not commonly used in EDs.[12]

▶ TRANSPORT ISSUES

Transporting the critically ill, intubated patient poses several challenges. The following airway issues should be considered prior to transport:

A. Proper placement of the ETT in the trachea and above the carina should be reconfirmed.

B. Accidental extubation is obviously a major risk to the patient *en route*. As difficult as it may have been to intubate the patient in the ED, it will be more difficult in the confined space of an ambulance or helicopter. Meticulous attention should be paid to securing the tube, as deaths have followed accidental extubation.

C. Paralysis should be strongly considered to help prevent extubation during transport. A single dose of nondepolarizing muscle relaxant, with accompanying sedation, is appropriate for anticipated transport times of under an hour. Longer transports may require additional doses to ensure adequate relaxation.

D. For short trips, a bolus of sedative/amnestic can be given prior to transport. Longer trips will require additional doses or an infusion.

E. If the patient is receiving positive pressure ventilation and is at risk for pneumothorax

---

▶ TABLE 10–1 THE EFFECT OF ALTITUDE ON PARTIAL PRESSURES OF OXYGEN

It is important to remember that the partial pressure of inspired oxygen decreases with altitude. The cabins of commercial aircraft are usually pressurized to the equivalent of 8000 feet, which translates to a patient alveolar PO_2 of 75 mm Hg and an O_2 saturation of 92%–93%. Clinicians who live at altitudes significantly above sea level and those who must transport critically ill patients by air (or those who think they can relax on a commercial flight!) need to be aware of Boyle's law, which simply states that as ambient pressure decreases, gas volume increases and therefore the density of that gas decreases.

Partial pressures of oxygen in dry air for representative pressure altitudes

Altitude (ft)	Atmospheric Pressure (mm Hg)	Ambient O_2 (mm Hg)
0	760	159
5000	632	133
10000	523	110
12000	483	101
13000	465	97
14000	447	94
15000	429	90
20000	350	73
25000	282	59

(e.g., rib fractures; significant pulmonary contusion), serious consideration should be given to placement of a chest tube prior to transport.

F. During patient transport, the administered FiO_2 should be 100%. This high FiO_2 will provide an extra margin of safety in case of an accidental extubation, and if the transport is by air, it will help compensate for the decrease in ambient partial pressure of oxygen with altitude (Table 10-1).

G. Water should be considered for ETT cuff inflation for an air transport if cabin pressure will be an issue, as air-filled cuffs can expand at altitude.

► SUMMARY

Tracheal intubation alone does not define an endpoint in airway management. Although a priority, airway management is just one component in the resuscitation of the acutely ill patient. The managing clinician should remain vigilant throughout the process of care and pay close attention to the postintubation period. Hypotension is common and often requires intervention. Sedation is almost always indicated and paralysis should be used when needed to optimize gas exchange, or protect the patient from accidental extubation.

REFERENCES

1. Benumof JL, Dagg R, Benumof R. Critical hemoglobin desaturation will occur before return to an unparalyzed state following 1 mg/kg intravenous succinylcholine. *Anesthesiology.* 1997;87(4):979–982.

2. Szekely SM, Webb RK, Williamson JA, et al. The Australian Incident Monitoring Study. Problems related to the endotracheal tube: an analysis of 2000 incident reports. *Anaesth Intensive Care.* 1993;21(5):611–616.

3. McCoy EP, Russell WJ, Webb RK. Accidental bronchial intubation. An analysis of AIMS incident reports from 1988 to 1994 inclusive. *Anaesthesia.* 1997;52(1):24–31.

4. Lovett PB, Flaxman A, Sturmann KM, et al. The insecure airway: a comparison of knots and commercial devices for securing endotracheal tubes. *BMC Emerg Med.* 2006;6:7.

5. Franklin C, Samuel J, Hu TC. Life-threatening hypotension associated with emergency intubation and the initiation of mechanical ventilation. *Am J Emerg Med.* 1994;12(4):425–428.

6. Shafi S, Gentilello L. Pre-hospital endotracheal intubation and positive pressure ventilation is associated with hypotension and decreased survival in hypovolemic trauma patients: an analysis of the National Trauma Data Bank. *J Trauma.* 2005;59(5):1140–1145; discussion 1145–1147.

7. Horak J, Weiss S. Emergent management of the airway. New pharmacology and the control of comorbidities in cardiac disease, ischemia, and valvular heart disease. *Crit Care Clin.* 2000;16(3): 411–427.

8. Brain Trauma Foundation; American Association of Neurological Surgeons; Joint Section on Neurotrauma and Critical Care. Resuscitation of blood pressure and oxygenation. *J Neurotrauma.* 2000;17(6–7):471–478.

9. Carroll GC, Tuman KJ, Braverman B, et al. Minimal positive end-expiratory pressure (PEEP) may be "best PEEP". *Chest.* 1988;93(5):1020–1025.

10. Mackersie RC, Karagianes TG. Use of end-tidal carbon dioxide tension for monitoring induced hypocapnia in head-injured patients. *Crit Care Med.* 1990;18(7):764–765.

11. Kerr ME, Zempsky J, Sereika S, et al. Relationship between arterial carbon dioxide and end-tidal carbon dioxide in mechanically ventilated adults with severe head trauma. *Crit Care Med.* 1996;24(5): 785–790.

12. Deiorio NM. Continuous end-tidal carbon dioxide monitoring for confirmation of endotracheal tube placement is neither widely available nor consistently applied by emergency physicians. *Emerg Med J.* 2005;22(7):490–493.

CHAPTER 11

Approach to Tracheal Intubation

▶ KEY POINTS

- The risk for the inexperienced clinician of proceeding with intubation must be balanced against the benefit of awaiting the arrival of more experienced help, especially if difficulty is anticipated.
- Difficult laryngoscopy in one clinician's hands may be less difficult in another's.
- Whatever the makeup of the assembled team, there needs to be a common understanding of the language of airway management.
- Recognizing the potential for difficult intubation should trigger appropriate early calls for help, heightened vigilance, and improved preparedness.
- The uncooperative patient will often need a rapid-sequence intubation (RSI), even in face of predictors of difficult laryngoscopy.
- Relatively large doses of a sedative-hypnotic agent alone do not create intubating conditions as favorable as those using RSI with neuromuscular blockade.
- Proceeding with RSI in the uncooperative patient with predictors of both difficult intubation and difficult bag-mask ventilation (BMV) is risky. Extra preparations are needed.
- Obtaining a view of the epiglottis as part of an "awake look" laryngoscopy may

impart useful information, but does not guarantee a subsequent view of the laryngeal inlet in the anesthetized patient.

▶ INTRODUCTION

The indications for endotracheal intubation have been reviewed in Chap. 2. For the patient requiring intubation in an emergency, assuming an attending clinician with requisite knowledge and skills, the next step is to decide how best to proceed with the intubation. This decision will be predicated upon the following factors:

A. **The airway evaluation.** Evaluating the patient for predictors of difficulty with laryngoscopic intubation, bag-mask ventilation and rescue oxygenation (referring to use of an extraglottic device [EGD] or cricothyrotomy) is of primary importance in deciding how to proceed.

B. **Presenting system pathophysiology.** Anticipated patient response to drugs used for rapid-sequence intubation (RSI) may also impact the decision.

C. **Patient cooperation.** The overtly uncooperative patient will usually require an RSI, whereas a more cooperative patient may be able to tolerate an awake intubation, if difficulty is predicted.

▶ THE AIRWAY EVALUATION

General Comments

Most patients requiring airway management in emergencies will need to be intubated. Most intubations in emergencies are facilitated by direct laryngoscopy, so a good starting point for the airway evaluation is to seek predictors of **difficult direct laryngoscopy**. This has been discussed in more detail in Chap. 5, but as a review, these predictors appear in Table 11–1. The airway evaluation should not stop there, however. **Bag-mask ventilation** (BMV) may be needed prior to, or between intubation attempts, so a formal assessment of predictors of difficulty with BMV should also be undertaken. These predictors appear in Table 11–2 and have been discussed in more detail in Chap. 4. Finally, if a failed airway is encountered at any point, **rescue oxygenation** may need to be undertaken with placement of an EGD or cricothyrotomy, so the patient should also be evaluated for the predicted success of these maneuvers. Predictors

▶ **TABLE 11–2** PREDICTING DIFFICULT BAG-MASK VENTILATION

Consider whether there may be difficulty with attaining a **mask seal** on the patient's face, or, if a mask seal is attained, if there will be difficulty controlling **collapsing soft tissues** in the naso-, oro-, or laryngopharynx, or, if a patent upper airway has been obtained, whether **obstructing pathology** at or below the cords, or **poor compliance** of the lungs/chest wall will cause difficulty. Alternatively, the mnemonic "BOOTS" can be used:
B—Beard and other mask seal issues
O—Obesity
O—Older (age >55 years)
T—Toothless
S—Sounds: Snoring; Stridor (obstructing airway pathology); Stiff lungs (wheezing; rales)

of difficulty with rescue oxygenation are reviewed in Table 11–3 and Chap. 7.

Note that predicted difficult intubation by **direct laryngoscopy** (DL) may not equate to predicted difficult intubation using a different device. **For those familiar with their use,** alternative intubation devices such as the LMA-Fastrach, lightwand, or rigid fiberoptic- or video-based instruments may enable successful intubation of the patient with traditional predictors of difficult direct laryngoscopy. While most emergency intubations are in fact facilitated by direct laryngoscopy, proceeding with RSI in the patient with predicted difficulty will be less intimidating if alternatives to DL are predicted to succeed, and the clinician is skilled in their use.

The Dimensions of Difficulty Triangle

The concept of evaluating the patient in all three "dimensions[1] of difficulty" in airway management can be represented by the three apices of a triangle[2] (Fig. 11–1). This visually illustrates the concept that **if difficulty is anticipated in**

▶ **TABLE 11–1** PREDICTING DIFFICULT DIRECT LARYNGOSCOPY

Consider whether there will be a problem **inserting the laryngoscope blade** into the patient's mouth, or once inserted, if difficulty will be encountered **displacing the tongue** out of the line-of-sight, or if the tongue has been controlled, whether the larynx will be in an **abnormal location,** or **unrecognizable**.
Alternatively, the mnemonic "MMAP" can be used:
M—Mallampati classification
M—Measurements: minimum of **3** finger-breadths of mouth opening; **3** of thyromental span, and **1 cm** of jaw protrusion
A—Atlantooccipital (i.e., head and upper neck) extension
P—Obstructing airway pathology

▶ **TABLE 11-3** PREDICTING DIFFICULT RESCUE OXYGENATION

Difficult Extraglottic Device Use	Difficult Cricothyrotomy
Consider whether there may be difficulty **inserting** the device through the patient's mouth, or having inserted it, whether there will be a problem **seating** the device in front of the laryngeal inlet, or even if well seated, whether obstructing pathology at the cords, or **poor compliance** of the lungs or chest wall will preclude effective ventilation due to "pop-off" pressure being exceeded. Alternatively, the mnemonic "MOODS" can be used: **MO**—Mouth opening limited **O**—Obstructing pathology at or below the cords **D**—Displacement, Distortion or Disruption of the upper or lower airway **S**—Stiff lungs or chest wall	Consider whether there will be difficulty with **identification** of the cricothyroid membrane, or having identified its location, whether there will be **trouble accessing the trachea** through it. The mnemonic "DART" can also be used: **D**—Distortion of the overlying anatomy due to blunt trauma, hematoma or infection **A**—Access issues due to obesity, or inability to extend head and neck **R**—History of neck radiation **T**—Tumor

any one apex, before proceeding with an intubation technique that ablates the patient's spontaneous respirations, success must be predicted with oxygenation in at least one, and preferably both other apices.

It should be emphasized that predicted difficulty with airway management lies on a spectrum from "moderately difficult" to "very difficult or impossible." Moderate difficulty should be overcome by fairly routine techniques. For example, although difficult laryngoscopy may

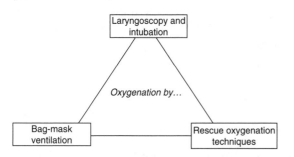

Figure 11-1. The three "dimensions of difficulty" of airway management. An adaptation of Sakles' triangle.[2]

be predicted in a C-spine immobilized patient, successful intubation should be possible with basic maneuvers such as external laryngeal manipulation (ELM) and use of the bougie. In this same patient, BMV and rescue oxygenation with an EGD should be nonproblematic. In contrast, the patient with obstructing upper airway pathology presents a very difficult situation. Here, all three points on the "dimensions of difficulty" triangle (BMV, laryngoscopy and intubation, and rescue oxygenation with an EGD) may fail if RSI is undertaken. This suggests the need to consider an awake intubation.

A NOTE ON THE LIMITATIONS TO PREDICTIONS When encountered, many difficult airways are reported as unanticipated. With the prediction of an "easy ride" never being guaranteed, the clinician should be prepared for difficulty during *every* emergency intubation. Indeed, the value of even *trying* to predict difficulty in emergencies has been questioned, on this basis.[3–7] However, the airway assessment is still important and should be done, for two reasons:

- Information yielded from the airway assessment will help point to the safest method for proceeding with the intubation.
- Doing an active and deliberate airway assessment becomes a "cognitive forcing strategy."[8] Even if no difficulty is predicted as a result of the assessment, it will help heighten vigilance and improve preparedness. The literature supports the use of such cognitive forcing strategies as a means of reducing medical error in emergency situations.[8]

▶ PRESENTING SYSTEM PHYSIOLOGY

The airway assessment, as outlined above, attempts to identify anatomic obstacles to physically securing the airway. However, system physiology issues should also be considered. Specifically, attention should be directed to two areas:

- Hemodynamic status
- System at risk

Hemodynamic Status

One of the most common adverse responses to intubation of the acutely ill patient is hypotension. This is most commonly due to direct effects of induction or sedative drugs, in addition to the relief of high sympathetic tone and adverse effects of positive pressure ventilation on venous return. The clinician must consider and prepare for these predictable effects prior to proceeding. In most cases, this translates to a preintubation fluid bolus and judicious drug dosing. However, in certain situations (e.g., the profoundly hypotensive or hypovolemic patient) it *may* be appropriate to consider avoiding systemic drugs altogether in favor of proceeding with an "awake" (i.e., non-RSI) intubation.

System at Risk

Occasionally, the presenting patient pathophysiology impacts the decision-making process. For example, the patient presenting with suspected increased intracranial pressure (ICP) may best be intubated by RSI, as induction medications may help attenuate adverse effects of laryngoscopy and intubation on ICP. A second example is the patient in *status asthmaticus,* in whom RSI using higher dose ketamine as an induction agent may aid with bronchodilation.

▶ PATIENT COOPERATION

Especially with predictors of a difficult airway, an assessment of the patient's ability to cooperate should be made, as an awake intubation generally requires an element of cooperation. Commonly, because of toxicologic, pathophysiologic (including hypoxia) or neuroanatomic derangement, patients requiring emergency intubation are not able to cooperate. However, patient cooperation should be perceived as a continuum.

As depicted in Fig. 11–2, at one end of the spectrum is the actively uncooperative patient, and at the other, the awake and cooperative patient.

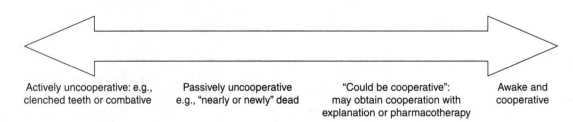

Actively uncooperative: e.g., clenched teeth or combative

Passively uncooperative e.g., "nearly or newly" dead

"Could be cooperative": may obtain cooperation with explanation or pharmacotherapy

Awake and cooperative

Figure 11–2. The continuum of patient cooperation.

A. The **actively uncooperative** patient may be physically combative, or may have **clenched teeth** secondary to a decreased level of consciousness (LOC). For the physically combative patient, an awake approach will not be feasible without varying degrees of physical restraint, which is rarely indicated. The patient deemed actively uncooperative on the sole basis of clenched teeth may tolerate an attempt at blind nasal intubation. However, such a patient will usually require an RSI, even with predictors of difficult laryngoscopy. In this situation, however, predicted ease of BMV and/or rescue oxygenation is imperative. Balancing the risk of a failed airway (i.e., can't intubate, or can't intubate, can't oxygenate) against the benefit of rapidly securing the airway is at the crux of this difficult decision.

B. The **passively uncooperative** patient will exhibit little or no resistance to an attempted airway maneuver, but neither is cooperation offered. Two categories exist: (a) the arrested, or nearly dead patient requiring no pharmacologic adjuncts to facilitate intubation, and (b) the intrinsically sedated patient. An example of the latter category would be a patient hypercarbic due to respiratory failure. Topical airway anesthesia, combined with the patient's drowsiness may allow a non-RSI approach, even if not truly "awake" or cooperative.

C. The **"could be cooperative"** patient may in fact cooperate with an awake intubation when an explanation is presented (bluntly or with sympathy). Alternatively, the patient may be controllable with medications such as ketamine or haloperidol:

- Ketamine can be used in titrated doses of 0.25–0.5 mg/kg IV. Ketamine's advantage lies in its tendency to not interfere with maintenance of spontaneous ventilation. Detractors point to increased secretions and propensity to laryngospasm. However, the risk of laryngospasm is low (<1%), and it occurs predominantly in young children.[9]

- Haloperidol, titrated to effect, can be used in divided doses of 2.5–5 mg IV.
- Other agents may prove useful in this context in the future, including the newer alpha-2 receptor agonist dexmedetomidine.

These agents are discussed further in Chap. 13. Failure to respond to such medications would place the patient in the more actively uncooperative category.

D. The **awake and cooperative** patient. Many patients with difficult airways present in this state, including those with upper airway pathology.

All except the "actively uncooperative" patient may allow the option of awake (i.e., non-RSI) intubation. It goes without saying that waiting for an actively uncooperative patient to medically deteriorate to the point of being moribund and only passively uncooperative is not good practice!

▶ PROCEEDING WITH INTUBATION: A REVIEW OF THE CHOICES

Most emergency intubations are performed awake, or using RSI. Advantages and disadvantages of each route, together with a more detailed description of the techniques have been presented in Chaps. 8 and 9. However, to redefine the terms for consideration in this chapter, the following choices are available:

A. **Awake intubation.** Although the term is poor, "awake" describes a technique in which the mainstays of patient preparation for intubation include topical airway anesthesia and light (if any) sedation. Although rarely used in contemporary practice, blind nasal intubation would be included in this category.

B. **Rapid-sequence intubation (RSI).** Following appropriate preparation, RSI involves the administration of predetermined doses of an induction agent and muscle relaxant in rapid succession, application of cricoid pressure and quick placement of an endotracheal tube.

C. **Primary surgical airway.** Primary cricothyrotomy or tracheotomy may occasionally be necessary in certain airway emergencies (e.g., severe facial trauma, or advanced airway infections).

As previously mentioned, a relatively large dose of a sedative agent by itself does not create intubating conditions as favorable as those obtained with RSI using neuromuscular blockade,[10–13] nor is this approach safer than RSI. In fact, deep sedation used alone significantly decreases protective reflexes and can be detrimental to the hemodynamic status of the patient, without necessarily improving ease of intubation. Most contemporary airway management education programs are discouraging the sole use of deep sedation to facilitate intubation.

▶ PROCEEDING WITH INTUBATION: THE APPROACH TO TRACHEAL INTUBATION ALGORITHM

Choosing how to proceed is predicated upon identifying predictors of difficulty during patient assessment. Identified difficulty represents the first branch point in the "Approach to Tracheal Intubation" algorithm (Fig. 11–3), to which the reader is invited to refer during the ensuing discussion. Note that this algorithm is presented as a guide (not doctrine), and is meant to facilitate safe decision-making *before* the procedure has begun.

No Difficulty Predicted

Cooperative Patient

If no difficulty is predicted in any facet of airway management, most clinicians would choose to proceed with an RSI for emergency intubations. However, this assumes familiarity with the technique, availability of equipment and drugs, and trained assistants. For the clinician less comfortable with RSI, an assessment of **patient cooperation** should be made. As long as the patient is not actively uncooperative, this may add the option of an awake intubation (Fig. 11–3, **track 1**).

Uncooperative Patient

For the actively uncooperative patient with no predictors of difficulty, RSI is indicated for rapid control of the patient and optimal intubating conditions (Fig. 11–3, **track 2**).

Difficulty Predicted

Preamble

Algorithms developed for the elective surgical setting often suggest simply proceeding with awake intubation if difficulty is predicted. However, for the emergency, out-of-operating room (OR) environment, these algorithms often fail to account for situation acuity, or whether the patient is able to cooperate with an awake intubation attempt. **Patient cooperation** is the next algorithm branch point requiring consideration for the patient with predictors of difficulty.

Difficulty Predicted: Cooperative Patient

A. **The decision.** Especially in the patient with an airway exam suggesting possible difficulty with BMV as well as laryngoscopic intubation, an awake approach should be considered, if patient cooperation permits (Fig. 11–3, **track 3**). This is the "gold standard" in such patients: the adage "no bridges have been burned" applies, in that these patients continue to breathe for themselves, and can maintain and protect their own airways. This is definitely the preferred route with obstructing airway pathology, as proceeding with RSI runs the risk of creating a "can't intubate, can't oxygenate" situation. It may also include the patient with *no*

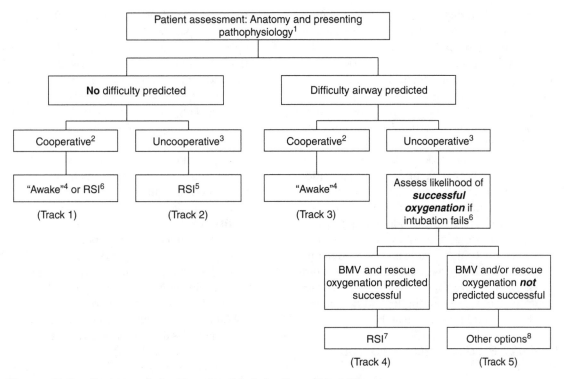

Figure 11–3. Approach to Tracheal Intubation Algorithm.

(1) Patient assessment includes an evaluation of anticipated difficulty with (a) laryngoscopy and intubation; (b) bag-mask ventilation; and (c) rescue oxygenation with an extraglottic device (EGD) or cricothyrotomy. The patient's physiologic status should also be considered, including hemodynamic status and the primary underlying presenting condition (heart, head, lungs etc.)

(2) The 'cooperative' patient in this context may be fully awake and cooperative; 'could be' cooperative with pharmacologic agents or a reassuring explanation; or passively uncooperative, whereby no significant resistance will be offered to a non-RSI technique.

(3) For the uncooperative patient with an anticipated difficult airway, help should be sought early. Can the patient be 'bridge' oxygenated until help comes? The actively uncooperative patient presents very different considerations than the passively uncooperative patient.

(4) An 'awake' intubation refers merely to an intubation facilitated by topical airway anesthesia with, or without small amounts of sedative agent, as distinct from rapid-sequence intubation. Thus, the term 'awake' in this context may also refer to the intubation of a deeply obtunded patient, as long as a formal RSI, facilitated by muscle relaxants, is not being undertaken.

(5) Both RSI and awake techniques require similar manual skills. RSI additionally requires a sound knowledge of airway pharmacology and a clear plan for dealing with the difficult airway. Any RSI undertaken in the face of predicted difficulty should be done with adequate preparation including availability and briefing of extra helpers, and alternative intubation techniques and rescue oxygenation devices, and the skill to use them.

(6) This should include an assessment of whether BMV and ideally *both* of a rescue EGD and cricothyrotomy are predicted to succeed in achieving oxygenation.

(7) This situation is far from ideal and is only done if the benefit of expeditious intubation outweighs the risk of a failed airway with attendant need for cricothyrotomy. RSI undertaken in the face of predicted difficulty should ideally be undertaken when additional help and equipment are available, with the expectation to proceed to EGD placement or cricothyrotomy. In general, RSI should only be undertaken if moderate difficulty with DL is expected, and is **not** a recommended first-line approach when upper airway pathology is suspected.

(8) Other options: see discussion in text.

anatomic predictors of difficult intubation, but simply difficult physiology (e.g., significant hypotension), in whom avoiding destabilizing induction agents may be desirable.

B. **Preparation and Execution.** For the awake intubation, communication should be established with the patient, topical airway anesthesia should be administered, and the patient positioned as comfortably as possible. In general, the procedure should employ an alternative (e.g., fiberoptic) intubation approach, especially if significant difficulty is anticipated with direct laryngoscopy.[14] Conversely, the patient undergoing an awake intubation for any other aspect of predicted difficulty (e.g. significant hemodynamic instability) may well be successfully intubated with direct laryngoscopy. The chosen approach will obviously depend on clinician skill and equipment availability.

Difficulty Predicted: Uncooperative Patient

The question in this situation is "...faced with a patient in whom I have predicted difficulty, but who is unable to cooperate with an awake intubation, can I safely proceed with RSI?" The patient with predictors of difficult airway management who is actively uncooperative presents a therapeutic conundrum. Use of RSI is obviously desirable in such a patient to gain control of the situation. However, before proceeding with RSI and rendering a breathing patient apneic, one must be reasonably certain that if intubation fails, one can take over oxygenation with BMV, or if BMV fails, that rescue oxygen will succeed with EGD placement or cricothyrotomy. Thus, based on the bedside airway evaluation, a judgment of predicted success of all these maneuvers is crucial.

OXYGENATION PREDICTED TO SUCCEED
IF INTUBATION FAILS

A. **The Decision.** In the uncooperative patient in whom difficult laryngoscopy is anticipated, but in whom BMV and rescue oxygenation

(with EGD and/or cricothyrotomy) are predicted to succeed, RSI may be the most appropriate option (Fig. 11–3, **track 4**). Note that the margin of safety of this route includes a favorable assessment of two of the three apices of the dimensions of difficulty triangle (Fig. 11–1) predicting successful oxygenation (i.e., BMV and rescue oxygenation). Extra preparations will have to be undertaken (see below). Two provisos apply to using RSI in this situation:

- Proceeding with RSI is only appropriate for the patient with predicted **moderately difficult** laryngoscopy. Practically speaking, this refers to the patient in whom there is still a reasonably good chance that 'best look' laryngoscopic intubation (Table 12–2), including ELM, head lift, adjunctive use of a bougie or fiberoptic stylet, or a blade change will succeed. An additional margin of safety is provided by the clinician skilled in the use of an alternative intubation device, such as the LMA Fastrach, lightwand, or fiberoptic- or video-based instrument.

- Secondly, it is critical to determine whether any signs or symptoms of **obstructing airway pathology** are present. In addition to dyspnea, signs of pathological upper airway obstruction often include stridor and/ or altered voice. Stridor in particular indicates an airway that is already critically narrowed. The concern in these patients is that by administering sedative or induction agents, a tenuous airway being maintained by patient effort will be lost: with obstructing pathology, landmarks can be obscured at laryngoscopy, and BMV can be impossible. **Thus, the patient population with obstructing airway pathology should generally not undergo RSI.**

B. **Preparation and Execution.** Despite the prediction of easy BMV, laryngoscopy has been assessed as being at least moderately difficult. If RSI is undertaken, the following preparations should occur:

- Extra help should be summoned.
- A variety of blades should be available, and a styleted, small endotracheal tube (ETT) prepared. The patient should be well preoxygenated. "Best Look" laryngoscopy should be employed, including optimal allowable positioning and ELM.
- A bougie or fiberoptic stylet should be available for immediate use.
- An alternative intubation device should be prepared for use in case direct laryngoscopy fails after one or two attempts.
- An EGD should be prepared for failed intubation or failed oxygenation situations (Chapter 12). Cricothyrotomy equipment should be available.
- All of the above-mentioned equipment should be appropriately sized for the patient, out of the package, lubricated, and physically arranged on a nearby work surface **in the order** of anticipated usage.
- Assistants should be briefed about the order of transition from direct laryngoscopy to alternative technique to rescue oxygenation device, both to clarify the plan in the clinician's mind and to inform the team.

OXYGENATION NOT PREDICTED TO EASILY SUCCEED IF INTUBATION FAILS

A. **The Decision.** The final situation to address is the difficult airway patient, who is uncooperative, and in whom oxygenation may be difficult if intubation fails (Fig. 11–3, **track 5**). This will be an unusual situation, and places the clinician "between a rock and a hard place," with only an array of suboptimal choices! Recognizing that the risk-benefit balance has now completely shifted, one of the following options may be appropriate:
- **Deferring intubation.** Not all indications for emergency intubation are of equal acuity. If significant difficulty is predicted in a patient with a lower priority indication for intubation (i.e., airway protection, or predicted clinical deterioration),

the risk of performing the intubation may outweigh its benefit. As such, the best course of action may be to await the arrival of additional expertise or equipment.
- **Calling for additional expertise.** Successful intubation is aided not only by favorable patient anatomy, but also the clinician's skill and experience: laryngoscopy which seems difficult in one person's hands may be less so in another's. The help of a colleague who has more expertise should be sought. If an uncooperative patient is not in *immediate* danger, then assisted positive pressure oxygenation (e.g., with BMV, noninvasive positive pressure ventilation or EGD such as the LMA or Combitube) may allow time for help to arrive. Conversely, if the situation allows, the patient may be transferred unintubated to a location where additional expertise or equipment is available. This may include transfer to an OR for intubation facilitated by **inhalational induction of anesthesia,** while maintaining spontaneous ventilation.
- **Seeking additional information.** It may be possible to obtain more objective information about ease of BMV or laryngoscopy. Especially in the "passively uncooperative" patient or with the assistance of small doses of a sedative agent, it may be possible to place a mask and gently assist the patient's spontaneous respirations with a manual resuscitator to get a feeling for ease of BMV. Secondly, if feasible, it may be possible to perform an "awake look" direct laryngoscopy, seeking additional information on the following:
  o Ease of blade insertion and tongue control (can the entire epiglottis, and even the posterior cartilages be easily seen or is only the tip of the epiglottis visible?).
  o Mobility of the epiglottis (is it easily elevated, or applied to the posterior pharyngeal wall?).

○ Location and state of the laryngeal inlet (is it in the expected midline location, or is it displaced? Is there evidence of edema of laryngeal inlet structures?). This last can also be assessed with nasopharyngoscopy.

The "awake look" should be interpreted with caution: no evidence backs the simplistic contention that "if the epiglottis can be seen, RSI can be performed, as the view should be better with a muscle relaxant." Finally, if by chance or skill, the laryngeal inlet happens to be visualized during an awake look, a small tube could potentially quickly be placed.

- **Pharmacologic restraint.** Sedative agents (e.g. ketamine) can be used in an attempt to render the patient cooperative enough to proceed with an awake intubation. However, this approach is not without risk, and in the patient uncooperative due to an underlying organic etiology, these agents may not reliably result in a sufficiently cooperative state to allow formal awake intubation or awake look laryngoscopy. Furthermore, sedating a patient with obstructing airway pathology may result in the loss of a marginally patent airway.

- **Blind nasal intubation.** Described and discussed in more detail in Chap. 8, blind nasal intubations, anecdotally, have bailed out many grateful clinicians over the years, faced with what initially appeared to be an impossible situation! Blind techniques, including blind nasal intubation, should generally not be attempted in the setting of inflammation, infection, or trauma at the level of the cords or epiglottis. It may, however, enable intubation in a patient whose lack of cooperation is limited to clenched teeth.

- **Proceeding with RSI with a reduced margin of safety.** On occasion, in the patient who is obstructing, actively uncooperative, and about to die, the only option may be to "give it your best shot." This *may* involve proceeding with RSI, with a "double set-up" (see B. Preparation and Execution, below), fully prepared and intending to proceed directly to cricothyrotomy if intubation is unsuccessful and failed oxygenation ensues. In this situation, one may be proceeding with RSI with only the cricothyrotomy option of the "rescue oxygenation" apex (Fig. 11–1) available. To do this, the clinician must be confident that the benefit of rapidly securing the airway by intubation outweighs the risk of encountering a failed airway.

- **Primary surgical airway**, be it cricothyrotomy or tracheostomy. An awake surgical airway (see next section), with continued spontaneous respirations, is theoretically an option. Generally, this will be difficult without an element of patient cooperation.

B. **Preparation and Execution.** Proceeding with RSI in the uncooperative patient with predictors of both difficult intubation and difficult BMV is risky. This risk is compounded if rescue oxygenation is also predicted to be difficult. Preparations should occur as described in the previous section. However, in addition, this is the situation where a **double set-up** may be appropriate, whereby the cricothyroid membrane has already been identified, marked, prepped, and an individual with appropriate equipment is ready to rapidly proceed to cricothyrotomy.

▶ PRIMARY SURGICAL AIRWAY

On rare occasions, intubation from above the cords will be impossible. Examples include patients with advanced airway infections, laryngeal tumors, thermal injury, or severe facial trauma. Awake primary cricothyrotomy or tracheostomy may be the best choice when a skilled set of hands is available at the bedside.

▶ **SUMMARY**

Patient assessment is crucial for deciding the best approach to the emergency intubation. If no difficulty is predicted, generally, RSI is the preferred technique. As presented in the Approach to Tracheal Intubation algorithm, for predicted difficulty with intubation, patient cooperation must be considered, as well as the likelihood of successful oxygenation using BMV or rescue techniques. The cooperative patient with predictors of difficult intubation may tolerate an awake intubation. The uncooperative patient with predictors of moderate difficulty with intubation, but in whom BMV and/or rescue oxygenation techniques (EGD or cricothyrotomy) are predicted to be successful, may require RSI. The unusual case where significant difficulty is predicted in all facets of airway management requires extra help and preparation. Although predictions are often fraught with error, an explicit cognitive attempt to identify such barriers may help the clinician to "expect the unexpected" during emergency airway management.

REFERENCES

1. Murphy M, Hung O, Launcelott G, et al. Predicting the difficult laryngoscopic intubation: are we on the right track? *Can J Anaesth*. 2005;52(3):231–235.
2. Walls RM, Murphy M. Identification of the difficult and failed airway. In: Walls RM, ed. *Manual of Emergency Airway Management*. 2nd ed. Philadelphia: Lippincott Willimas and Wilkins; 2004;70–81.
3. Merah NA, Wong DT, Ffoulkes-Crabbe DJ, et al. Modified Mallampati test, thyromental distance and inter-incisor gap are the best predictors of difficult laryngoscopy in West Africans. *Can J Anaesth*. 2005;52(3):291–296.
4. Randell T. Prediction of difficult intubation. *Acta Anaesthesiol Scand*. 1996;40(8 Pt 2): 1016–1023.
5. Rose DK, Cohen MM. The airway: problems and predictions in 18,500 patients. *Can J Anaesth*. 1994;41(5 Pt 1):372–383.
6. Shiga T, Wajima Z, Inoue T, et al. Predicting difficult intubation in apparently normal patients: a meta-analysis of bedside screening test performance. *Anesthesiology*. 2005;103(2):429–437.
7. Levitan RM, Everett WW, Ochroch EA. Limitations of difficult airway prediction in patients intubated in the emergency department. *Ann Emerg Med*. 2004;44(4):307–313.
8. Croskerry P. Cognitive forcing strategies in clinical decisionmaking. *Ann Emerg Med*. 2003;41(1): 110–120.
9. Green SM, Krauss B. Clinical practice guideline for emergency department ketamine dissociative sedation in children. *Ann Emerg Med*. 2004;44(5): 460–471.
10. Lieutaud T, Billard V, Khalaf H, et al. Muscle relaxation and increasing doses of propofol improve intubating conditions. *Can J Anaesth*. 2003;50(2): 121–126.
11. McNeil IA, Culbert B, Russell I. Comparison of intubating conditions following propofol and succinylcholine with propofol and remifentanil 2 micrograms kg-1 or 4 micrograms kg-1. *Br J Anaesth*. 2000;85(4):623–625.
12. McKeating K, Bali IM, Dundee JW. The effects of thiopentone and propofol on upper airway integrity. *Anaesthesia*. 1988;43(8):638–640.
13. Donati F. Tracheal intubation: unconsciousness, analgesia and muscle relaxation. *Can J Anaesth*. Feb 2003;50(2):99–103.
14. Kovacs G, Law JA, Petrie D. Awake fiberoptic intubation using an optical stylet in an anticipated difficult airway. *Ann Emerg Med*. 2007;49(1):81–83.

CHAPTER 12

Response to an Encountered Difficult Airway

▶ **KEY POINTS**

- The **failed airway** is defined in one of two ways: (a) **failed intubation** (*can't intubate, CAN oxygenate*) is defined simply by a failure to intubate after three attempts, or (b) **failed oxygenation** (*can't intubate, CANNOT oxygenate*), which is the failure to intubate in conjunction with a failure to oxygenate with bag-mask ventilation (BMV).

- Multiple intubation attempts (defined as three or more) have been associated with significant complications and poor patient outcomes.

- All too often in difficult or failed airway scenarios, fixation occurs on intubation attempts, at the expense of attention to maintaining oxygenation with bag-mask ventilation.

- *Before* the first attempt at laryngoscopy, a plan for encountered difficulty should have been mentally rehearsed, all equipment assembled, and assistants briefed.

- In response to a Grade 3 or 4 view at laryngoscopy, all components of "best look" laryngoscopy should be undertaken.

- A blade change need not be an automatic response to a difficult laryngoscopy situation, and should be undertaken only with a specific goal in mind.

- Which alternative intubation, "go to" device is chosen will depend on availability and clinician preference, skill, and experience.

- Some rescue oxygenation devices may provide more protection against aspiration of gastric contents than others, but none are as effective in this regard as a cuffed endotracheal tube, which is still the desired end point.

- In a failed oxygenation situation, the default maneuver is cricothyrotomy. Any attempt at rescue oxygenation with extraglottic device (EGD) placement must be brief, and must not delay the onset of cricothyrotomy.

▶ **INTRODUCTION TO THE ENCOUNTERED DIFFICULT AIRWAY**

The identification of, and approach to the patient with the anticipated difficult airway has been presented in Chap. 11. This chapter will review how to respond to the difficult airway **once encountered** at laryngoscopy or with attempted bag-mask ventilation (BMV). Airway management literature often refers to the situation where difficult laryngoscopy has been encountered as "unanticipated." However, especially for the emergency intubation of an actively uncooperative patient, rapid-sequence intubation (RSI) may need to be undertaken even with predictors of difficulty. Ensuing difficult laryngoscopy is thus *not* unanticipated, but rather, may be addressed by good preparation and a plan for an orderly approach to the situation.

▶ DEFINITIONS

The Difficult Airway

Clear definitions of both the difficult and failed airway are needed to help the clinician identify when different strategies must be employed. The American Society of Anesthesiologists (ASA) Task Force has used the term **difficult airway** to describe difficulty with mask ventilation, difficulty with tracheal intubation, or both.[1] This definition is broad and meant for a "conventionally trained anesthesiologist." For our purposes, a difficult airway can be similarly defined, but in the hands of the most experienced clinician at the bedside. However, it is important to keep in mind that when using this definition, the likelihood of encountering a difficult airway will often vary according to the experience of the clinician.

Other important definitions include the following:

A. **Difficult bag-mask ventilation (BMV)** occurs when "it is not possible for the unassisted clinician to maintain oxygen saturation (SaO_2) >90% using 100% oxygen and positive pressure mask ventilation in a patient whose SaO_2 was >90% before clinician intervention."[2]

B. **Difficult laryngoscopy** is a Grade 3 or 4 view according to Cormack and Lehane[3] grading, and does not necessarily imply difficult intubation.

C. **Difficult intubation** may be defined as "a situation where an experienced laryngoscopist, using direct laryngoscopy, requires:

- •. more than two attempts with the same blade;
- • a change in blade or use of an adjunct to a direct laryngoscope (e.g., bougie); or
- • use of an alternative intubation device or technique following failed intubation with direct laryngoscopy."[2]

The Failed Airway

Failure to intubate and/or failure to oxygenate with BMV represent decision nodes in airway management that require urgent action. There are two pathways that define the failed airway:

A. **Failed intubation** is defined by the failure to intubate the patient after three attempts by an experienced clinician (i.e., *can't intubate, CAN oxygenate*).

B. **Failed oxygenation** assumes that in addition to a failed attempt at intubation, the patient cannot be oxygenated (i.e., to an SaO_2 of 90% or more) with BMV (i.e., *can't intubate, CAN'T oxygenate*).

▶ INCIDENCE OF THE DIFFICULT AIRWAY

Difficult laryngoscopy (i.e., a Cormack Grade 3 or 4 view) has been reported to occur in 2%–8% of cases in the operating room (OR) setting.[2] Corresponding literature derived from out-of-OR settings such as the emergency department (ED) is limited. One study has reported an inability to visualize the cords in 14% of trauma patients,[4] while other reports have pegged the likelihood of a Grade 3 or worse view in patients undergoing manual in-line neck stabilization at closer to 25%.[5] First attempt failure occurs in between 10 and 23% of RSI cases in the ED, while the need for more than two attempts, at 3%, is significantly less.[4,6,7] It should be noted that the published incidence of difficult intubation is only a fraction of difficult laryngoscopy. While a "can't intubate, can't oxygenate" situation is very unusual in the OR (1–3/10,000),[2] failure to maintain SaO_2 above 90% with BMV as part of an RSI in the emergency setting is more common.[8] Fortunately, as the common end point of the failed airway, the incidence of ED cricothyrotomy is reported to be less than 1%.[6,7]

▶ THE DANGER OF MULTIPLE INTUBATION ATTEMPTS

Multiple intubation attempts (defined as three or more) have been associated with significant complications, and ultimately poor patient outcomes. Multiple attempts may result in failed oxygenation as trauma to the laryngeal inlet caused by laryngoscope blade manipulations or blind attempts at tube passage result in bleeding, laryngospasm, and edema. In a review of 2833 patients intubated in an emergency, out-of-OR setting, the need for three or more attempts was associated with severe hypoxemia (14 times that observed for fewer than three attempts); esophageal intubation (6 times); regurgitation (7 times); aspiration (4 times); bradycardia (4 times); and cardiac arrest (7 times).[9] Of note, only 20% of patients in this series had undergone intubation facilitated by RSI.

▶ RESPONSE TO DIFFICULT BAG-MASK VENTILATION

An appropriate response to difficult BMV is outlined in Table 12–1. The reader is referred to Chap. 4 for a more detailed review of the topic. However, it should be reemphasized that oxygenation by BMV is a core skill, and must be properly performed in a difficult situation. All too often in difficult or failed airway scenarios, fixation occurs on attempted intubation, at the expense of attention to maintaining oxygenation with BMV. Early placement of an oral airway, combined with two-person BMV will generally be effective in the difficult mask ventilation situation.

▶ **TABLE 12–1** STAGED RESPONSE TO DIFFICULT BAG-MASK VENTILATION

- **Perform exaggerated head tilt**/chin lift if not contraindicated by C-spine precautions.
- Do an **exaggerated jaw thrust**, lifting the mandible anteriorly into the mask.
- Consider insertion of **oral and/or nasopharyngeal airway.**
- Perform **two-person bag-mask technique**
- If **cricoid pressure** is being applied, ease up on, or release it.
- Consider a **mask change** (size or type) if seal is an issue.
- Rule out **foreign body** in the airway.
- Consider placing a **rescue oxygenation** device, e.g., extraglottic device such as an LMA.
- Consider an early attempt at **intubation**.

▶ RESPONSE TO DIFFICULT DIRECT LARYNGOSCOPY (DL)

For the reasons previously presented, total intubation attempts should be limited. As such, the clinician should maximize the chances of success with the first, and if needed, each succeeding attempt. *Before* the first attempt at laryngoscopy, a plan for difficult laryngoscopy should be mentally rehearsed, all equipment assembled, and assistants briefed on what to expect and how they can help (e.g., with immobilization, two-person BMV, cricoid pressure, external laryngeal manipulation [ELM] etc.). The position of both the patient and clinician should be optimized, and an appropriately sized blade selected. If a skeletal muscle relaxant is used, it must be given time to act.

Initial Response to Difficult DL

If a Grade 3 or 4 view is obtained at laryngoscopy, all components of "best look" laryngoscopy should be undertaken, as outlined in Table 12–2. In addition to optimal technique, ELM and adjunctive use of the bougie or fiberoptic stylet should be attempted. Further discussion on "best look" laryngoscopy is presented in Chap. 5. When properly prepared, *all* of the items in Table 12–2 can be performed during the *first* attempt at laryngoscopy. It should be noted that while the bougie is a useful adjunct in a Grade 3A (epiglottis elevated) case, it is less likely to be successful in a Grade 3B or Grade 4 situation (see Fig. 3–12). In these latter cases, a fiberoptic stylet may be a better adjunct to DL, or an alternative, non-DL technique can be used.

Before a second attempt, a few points should be noted:

- A call for help should be initiated as soon as difficulty has been encountered.
- The emergency patient should be bag-mask ventilated with 100% O_2 between attempts, even if an RSI is underway. Cricoid pressure, if in use, can be maintained. BMV re- and pre-oxygenates the patient for the second attempt and delivers vital information to the clinician: if the patient can be easily oxygenated with mask ventilation, the clinician may take comfort that a failed oxygenation situation does not yet exist, and time is available for another intubation attempt (Fig. 12–1).
- Consideration should be given to the status of the muscle relaxant, if in use: rocuronium or other nondepolarizing agent will act long enough for multiple attempts at laryngoscopy, whereas if succinylcholine is in use, the second attempt should not be excessively delayed, as the medication wears off quickly.
- If direct laryngoscopy (DL) has failed during an awake intubation, the need for additional topical airway anesthesia or (judicious) sedation should be assessed.

Second and Subsequent Attempts at DL

With experience, many clinicians will recognize after a single attempt that successful intubation using DL is unlikely, and may choose to move on to an alternative intubation technique. Given the increasing morbidity with multiple intubation attempts, a second or subsequent attempt at DL should be undertaken only if something *different* can be done, for example:

- To complete a previously untried component of best look DL.
- A muscle relaxant has been introduced, or redosed.
- Additional topical airway anesthesia or sedation has been added, for an awake intubation.
- A blade change is attempted.
- A more experienced colleague takes over.

A blade change need not be an automatic response to a difficult laryngoscopy situation, and should be undertaken only with a specific goal in mind. Such situations may include the following:

▶ **TABLE 12–2** COMPONENTS OF "BEST LOOK" DIRECT LARYNGOSCOPY

- **Patient positioning optimized**: Stretcher height appropriate; patient at head of bed; ear-sternum line optimized ("sniff" position) unless contraindicated.
- **Optimal muscle relaxation**, if used.
- **Laryngoscopist's positioning optimized**: Laryngoscope held at base of handle; back straight, arm modestly flexed or stabilized on trunk.
- **Appropriate blade tip location**: With indirect epiglottis lift, blade tip in vallecula is contacting hyo-epiglottic ligament.
- **Appropriate laryngoscope lift**: Occurs along axis of the handle, with use of a second hand if needed.
- **Head lift**: With use of the right hand (if not contraindicated) during laryngoscopy.
- **ELM**: To bring the laryngeal inlet into view.
- Consideration of whether **cricoid pressure** is adversely affecting the view.
- **Use of an adjunct to DL**, e.g., bougie (tracheal tube introducer) or fiberoptic optical stylet.

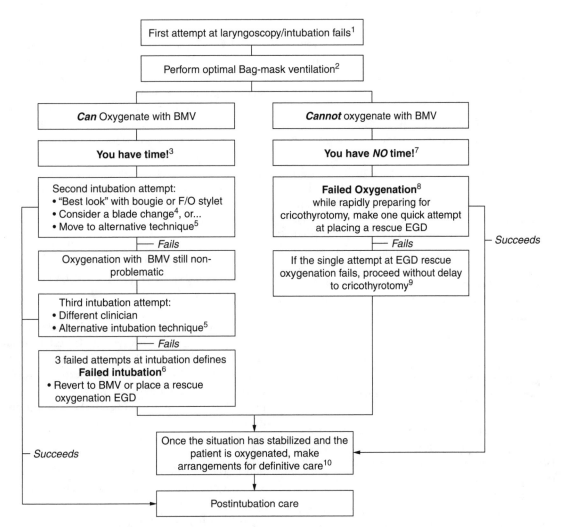

Figure 12–1. Encountered Difficult Airway algorithm.
(1) All components of 'Best Look' laryngoscopy should be performed during the first and any subsequent laryngoscopy attempts (Table 12–2).
(2) Optimal bag-mask ventilation (BMV) includes use of an oral airway, jaw lift, and two-person mask ventilation (Table 12–1).
(3) As long as oxygenation is possible via BMV between attempts, **you have time**. Consideration should occur as to why the first attempt failed, and how chances of success can be increased during a second attempt.
(4) A longer curved blade may be helpful to better engage the hyoepiglottic ligament or 'pick up' the epiglottis; a straight blade may help displace the tongue and directly lift the epiglottis, and a levering tip (e.g., McCoy or CLM) blade may help in C-spine precaution situations.
(5) Alternative intubation techniques include the LMA Fastrach, Lightwand, and indirect rigid or flexible fiberoptic or video devices.
(6) In the 'failed intubation ' routine, placement of a rescue oxygenation (e.g., extraglottic) device is considered after three attempts.
(7) The inability to oxygenate the patient with BMV, in conjunction with failed intubation, even after only a single attempt, defines **failed oxygenation. You have no time** for further intubation attempts.
(8) With **failed oxygenation,** the default action is cricothyrotomy. While preparations are being made for the cricothyrotomy, placement of a rescue extraglottic device may be quickly attempted.
(9) Cricothyrotomy may be performed by open surgical or percutaneous needle-guided cannula techniques.
(10) Definitive care must be arranged, by obtaining additional equipment or expertise from colleagues, or transferring the patient.

- If it is suspected that the blade was not long enough to control the epiglottis, (e.g., by failing to completely advance into the vallecula and engage the hyoepiglottic ligament) a longer blade can be used.
- If the epiglottis is long and "floppy," the tip of the laryngoscope blade (straight or curved) can be repositioned to directly lift it.
- A different blade may best handle certain anatomic conditions. As noted in Chap. 5, a straight blade used by a paraglossal route can convert a Grade 3 view to Grade 2 or better,[10] particularly in the patient with a small mandible, prominent upper central incisors, or a long floppy epiglottis. The levering-tip McCoy/CLM blade may also be useful in converting Grade 3 views to 1 or 2, particularly in the patient undergoing manual in-line neck stabilization.[11–13]

▶ MOVING ON TO AN ALTERNATIVE, NON-DL INTUBATION TECHNIQUE

Following a second failed attempt at intubation, the patient should again be oxygenated with BMV. As long as mask ventilation continues to be nonproblematic, a third attempt at intubation can be considered. However, after two failed attempts at intubation using best look DL, a third attempt at laryngoscopic intubation is rarely warranted, unless a more skilled clinician has arrived. Rather, an **alternative intubation technique** should now be considered. Alternative intubation devices and techniques have been discussed in more detail in Chap. 6. Which alternative, "go to" device is chosen will depend on availability and clinician preference, skill, and experience. The Fastrach LMA (ILMA) has the advantage of being both an alternative intubation and rescue oxygenation device. The Trachlight lighted stylet and increasingly, fiberoptic and video-based devices are also available. The latter devices have the advantage of allowing indirect visualization of the laryngeal inlet. Regardless of the instrument chosen, the clinician must (a) attain skill in use of the device

(e.g., by using it in anticipated easy intubations, or in the OR), and (b) move on to using the device early, while muscle relaxation, if used, is still acting, and the airway has not been bloodied or otherwise traumatized. The alternative intubation devices all have an associated learning curve: success rates will depend on the individual clinician's skill. However, in experienced hands, they will often succeed where DL has failed. All clinicians who regularly manage airways should have skills in using at least one alternative intubation technique.

▶ RECOGNITION OF AND RESPONSE TO THE FAILED AIRWAY

As previously outlined, the **failed airway** is defined in one of two ways: (a) **failed intubation,** defined simply by a failure to intubate after three attempts, or (b) **failed oxygenation**—failure to intubate *in conjunction with* a failure to oxygenate using BMV. Admittedly, these are two very different scenarios, sitting on two different arms of the Encountered Difficult Airway algorithm (Fig. 12–1). In the former situation (*can't intubate, CAN oxygenate*), one is still dealing with an oxygenated patient, and in the latter situation (*can't intubate, CAN'T oxygenate*), a hypoxic one.

Failed Airway (1): Failed Intubation

The **failed intubation** definition of the failed airway, represented on the left-hand arm of the Encountered Difficult Airway algorithm (Fig. 12–1) exists for the following reasons:

A. Failure to intubate after three attempts on the part of any one clinician should be a warning sign to stop, take stock, and reassess the situation. Otherwise, "fixation error" can set in, with a harried clinician focused excessively on the intubation, while losing sight of the "bigger picture" of ensuring patient oxygenation.

B. As previously presented, multiple intubation attempts are associated with increasing morbidity. At its worst, multiple attempts could eventually cause trauma, edema, and bleeding to the extent that mask ventilation now becomes impossible.

C. Neuromuscular blockade may have worn off, and a decision will have to be made about allowing the patient to resume spontaneous ventilation with no further doses of muscle relaxant or conversely, whether a second dose should be given.

After a third failed attempt, the patient should again be ventilated by BMV to reoxygenate and indeed, confirm that the patient can still be mask ventilated. At this point, although BMV can continue indefinitely, we espouse placing a rescue oxygenation device, in the form of an extraglottic device (EGD). These devices have been discussed in Chap. 7. They confer a number of advantages: once placed, they generally enable easier positive pressure ventilation of the patient, often with just one hand; they deliver positive pressure ventilation from just outside the laryngeal inlet, and thirdly, gastric insufflation is likely to be less than that incurred with BMV. Some devices (Combitube, King LTS-D, LMA ProSeal, or Supreme) may provide more protection against aspiration of gastric contents than others, although probably none are as effective in this regard as a cuffed endotracheal tube, which is still the ultimately desired end point. Although most extraglottic devices will require transient release of any applied cricoid pressure during their insertion, it can be reapplied following successful placement. Once oxygenation is confirmed and the situation has stabilized, definitive care should be arranged.

Note that clinical judgment should be applied to the directive to limit intubation attempts to three. For example, if a more experienced colleague has arrived, a fourth attempt may be warranted by that clinician, or similarly, if an adjunct such as a bougie has now become available, a further attempt may be undertaken. As always, common sense should prevail.

Failed Airway (2): Failed Oxygenation

The inability to oxygenate the patient with mask ventilation or via an endotracheal tube is an emergency situation. This scenario is represented on the right-hand side of the Encountered Difficult Airway Algorithm (Fig. 12–1). Without doubt, the default intervention for this **failed oxygenation** situation is **cricothyrotomy**. Too often, in can't intubate, can't oxygenate scenarios, a cricothyrotomy is started after the patient is no longer viable. This underscores the importance of recognizing a failed oxygenation situation, with its implication (cricothyrotomy). Access to the lower airway through the cricothyroid membrane can be by open surgical or percutaneous, needle-guided cannula techniques, as discussed in more detail in Chap. 7.

Two provisos apply to the failed oxygenation scenario:

A. Before declaring a failed oxygenation situation, an *aggressive* response to difficult BMV should have been undertaken. As mentioned earlier, this includes an oral airway and two-person technique (Table 12–1).

B. In most situations, before cricothyrotomy, a brief detour to EGD placement should be attempted. Many case reports and anecdotes attest to the effectiveness of extraglottic devices such as LMAs or the Combitube in establishing a patent airway in failed oxygenation situations, allowing successful reoxygenation of the patient. EGDs may succeed where BMV has failed for the following reasons:

• No mask-to-face seal issues.

• No clinician hand size to patient face size disparity issues.

• Positive pressure ventilation (PPV) is delivered from immediately in front of the cords, bypassing more proximal sites of functional obstruction.

• Improved delivery of PPV immediately in front of cords may help break laryngospasm, if contributory to the situation.

EGDs may not succeed in oxygenating and ventilating the patient with pathology or obstruction at or below the cords. However, sporadic case reports are emerging of successful oxygenation with EGDs even in such situations (e.g., airway burns, anaphylaxis, neck hematoma), where they may not have been anticipated to work.[14–17] If EGD placement is successful in a failed oxygenation situation, cricothyrotomy can be avoided, and definitive care should be arranged. It must be emphasized, however, that in the failed oxygenation situation, the EGD placement attempt must be brief, and **must not delay the onset of cricothyrotomy**. In practice, this translates to a single attempt at EGD insertion while the cricothyrotomy package is being opened.

Finally, the occasional patient may present with pathology rendering airway access from above the cords obviously impossible from the outset. These patients may require a primary cricothyrotomy or tracheostomy.

▶ "BARS"

The mnemonic "**BARS**" represents a simple reminder of the foregoing step-wise progression, once difficult laryngoscopy has been encountered:

Best look laryngoscopy, including *B*URP (ELM),
   *B*ougie and *B*lade change;
   Maximum 1-2 attempts, then proceed to...
Alternative intubation technique;
   Maximum total of three intubation attempts via any technique, then place...
Rescue oxygenation device, for example, EGD;
   For failed oxygenation at any point unrelieved by EGD placement, rapidly perform...
Surgical airway (cricothyrotomy).

▶ ARRANGING FOR DEFINITIVE CARE AFTER A FAILED AIRWAY

Generally, the desired endpoint in the failed airway situation will remain placement of a cuffed tracheal tube below the cords. Thus, following successful "rescue" of a failed airway situation with an EGD or cricothyrotomy, arrangements must be made for intubation or tracheostomy. This may involve bringing additional equipment and/or expertise to the now oxygenated patient, or moving the patient to the location of the expertise or equipment. Alternatively, the "breathing room" afforded the original clinician may allow for reevaluation of whether anything can be further optimized for another intubation attempt, or conversely, whether the intubation was really needed in the first place. Some of these points are expanded upon below:

• **Additional expertise:** No clinician, no matter how experienced or capable, can easily handle every situation. Consideration should be given to where help can be obtained. It may be a colleague or other health-care provider with equal or greater experience: for example, an emergency physician, intensivist, anesthesia provider, surgeon, respiratory therapist, or paramedic.

• **Additional equipment:** Other intubation devices not initially available may be obtainable from other areas of the hospital, such as the operating room. Flexible fiberoptic or video-bronchoscopes may enable intubation through or alongside an extraglottic device, or alongside a cricothyrotomy cannula. Other options include retrograde intubation or conversion to a formal tracheostomy.

• **Consideration of patient transfer unintubated:** After the situation has stabilized, risk/benefit analysis may now suggest transferring the patient unintubated. This is an intimidating concept, however, it may be better to transfer an unintubated, oxygenated patient with an EGD than one who has aspirated and has a bloodied and edematous airway from inappropriate multiple intubation attempts!

- **Reevaluation of the indication for intubation:** In an emergency, most often the patient will still require intubation, but occasionally, the risk of persisting with attempted intubation for a less pressing indication, such as airway protection, may now exceed its benefit, especially if the patient is anticipated to recover over the short term.
- **Consider the status of muscle relaxation:** Once the situation has stabilized with an oxygenated patient, if a muscle relaxant had been used, it may be appropriate to allow it to wear off, or to reverse it. This may allow resumption of spontaneous ventilation. Conversely, consideration can be given to the merits of giving an additional dose of relaxant.

▶ SUMMARY: FAILED AIRWAY

The appropriate identification of, and response to the failed airway is of paramount importance. Decisions revolve largely around the ability to oxygenate the patient with BMV, once again underscoring the importance of this seemingly basic skill. If a failed intubation is encountered in the setting of easy mask ventilation and oxygenation, up to two further attempts can be made at intubation, unless additional expertise or equipment has become available. Beyond this, the *failed intubation* definition of the failed airway applies, and oxygenation should be maintained with BMV or by placement of an EGD, while arrangements are made for definitive airway management. *Failed oxygenation* is defined by a failure to intubate, even after only a single attempt, if adequate oxygenation cannot be achieved with BMV. Immediate cricothyrotomy is the correct response to a failed oxygenation situation, with a single, brief attempt at EGD placement, while preparations are being made to proceed with the cricothyrotomy.

REFERENCES

1. Practice guidelines for management of the difficult airway: an updated report by the American Society of Anesthesiologists Task Force on Management of the Difficult Airway. *Anesthesiology.* 2003;98(5): 1269–1277.
2. Crosby ET, Cooper RM, Douglas MJ, et al. The unanticipated difficult airway with recommendations for management. *Can J Anaesth.* 1998;45(8): 757–776.
3. Cormack RS, Lehane J. Difficult tracheal intubation in obstetrics. *Anaesthesia.* 1984;39(11):1105–11.
4. Graham CA, Beard D, Henry JM, et al. Rapid sequence intubation of trauma patients in Scotland. *J Trauma.* 2004;56(5):1123–1126.
5. Heath KJ. The effect on laryngoscopy of different cervical spine immobilisation techniques. *Anaesthesia.* 1994;49(10):843–845.
6. Sagarin MJ, Barton ED, Chng YM, et al. Airway management by US and Canadian emergency medicine residents: a multicenter analysis of more than 6,000 endotracheal intubation attempts. *Ann Emerg Med.* 2005;46(4):328–336.
7. Levitan RM, Rosenblatt B, Meiner EM, et al. Alternating day emergency medicine and anesthesia resident responsibility for management of the trauma airway: a study of laryngoscopy performance and intubation success. *Ann Emerg Med.* 2004;43(1):48–53.
8. Simpson J, Munro PT, Graham CA. Rapid sequence intubation in the emergency department: 5 year trends. *Emerg Med J.* 2006;23(1):54–56.
9. Mort TC. Emergency tracheal intubation: complications associated with repeated laryngoscopic attempts. *Anesth Analg.* 2004;99(2):607–613.
10. Henderson JJ. The use of paraglossal straight blade laryngoscopy in difficult tracheal intubation. *Anaesthesia.* 1997;52(6):552–560.
11. Uchida T, Hikawa Y, Saito Y, et al. The McCoy levering laryngoscope in patients with limited neck extension. *Can J Anaesth.* 1997;44(6): 674–676.
12. Laurent SC, de Melo AE, Alexander-Williams JM. The use of the McCoy laryngoscope in patients with simulated cervical spine injuries. *Anaesthesia.* 1996;51(1):74–75.
13. Gabbott DA. Laryngoscopy using the McCoy laryngoscope after application of a cervical collar. *Anaesthesia.* 1996;51(9):812–814.

14. Martin R, Girouard Y, Cote DJ. Use of a laryngeal mask in acute airway obstruction after carotid endarterectomy. *Can J Anaesth*. 2002;49(8): 890.

15. Jones DA, Geraghty IF. Emergency management of upper airway obstruction due to a rapidly expanding haematoma in the neck. *Br J Hosp Med*.7–20 1995;53(11):589–590.

16. King CJ, Davey AJ, Chandradeva K. Emergency use of the laryngeal mask airway in severe upper airway obstruction caused by supraglottic oedema. *Br J Anaesth*. 1995;75(6):785–786.

17. Shaw IC, Welchew EA, Harrison BJ, et al. Complete airway obstruction during awake fibreoptic intubation. *Anaesthesia*. 1997;52(6):582–585.

18. Levitan RM, Kush S, Hollander JE. Devices for difficult airway management in academic emergency departments: results of a national survey. *Ann Emerg Med*. 1999;33(6):694–698.

19. McGuire GP, Wong DT. Airway management: contents of a difficult intubation cart. *Can J Anaesth*. 1999;46(2):190–191.

▶ APPENDIX: CONTENTS OF AN EMERGENCY AIRWAY AND/OR DIFFICULT AIRWAY CART

It makes sense to have a dedicated airway cart[18,19] incorporating all equipment that could possibly be needed for emergency airway management. Organization of the cart is at the discretion of the unit in question, however a logical means of storage will help locate needed equipment in a hurry. Consideration should be given to standardizing cart organization with units elsewhere in the hospital, for example, the intensive care unit (ICU) or the OR.

Sample adult airway cart contents

A. Mask ventilation:
  - Oxygen tank
  - Oxygen tubing
  - Oxygen face masks, simple and nonrebreathing
  - Manual resuscitator with reservoir bag
  - Manual resuscitator face masks, #3–6
  - Nasopharyngeal airways, #7, 8, 9
  - Oropharyngeal airways: 8, 9, 10 cm
  - Water-soluble lubricant

B. Nasal intubation:
  - Endotrol tubes, #6.0–8.0, for blind nasal intubation
  - Phenylephrine 0.5% nasal spray; lidocaine 4% liquid; lidocaine 2% gel

C. Oral Intubation:
  - Endotracheal tubes, (cuffed) 5.0, 5.5, 6.0, 6.5, 7.0, 7.5, 8.0, 8.5 mm internal diameter
  - Stylets, size 14 French
  - Laryngoscope handles, regular and short length
  - Laryngoscope blades, curved (Macintosh) #3 and 4; straight (e.g., Miller) #2 and 3; +/– levering tip blades (e.g., CLM/McCoy) #3 and 4
  - Laryngoscope charger and/or spare batteries
  - Tracheal tube introducer ("bougie")
  - +/– Fiberoptic optical stylet (e.g., Levitan FPS, Shikani, or Bonfils)

D. *Alternative* Intubation Techniques:
  - At least one of:
    - LMA Fastrach (Intubating Laryngeal Mask Airway), #3,4,5 (with manufacturer sizing card). Dedicated LMA Fastrach tubes, sizes 6.0, 6.5, 7.0, 7.5, 8.0 (and stabilizer)
    - Lightwand (e.g., Trachlight): handle and wands
    - Other fiberoptic or video-based intubation device
  - Trachlight and fiberoptic or video-based device batteries and battery compartment access tools.

E. *Rescue* ventilation devices:
  - At least one of:
    - Combitube, #37 and #41
    - Laryngeal Masks (e.g., Classic, Unique, Proseal, or Supreme #3, 4, 5 (manufacturer sizing card)

○ Other extraglottic device, according to institutional preference

F. Surgical:
- Needle-guided percutaneous cricothyrotomy set, for example, Melker or PCK, with cuffed cannula
- Surgical cricothyrotomy equipment: scalpel handle, #11 blade, tracheal hook, Trousseau dilator, #6.0 ETT, Shiley cuffed tracheostomy (#4) tubes

G. Other Equipment:
- End-tidal CO_2 ($ETCO_2$) detector
- Twill tape
- Esophageal detector device (EDD), for example, 60 cc catheter-tip (Toomey) syringe
- 10 cc syringes for cuff inflation
- Suction catheters: rigid tonsillar (e.g., Yankauer) and flexible endotracheal tube suction catheters
- Magill forceps
- Bite blocks
- Adult airway exchange catheter
- Materials for application of topical airway anesthesia: tongue depressors; Mucosal Atomization Device (e.g., MADgic®) or DeVilbiss atomizer; Jackson forceps; cotton pledgelets; Lidocaine 10% spray, 2% gel, 5% ointment, 4% liquid

Sample Pediatric Equipment

Note: Departments with significant pediatric volumes may wish to consider organizing equipment in a color-coded fashion according to Broselow tape sizes.

- Broselow tape
- Oxygen masks: newborn, pediatric
- Manual resuscitator with infant and child-sized masks
- Oral airways: 3.5, 5, 6, 7 cm
- Laryngoscope blades: straight (e.g., Miller) 0, 1, 2; & curved (Macintosh) 1,2, and 3
- ETT: uncuffed—2, 2.5; cuffed and uncuffed—3, 3.5, 4, 4.5; cuffed—5, 5.5, 6, 6.5, 7
- Stylet: 6 Fr, 8 Fr
- Bougie: pediatric
- LMA: 1, 1.5, 2, 2.5, 3; or other pediatric extraglottic devices
- +/- Lightwand: infant and child sizes
- +/- Pediatric fiberoptic stylet: Shikani or Brambrinck
- Small Magill forceps
- $ETCO_2$ detector, pediatric size
- #18, #16, and #14 G IV catheters for cricothyrotomy

Finally, the presence of an "airway drug kit" with all the necessary pharmacologic agents, in one location, is highly recommended.

CHAPTER 13

Airway Pharmacology

▶ KEY POINTS

- For the patient requiring emergency airway management, *preservation* of oxygenation and blood pressure often takes priority over *attenuation* of undesirable reflexes.
- There is strong evidence that in the head-injured patient, hypoxia or hypotension occurring during patient resuscitation can significantly increase mortality.
- Ketamine produces excellent amnesia and is the only induction agent to also provide analgesia.
- Although ketamine can indirectly raise blood pressure by sympathetic nervous system stimulation, intrinsically, it is a myocardial depressant.
- Etomidate is remarkable for its stable hemodynamic effects and has become the induction agent of choice in many North American emergency departments.
- Etomidate does cause adrenal suppression. Unless risk/benefit assessment suggests otherwise, an alternative agent should be used for induction in the septic patient.
- In airway management, the primary role of midazolam is as a light sedative for the patient undergoing an awake intubation.
- The advantageous effects of pretreatment agents must be balanced against their potential adverse hemodynamic

and respiratory consequences, in the at-risk patient.
- Succinylcholine remains in widespread use for several reasons: (a) it has a very rapid onset; (b) it usually has a very short duration of action; and (c) clinicians are familiar with its use.
- Rocuronium use avoids the need to consider many of the contraindications to, and precautions associated with succinylcholine use.
- A decrease in blood pressure is common following induction and intubation.
- The initial response to hypotension from almost any cause should be circulatory volume expansion. However, clinicians should also be comfortable with the indications for, and use of short-acting vasopressors.

▶ INTRODUCTION

Airway management, including endotracheal intubation, requires a competent understanding of airway pharmacology. A small number of medications are used to facilitate airway management, for various indications as shown in Table 13–1. Successful airway intervention without patient compromise requires a good working knowledge of these agents, together with an appreciation of expected physiological responses to manipulation of the airway.

▶ **TABLE 13–1** MEDICATIONS COMMONLY USED FOR AIRWAY MANAGEMENT

Procedure	Medication Type	Indication	Sample Medications
Awake intubation	Topically applied or regionally injected local anesthetic agents	Airway anesthesia for awake intubation	Lidocaine spray, jelly, ointment, injectable
Awake intubation	Adjuvant sedative agents	Anxiolysis, analgesia, and sedation during awake intubation	Benzodiazepines, Opioids, Buty rophenones, Propofol, Ketamine
Awake intubation	Opioid and benzodiazepine anatogonists	Use in case of overdose of opioid or benzodiazepine	Naloxone, Flumazenil
Rapid-sequence intubation	"Pretreatment" agents	Attenuation of undesirable physiologic reflexes during laryngoscopy and intubation	Atropine, Lidocaine, Opioids, Neuromuscular blockers
Rapid-sequence intubation	Induction agents and neuromuscular blockers	Induction of unconsciousness (control of ICP), and subsequent skeletal muscle relaxation to facilitate laryngoscopy	Etomidate, Propofol, Thiopental, Ketamine. Succinylcholine, Rocuronium
Rapid-sequence intubation	Miscellaneous rescue agents	Treatment of succinylcholine-induced malignant hyperthermia	Dantrolene
Awake or rapid-sequence intubation	Rescue vasopressor and other agents	Treatment of postintubation hypotension	Ephedrine, Phenylephrine

▶ THE PHYSIOLOGIC RESPONSE TO LARYNGOSCOPY AND INTUBATION

Laryngoscopy and intubation are powerful stimuli that can provoke intense physiologic responses from multiple body systems.[1,2] These responses, including hypertension, tachycardia, increased intracranial pressure (ICP), and bronchoconstriction, are generally transient, and of little consequence in most individuals. However, for some patients, if these responses are not attenuated, significant morbidity may ensue. It should be appreciated that most of the data supporting the attenuation of these adverse physiologic responses has been gathered from generally healthier, elective surgical patients. For the patient requiring emergency airway management, *preservation* of oxygenation and blood pressure often takes priority over *attenuation* of undesirable reflexes.

Stimulation of the oropharynx and upper airway activates both arms of the autonomic nervous system. In adults, the sympathetic response usually predominates, with an increase in circulating levels of catecholamines. In young children (and some adults) airway instrumentation may cause a predominately vagal response, including bradycardia.

It is important to note that intubation techniques other than direct laryngoscopy will still elicit these responses.[3] Systems primarily affected by direct laryngoscopy and/or intubation include the **cardiovascular, respiratory, and central nervous systems.** When indicated, local anesthesia and systemic medications can be used to minimize these undesirable effects. The following sections will review the responses in question.

Cardiovascular Response to Laryngoscopy and Intubation

Laryngoscopy and intubation causes an increase in both sympathetic and sympathoadrenal activity. This usually results in transient hypertension and tachycardia, correlating with a rise in catecholamine levels. Under "light general anesthesia," systolic blood pressure has been shown to rise an average of 53 mm Hg in response to laryngoscopy and intubation, while the heart rate increases by 23 beats per minute.[1] In smokers and individuals with preexisting hypertension, the rise in blood pressure can be more pronounced.[4] In healthy patients, these hemodynamic effects are usually of little consequence. However, patients in whom attenuation of this pressor response may be important include:

- The patient with **coronary artery disease**. Significant rises in heart rate and blood pressure (BP) could result in myocardial ischemia due to increased myocardial oxygen demand.
- The patient with an **unruptured cerebral or aortic aneurysm, or aortic dissection**. A dramatic increase in mean arterial pressure (MAP) could lead to aneurysm rupture or worsening dissection, respectively.
- Patients with **significant preexisting hypertension,** including women with pregnancy-induced hypertension. Further increases in BP could overcome the limits of cerebral autoregulation and potentially lead to increased ICP or cerebral hemorrhage

The pressor response to laryngoscopy and intubation can be attenuated by one of a number of drug regimens, including deep anesthesia and/or vasoactive agents. However, in the volume-depleted emergency patient, any pressor response to laryngoscopy and intubation may by counteracted by the vasodilating and negative inotropic effects of induction agents. Such a drop in blood pressure during a resuscitation can be associated with increased morbidity and mortality.[5] The best approach must take into consideration the individual patient, the experience of the physician, and the available medications.

Respiratory System Response to Laryngoscopy and Intubation

Coughing, laryngospasm, and bronchospasm are all potential responses to airway manipulation. Laryngospasm may be more common in the pediatric population. Gagging may lead to vomiting and potential aspiration. All of these responses are more likely in the inadequately anesthetized patient and those with underlying respiratory pathology.

Coughing, gagging, and laryngospasm can be abolished with the use of neuromuscular blocking agents. Bronchospasm does not respond to muscle relaxants since these agents do not block smooth muscle receptors in the airways. Bronchoconstriction can be attenuated by deep anesthesia and the use of drugs that promote bronchial smooth muscle relaxation.

Obviously, hypoxia and hypercarbia are potential complications of laryngoscopy and intubation, especially if prolonged attempts at intubation are made without intervening bag-mask ventilation (BMV).

Central Nervous System Response to Laryngoscopy and Intubation

Laryngoscopy and intubation results in a transient rise in ICP.[1] This increase in ICP may be a direct response to central nervous system (CNS) stimulation, causing an increase in cerebral blood flow (CBF). ICP may also rise if systemic blood pressure is profoundly raised and/or venous outflow is obstructed (e.g., by straining or coughing). Although this is of little consequence in most individuals, in patients in whom ICP is already elevated or in whom cerebral autoregulation is impaired, these effects could complicate an already dangerous situation.

As discussed in more detail in Chap. 14, the focus in management of the patient with traumatic brain injury has shifted from simply preventing an ICP rise with endotracheal intubation, to maintenance of cerebral perfusion pressure (CPP). CPP is determined by the difference between mean arterial pressure (MAP) and the ICP, that is, CPP = MAP – ICP. There is now evidence that **in the head-injured patient, hypoxia or hypotension occurring during patient resuscitation can significantly increase mortality.**[6] Therefore, the importance of avoiding a lowered MAP during intubation may assume greater clinical significance than a transient increase in ICP.

Although deep anesthesia can block the direct effect of laryngoscopy and intubation on ICP, this approach can also result in a significant decrease in MAP and CPP. In the head-injured patient, a pre-intubation fluid bolus and special care in choosing the dosage of induction medication is needed to help avoid significant drops in CPP.

▶ INDUCTION SEDATIVE/ HYPNOTICS

Induction sedative/hypnotics are used primarily to induce unconsciousness in the patient as part of an RSI. In lower doses, some can also be used as sedative agents. In modern practice it is accepted that, except in unusual circumstances, the use of muscle relaxants requires the concomitant use of an induction agent to ensure lack of awareness. To this extent, induction sedative/hypnotics are generally considered a mandatory component of RSI, at all ages.

There is some evidence suggesting that use of induction sedative/hypnotics as part of an RSI actually improves intubating conditions and decreases time needed to perform RSI.[7,8] However, this data is difficult to interpret and may in part simply reflect the rapid onset and potency of the sedative/hypnotic compensating for attempted intubation before full onset of neuromuscular blockade.

In determining the appropriate dosage of induction agent, several factors must be considered. These include:

A. **Patient weight:** Drug dosing is based primarily on patient weight. The appropriate loading dose of an agent is largely dependent on the volume of distribution. The volume of distribution reflects the medication's lipid solubility. How the drug is distributed in turn impacts the decision to dose based on ideal body weight (IBW) or total body weight (TBW).[9] With obesity, both lean and fat mass increase, but fat increases proportionally more. Clinical data on how to dose induction sedative/hypnotics in obese patients is limited. For propofol and thiopental, the recommendation is for dosing based on TBW.[9] However, for many drugs, the situation is indefinite. For this reason, many clinicians dose agents based on a weight that lies somewhere between IBW and TBW.

B. **Age:** With the exception of neonates, anesthetic requirements decrease with advancing age. An 80-year old will typically require only half the induction dose of a 20-year old.

C. **Hemodynamics:** Hypotension is common following intubation. One study quotes a 25% incidence of life-threatening hypotension in the initial phase of mechanical ventilation.[10] It is important to note that *all* induction sedative/hypnotics can cause a drop in blood pressure. As this is more dramatic in patients with preexisting hypovolemia, volume status must be taken into account when determining the dose of induction agent.

D. **Level of Consciousness:** The purpose of using an induction sedative/hypnotic is to induce a state of unconsciousness and amnesia. If this is already present, either from drugs (e.g., the overdose patient) or pathology (e.g., the head-injured, hypotensive, or arrested patient), the need for additional induction agent is diminished (but often still necessary). This can sometimes be a difficult decision, as airway manipulation is intensely stimulating and especially in an overdose situation may "awaken" an apparently unconscious patient. Provided the hemodynamics will tolerate it, the authors would generally recommend administration of an induction sedative/hypnotic (even to the unconscious patient) whenever muscle relaxants are used.

Propofol

Propofol is an intravenous sedative/hypnotic agent that works primarily via gamma amino butyric acid (GABA) receptors to produce hypnosis.[11,12] Propofol has become popular because of its **rapid onset and short clinical duration**. Recovery from the effects of propofol is notable for the **lack of residual sedation**.

Propofol causes a dose-dependent decrease in level of consciousness. Small doses (0.25–0.5 mg/kg) result in sedation while larger doses (1–3 mg/kg) are used to induce unconsciousness. **Propofol does not possess intrinsic analgesic properties** and although it may produce amnesia, this effect is not as reliable as that seen with the benzodiazepines. Following a bolus of 2 mg/kg to a healthy adult, unconsciousness is generally produced within 30 seconds, with recovery taking 5–15 minutes. As a potent respiratory depressant, apnea is common following an induction dose. Propofol decreases airway reflexes to intubation in a dose-dependent manner.

Propofol is a myocardial depressant and also results in peripheral vasodilation. This results in **a decrease in blood pressure following a bolus dose.** For this reason, a fluid bolus is commonly given before its administration. In patients with hypovolemia or impaired heart function, this drop in blood pressure can be quite marked. The hemodynamic effects are more pronounced in the elderly, in whom the dose should also be lowered.

Although propofol lowers ICP, a decrease in CPP can still result from its administration, because of its adverse effect on blood pressure. This decrease in CPP may be particularly detrimental in the head-injured patient who is also hypovolemic and has impaired autoregulation. Propofol may offer a degree of cerebral protection,[13] but the clinical significance of this is unknown.

Prolonged high-dose propofol infusions have been associated with poor outcomes in the ICU setting. This phenomenon, called "propofol infusion syndrome" has been described mainly in children but recently also in adults.[12] As such, caution should be exercised when propofol infusions are to be administered in high doses for more than 48 hours. The manufacturer does not recommend propofol for long-term sedation in pediatric ICU patients.[14] For emergency intubations and to facilitate procedures, however, even in children, propofol has been safely used outside the OR.[15]

Propofol may cause pain on injection. This can be minimized by injecting into a large vein. The addition of 1–2 cc of 1% lidocaine to the syringe of propofol just prior to injection may also decrease discomfort.

Propofol is supplied as a 10 mg/mL emulsion containing 10% soybean oil and 1.2% purified egg phosphatide. In theory, individuals with egg or soybean allergies could be sensitive, but in practice, allergic reactions to propofol are exceedingly rare. This preparation has been shown to be a growth medium for certain microorganisms, so that sterile technique should be utilized when handling propofol: it should be drawn up immediately before use and unused portions discarded.[14]

PROPOFOL AS A SEDATIVE AGENT

Propofol can be used as an agent to blunt awareness for an 'awake' intubation, but does not address anxiety or discomfort associated with the procedure in the way that benzodiazepines or narcotics, respectively, are able to do. If used for sedation, propofol should be administered in small doses (e.g., 0.25 mg/kg), maintaining verbal contact with the patient. In the critically ill patient, even when used in small doses, it can cause loss of consciousness and hypotension. Use of propofol to achieve a state of deep sedation for intubation will impair protective airway reflexes, while not providing the facilitated conditions provided by RSI with a muscle relaxant.

SUMMARY

Drug: Propofol.

Drug type: Anesthetic induction sedative/ hypnotic.

Indication: Induction of unconsciousness; sedation.

Contraindications: Uncorrected shock states are relative contraindications, at least requiring a significant decrease in dose. Pediatric long-term infusions are contraindicated.

Dose: Induction dose is 1–3 mg/kg (average 75 kg = 150 mg). Dosage should be decreased in the elderly and volume-depleted patient.

Onset/Duration: Onset is ~30 seconds. Clinical duration is 5–15 minutes.

Potential Complications: Hypotension and apnea; pain on injection.

Thiopental

Thiopental is a barbiturate sedative/hypnotic, and until the introduction of propofol, it was the primary agent used for induction of general anesthesia. Despite the popularity of propofol, thiopental is still widely used in many operating rooms (ORs) and emergency departments (EDs).

The barbiturates exert their main effect by binding to and potentiating GABA receptors in the central nervous system (CNS). They produce a dose-dependent CNS depression, ranging from sedation to pharmacologic coma. Thiopental has a rapid onset with clinical effects seen within about 30 seconds. Following a single dose, recovery generally takes 5–10 minutes. Recovery may be substantially longer following repeated doses or infusions.

Thiopental is a potent respiratory depressant, and apnea is the norm following an induction dose. This agent has also been associated with clinically relevant histamine release, which may induce bronchospasm. In fact, the manufacturer lists *status asthmaticus* as an absolute contraindication.[16] Despite this, thiopental has been used successfully in the management of severe asthma.[17]

Thiopental, like propofol, causes a decrease in ICP and cerebral oxygen consumption, theoretically making it an attractive choice for use in the brain-injured patient. As with propofol, however, care must be taken to not lower ICP at the expense of a profound reduction in blood pressure, as thiopental is also a potent myocardial depressant. In the presence of hypovolemia, a significant drop in blood pressure can result.

The dose of thiopental for RSI is 3–5 mg/kg, although this dose should be lowered in elderly or hypovolemic patients. It is supplied as a powder, which must be dissolved in sterile water to produce a 2.5% solution (25 mg/mL). The resulting solution is highly alkaline and care must be taken to avoid interstitial or intraarterial injection. Care must also be taken to avoid direct interaction with acidic solutions (e.g., most of the neuromuscular blockers) as this may result in precipitation and loss of intravenous (IV) access.

THIOPENTAL AS A SEDATIVE AGENT

Thiopental is not generally used as a sedative agent to facilitate awake intubations.

SUMMARY

Drug: Thiopental.

Drug type: Anesthetic induction agent; sedative/ hypnotic.

Indication: Induction of unconsciousness.

Contraindications: Uncorrected shock states are relative contraindications that require a marked decrease in dose.

Dose: Dose is 3–5 mg/kg (average 75 kg = 250 mg), depending on hemodynamics.

Onset/Duration: Onset is about 30 seconds. Clinical duration is 5–10 minutes.

Potential complications: Hypotension and apnea.

Ketamine

Ketamine is unique among the sedative/hypnotic agents in both its mechanism of action and its clinical effects. Ketamine produces a state of "**dissociative amnesia,**" referring to a dissociation occuring between the thalamocortical and limbic systems on electroencephalogram (EEG). Clinically, the result is a catatonic state in which the eyes often remain open, with obvious nystagmus. The patient may sporadically move, but nonpurposefully, and not generally in reaction to painful stimuli. **Ketamine produces excellent amnesia and is the only induction agent to also provide analgesia**. Ketamine may exert some of its analgesic properties via opioid receptors, although these effects are not consistently antagonized by naloxone.[18]

Ketamine has a centrally stimulating effect on the sympathetic nervous system (SNS) by decreasing catecholamine reuptake. These effects are responsible for many of the observed clinical effects. For example, via SNS stimulation, ketamine relaxes bronchial smooth muscle, in turn causing a decrease in airway resistance and improved pulmonary compliance. At higher doses, ketamine may also act **directly** to relax bronchial smooth muscle, although clinical benefit has not been clearly demonstrated.[18,19] These effects make ketamine a particularly **attractive agent for induction of the patient with acute bronchospasm**.

Ketamine tends to preserve ventilatory drive, although a large, rapidly administered bolus dose may still result in apnea. Ketamine may result in an increase in secretions, an effect which can be managed (although rarely indicated) by pretreatment with a drying agent such as glycopyrrolate or atropine. In addition, ketamine when used alone (i.e., not part of an RSI) has been associated with laryngospasm.[18,20] This may be more common in infants, to the extent that ketamine sedation may be contraindicated under 3 months of age.[20]

SNS stimulation is also responsible for an increase in heart rate (by about 20%) and blood pressure (a rise of around 25 mm Hg) with ketamine use. **Care should thus be exercised in patients with coronary artery disease,** as ketamine has the potential to aggravate myocardial ischemia. Due to its ability to raise blood pressure, it has been suggested that ketamine would be particularly suited for use in patients with unstable hemodynamics. It must be remembered, however, that the hemodynamic effects are secondary to SNS stimulation and that intrinsically, ketamine is in fact a myocardial depressant. Thus, ketamine could theoretically lower blood pressure in patients who are already maximally sympathetically stimulated. **Therefore, as with all induction sedative/hypnotics, caution should be used in patients with severe shock, and the induction dosage reduced.**

Much controversy has centered around the use of ketamine in patients with intracranial pathology. Historically, ketamine has been considered to be contraindicated in patients with decreased intracranial compliance due to reports that it could increase ICP and increase cerebral oxygen demand. However, the data upon which these recommendations were made did not involve patients with traumatic brain injury.[21] Indeed, more recent data using human and animal subjects suggest that low-dose bolus ketamine may have a beneficial effect on CPP in this setting.[21,22] When used in conjunction with a GABA agonist (such as propofol or midazolam), ketamine has actually been shown to lower ICP.[23] A cerebral protective effect has been shown with ketamine use in animals, possibly mediated through NMDA receptor blockade, and a similar effect is being investigated in humans and appears to show promise.[22] However, at this time, ketamine cannot be recommended for routine use in patients at risk of increased ICP, unless they also are also hypotensive (in relative or absolute terms), in which case ketamine's hemodynamic effects may help preserve CPP.

Ketamine has been associated with unpleasant emergence reactions characterized by "bad dreams," disorientation and perceptual disturbances.[18] This is relatively uncommon in children and seems in part to be related to the "state of mind" at the time of the drug's administration.[18,20,24] At least in children, this phenomenon is not reduced by concomitant administration of benzodiazepines.[18,20,24,25] Emergence reactions are not generally a consideration in the patient requiring RSI in emergencies.

Ketamine is supplied as either a 10 or 50 mg/mL solution. The induction dose of ketamine is 1-2 mg/kg as an IV bolus. Onset time is generally within 1 minute and clinical duration is 15–20 minutes. A lower dose should be used for the patient in profound shock. Conversely, the higher end of the dose range should be used if bronchodilation is the goal.

An "off-label" combination of ketamine with propofol (each in 10 mg/mL concentrations) drawn up in a single syringe ("ketafol") has been used in recent years, primarily for procedural sedation in emergency departments.[26,27] The mixture has also been used as an induction agent for RSI, with at least a theoretic advantage of maintenance of stable hemodynamics.

KETAMINE AS A SEDATIVE AGENT

Ketamine is usually administered as a single predetermined dose to achieve a state of disassociation. However, smaller doses of ketamine can be used as a sedative for awake intubation or "awake look" laryngoscopy in the uncooperative patient. Used in this way, in divided doses of 0.25–0.5 mg/kg, it has the advantage of maintained respiratory drive and good analgesia. However, it can also increase secretions, which as mentioned can increase the risk of laryngospasm, particularly in the pediatric patient. A theoretical risk of under-dosing relates to ketamine's use as a "street drug," where it may induce, or worsen an intoxicated, uncooperative state.

SUMMARY

Drug: Ketamine.

Drug type: Anesthetic induction agent, sedative/hypnotic, analgesic.

Indication: Induction of unconsciousness, especially for patients with severe bronchospasm or unstable hemodynamics. Sedative to facilitate non-RSI intubations.

Contraindications: Known coronary artery disease or an elevated ICP are relative contraindications (see text).

Dose: Dose is 1–2 mg/kg IV (average 75 kg = 100 mg).

Onset/Duration: Onset is within 60 seconds. Clinical duration is 15–20 minutes.

Potential Complications: Increase in heart rate (HR) and BP, with potential myocardial ischemia. Increase in ICP. Emergence reactions.

Etomidate

Etomidate is a sedative-hypnotic which has been available for use in the United States since 1983. Its mechanism of action probably involves GABA receptors, although it has a different drug-receptor interaction than that seen with the barbiturates and propofol. As with other induction agents, it has a predictably rapid onset and short duration of action (5–15 minutes following a standard induction dose). Etomidate has become the induction sedative/hypnotic of choice in many EDs throughout North America.[28]

Etomidate is remarkable for its hemodynamic stability.[29,30] This makes it particularly suited for RSI in the multitrauma patient. With the usual induction dose of 0.2–0.3 mg/kg there is generally no significant change in heart rate or reduction in blood pressure (BP). Even in the patient presenting with a systolic blood pressure below 100, use of etomidate for RSI appears to result in considerable hemodynamic stability.[30] Hypotension can occur, but does so with much less frequency compared to other agents, including midazolam.[31] In situations of extreme hypovolemia and/or hypotension, the dose of etomidate (as with all induction agents) should be reduced.

Spontaneous ventilation is better preserved with etomidate use than with the barbiturates, but apnea is still common after an induction dose. Ventilatory depression is more common when adjuvant agents (especially opioids) are used with etomidate. This is of little concern during an RSI.

Etomidate will lower ICP and decrease cerebral oxygen requirements. However, of some concern are a few studies indicating a worsening of cerebral ischemia with etomidate administration in operative patients undergoing subsequent temporary cerebral arterial occlusion.[13,32,33] These results at best suggest that etomidate does not have a neuroprotective effect. In the patient at risk for cerebral ischemia, this knowledge must be balanced against etomidate's upside of hemodynamic stability and potential for maintenance of cerebral perfusion pressure.

Etomidate can cause myoclonus but has not been shown to induce seizures.[34] It does not have any analgesic properties and does not block the pressor response to intubation. In patients in whom a blood pressure increase is a concern (e.g., the patient with a cerebral aneurysm) use of adjunctive agents may be considered to block this response. Other side effects may include pain on injection and nausea and vomiting on emergence.[34]

Much of the debate surrounding etomidate use in the critically ill patient surrounds its potential to cause adrenal suppression. Initially thought to be relevant only in patients receiving maintenance infusions, it has now been clearly demonstrated, lasting from 12–24 hours, following a single dose.[35] Historically, the clinical relevance of this was not clear, and proponents of etomidate argued that the benefits of hemodynamic stability during RSI outweighed the risks of adrenal suppression. However, the debate has been rekindled by the potential clinical significance of adrenal suppression in the septic patient.[36,37] In this population, steroid replacement therapy has been shown to have a survival benefit.[39] As such, concern has been raised that additional adrenal suppression caused by etomidate in already suppressed septic patients could lead to a worse outcome.[40] Conflicting data exists on the induction agent choice in patients with septic shock.[38] Until further evidence is available, it appears prudent to avoid etomidate use in the sepsis population as long as appropriate alternative agents are available. If etomidate *is* used in a septic patient, this should be communicated to the critical care team. In such cases a baseline cortisol level and a cosyntropin stimulation test (CST) should be performed to guide subsequent critical care decisions on replacement therapy.[33] Although the suggestion has been made that steroids be empirically administered in replacement doses until these laboratory results are available, there is little prospective evidence to support the practice at this time.[36,41]

Clinicians should be aware of these risk/benefit issues when considering the use of etomidate. As the status of etomidate as a "one drug fits all" induction agent has been questioned, further study of its safety in the critically ill patient is needed.

ETOMIDATE AS A SEDATIVE AGENT

Etomidate is being used increasingly as an alternative to propofol for sedation in the ED.[42] However, even in low doses, it can cause vomiting and myoclonus. As with propofol, use of etomidate for deep sedation to facilitate endotracheal intubation will not provide conditions as favorable as those using RSI with a muscle relaxant.

SUMMARY

Drug: Etomidate.

Drug type: Anesthetic induction agent, sedative/hypnotic.

Indication: Induction of unconsciousness, especially in patients with unstable hemodynamics.

Contraindications: Known hypersensitivity. Septic shock is a relative contraindication.

Dose: Dose is 0.2–0.3 mg/kg IV (average 75 kg = 20mg).

Onset/Duration: Onset is within 30 seconds. Clinical duration is 5–10 minutes.

Potential Complications: Hypotension and apnea. Adrenal suppression.

▶ ADJUNCTIVE AGENTS

Adjunctive agents are usually given in the "pretreatment" phase of an RSI, or used to facilitate an awake intubation (or "awake look" laryngoscopy). The evidence supporting use of these pretreatment agents in RSI is relatively poor. When performing an RSI, it is important to keep in mind that the pharmacologic goal is to rapidly and safely induce a state of unconsciousness and paralysis to facilitate endotracheal intubation. The use of additional medications may or may not always be necessary, warranted, or desirable.

Benzodiazepines

The benzodiazepines (BDZs) are sedative-hypnotic drugs that exert their main effect via GABA receptors in the CNS. The effect of this binding is dose-related and includes sedation, anxiolysis, amnesia, and centrally mediated muscle relaxation. At low doses the effect is mainly sedation, anxiolysis and amnesia, while higher doses can be employed to induce general anesthesia. Of note, the BDZs do not have primary analgesic properties. All BDZs act in a similar manner, with the main differences related to their individual pharmacokinetic properties. The effects of the BDZs may be reversed by **Flumazenil** (Anexate®), a specific BDZ receptor antagonist.

Used alone and in low doses, BDZs usually have minimal effect on hemodynamics. However, although they do not appear to act directly as myocardial depressants, they may reduce SNS tone and secondarily result in a blood pressure drop. This effect may be significant if high sympathetic tone is a predominant factor in preserving blood pressure.

The BDZs may also cause respiratory depression. This is rarely a problem if used alone in low doses for sedation, although higher doses can result in apnea. Both the cardiovascular and respiratory side effects are more pronounced if BDZs are used in conjunction with other agents, such as opioids.

Clinician familiarity with these drugs has made them a common choice for sedation in patients undergoing airway management.

Midazolam

Midazolam has become a popular agent for sedation in the setting of emergency airway management. It has also been used as an induction agent to facilitate RSI both in the ED and the prehospital setting.[31,43,44]

Compared to its predecessor diazepam (Valium®), midazolam is 2–3 times more potent, has a faster onset and shorter time to recovery. Clinical effect is generally seen approximately 1–2 minutes following an IV bolus. Onset time is dose-dependent and can be shortened by using larger doses. Although quick, midazolam's onset time is still substantially slower than that of the induction sedative/hypnotics previously discussed.[45] In addition, compared to other induction agents, midazolam does not produce unconsciousness with the same degree of predictability.[45] These reasons, together with potential adverse effects on blood pressure, limit the usefulness of midazolam as an induction agent.

The general anesthetic induction dose of midazolam is 0.1–0.3 mg/kg. This equates to 7–21 mg of midazolam for a 70-kg adult. At these higher doses, the onset time is quicker, but still not as rapid as the previously discussed induction agents. Clinicians frequently under-dose midazolam when using it as an induction agent.[44]

There is a misconception that midazolam is hemodynamically benign. In fact, data exists showing that midazolam causes dose-related hypotension when used for RSI.[46] Even at low doses, compared with etomidate, hypotension occurs much more frequently with midazolam use for RSI.[31]

Smaller doses of midazolam may be used for sedation, especially if used in conjunction with other drugs. The recommended dose range for light sedation is 0.025–0.05 mg/kg, with the higher doses used to sedate the already intubated patient (e.g., 2–5 mg for the average adult). To avoid oversedation, one should wait *at least* 2 minutes between doses.

In airway management, the primary role of midazolam is as a light sedative for the patient undergoing an awake intubation. Although its slower onset time limits the drug's usefulness as a primary induction agent for RSI, it can be used as a co-induction agent to help ensure amnesia. Midazolam may also be useful in providing post-intubation sedation and amnesia.

Midazolam is supplied as either 1 mg/mL or 5 mg/mL concentrations, in a variety of vial sizes. **Flumazenil** can be used to reverse the effect of benzodiazepines (e.g., 0.3 mg, repeating 0.5 mg q 1 minute to maximum of 3 mg). Flumazenil should be avoided in conditions that predispose the patient to seizures.

SUMMARY

Drug: Midazolam.

Drug type: Benzodiazepine. Sedative, anxiolytic, hypnotic.

Indications: Sedation, amnesia, anxiolysis, co-induction agent.

Contraindications: Uncorrected shock states are relative contraindications that require a decrease in dose.

Dose: Dose is 0.025–0.05 mg/kg IV for sedation, and 0.1–0.3 mg/kg IV for induction.

Onset/Duration: Onset is 1–2 minutes. Clinical duration is 15–20 minutes.

Potential Complications: Hypotension and apnea.

Butyrophenones

Butyrophenones, including **haloperidol** and **droperidol** are phenothiazine-like agents with a long history of clinical use. In the context of airway management, they can sometimes be used for "chemical restraint," whereby an otherwise mildly uncooperative patient may be rendered outwardly tranquil, immobile, and apparently indifferent to the surroundings. Although theoretically of use in facilitating an "awake" intubation, these agents are less likely to be successful in the actively uncooperative, critically ill patient in need of emergency airway management.

Haloperidol

Haloperidol can be used by intravenous or intramuscular routes. To help control an unruly patient, it is commonly used in combination with a benzodiazepine.

SUMMARY

Drug: Haloperidol.

Drug type: Antipsychotic/sedative.

Indication: Chemical restraint.

Contraindications: Hypersensitivity; Parkinson's disease.

Dose: Dose is 2–5 mg IV, repeated *prn*. Intramuscular (IM) dose is 5–10 mg. May be combined with midazolam or lorazepam in a ratio of 5:1 (e.g., haloperidol 5 mg/ lorazepam 1 mg).

Onset/Duration: Onset is within 5 minutes (intravenous) or 20 minutes (intramuscular). Clinical duration is 1–2 hours.

Potential Complications: Extrapyramidal effects; hypotension and dysrhythmias (rarely).

Dexmedetomidine

Dexmedetomidine is a relatively new alpha-2 receptor agonist, currently approved for sedation in an intensive care setting. Delivered by infusion in an initial dose of 1 μg/kg over 10 minutes, followed by ongoing infusion at 0.2–0.7 μg/kg/h, it is remarkable for not significantly suppressing ventilatory drive. Case reports and series[47, 48] are appearing on its use to facilitate awake intubations in the OR setting. In time, its use for this indication may expand to the uncooperative patient outside the OR.

Opioids

The term *opiate* refers to the group of drugs derived from opium, while *opioid* refers to all exogenous substances that bind to opioid receptors. There are four main classes of opioid receptor, and multiple subclasses within each class.

The major effect of opioids is to produce dose-dependent analgesia and sedation. The major side effects are also mediated by receptor binding and include respiratory depression, pruritis, and ileus. Nausea and vomiting are also important side effects of the opioids, but may not necessarily be related to specific receptor binding. It is important to remember that the **opioids do not possess intrinsic amnestic properties, nor do they cause muscle relaxation.**

Opioid medications cause a dose-dependent decrease in minute ventilation, primarily by a decrease in respiratory rate. Large or bolus doses may result in apnea, especially when used in conjunction with other sedatives. Opioids blunt airway reflexes (especially the cough reflex) in a dose-dependent fashion.

Opioids do not decrease myocardial contractility, nor do they directly cause a decrease in blood pressure. They may, however, result in hypotension secondary to a decrease in sympathetic tone. As with the BDZs, caution should be exercised in the patient running on "sympathetic overdrive."

Although opioids blunt the hemodynamic response to intubation, the dosages required for complete blunting tend to be large. Opioids do not intrinsically raise ICP, however by causing the spontaneously breathing patient to hypoventilate, they can cause a secondary rise in $PaCO_2$, in turn resulting in a rise in ICP. The effects of the opioids can be reversed with **naloxone**, a specific opioid receptor antagonist.

Narcotics as an Adjunct to Awake Intubation

Small doses of narcotics such as fentanyl may be a useful adjunct to "awake" intubation. As potent analgesics, narcotics help attenuate the discomfort associated with laryngoscopy, and also help obtund the cough reflex to insertion of the endotracheal tube in the trachea. Fentanyl used in this capacity can be given in doses of 25–50 μg (in an average-sized adult) at a time, repeated as needed. The newer short-acting narcotic **Remifentanil** is making inroads as an adjunct to awake intubation in the OR, delivered in small bolus doses and/or by infusion.

Morphine

Morphine is the prototypical opioid agent. Although it is an excellent analgesic, it has several features that make it unattractive as a pharmacologic aid in airway management. It has a relatively slow onset time, taking up to 15 minutes for peak effect following an IV injection. In addition, morphine can result in histamine release, making it undesirable for use in patients with asthma, and contributing to a tendency to drop blood pressure. Morphine's role in airway management is essentially limited to postintubation sedation and analgesia.

SUMMARY
Drug: Morphine.
Drug type: Opioid analgesic.
Indication: Analgesia.
Contraindications: Uncorrected shock states are relative contraindications; if used, a decrease in dose will be required.
Dose: Dose is 0.05–0.1 mg/kg IV (average 75 kg = 5 mg).
Onset/Duration: Onset is within 5–15 minutes. Clinical duration is 1–2 hours.
Potential Complications: Hypotension and apnea. Histamine release.

Fentanyl

Fentanyl is a synthetic opioid agent that is significantly more potent than morphine. It results in minimal histamine release and has a rapid onset (30–60 seconds after an IV bolus) and relatively short duration of action. These features make it a suitable adjunct for RSI.

To completely block the pressor response to laryngoscopy and intubation, relatively large doses (≥6 µg/kg[49–51]) of fentanyl are needed. These larger doses are rarely used for emergency intubations, due to concerns of potential hemodynamic compromise. Large doses of fentanyl may also cause bradycardia secondary to a blunting of the baroreceptor heart rate reflex, although this bradycardia will respond to atropine, if necessary. If used as an adjunctive medication for RSI, fentanyl is generally given in the pretreatment phase, before administration of the induction sedative/hypnotic. In this context, 1–3 µg/kg of fentanyl has been shown to somewhat attenuate the hemodynamic and respiratory responses to intubation.[49, 51, 52] The theoretic value of this pretreatment effect must be balanced against the potential hemodynamic and respiratory consequences (e.g., premature hypoxia) in the at-risk patient. Fentanyl is supplied as a 50 µg/mL solution and is available in a variety of vial sizes.

SUMMARY
Drug: Fentanyl.
Drug type: Opioid analgesic.
Indication: Analgesia. Sedation.
Contraindications: Uncorrected shock states are relative contraindications; if used, a decrease in dose is required.
Dose: Dose is 1–3 µg/kg IV. (Average pretreatment dose 75 kg = 150 µg)
Onset/Duration: Onset is less than 1 minute. Clinical duration is 1 hour.
Potential complications: Apnea. Hypotension.

Lidocaine

Lidocaine as Pretreatment Agent

Intravenous lidocaine has been espoused as a pretreatment agent to block the pressor response, attenuate the rise in ICP, and suppress the cough or bronchospastic reflex that may accompany laryngoscopy and intubation.[53] However, a number of reports have questioned the benefit of IV lidocaine for these indications.[54–56] Certainly there is no clear evidence of its benefit as a pretreatment agent for RSI in head-injured patients,[56] although it is possible that future work may reveal a neuroprotective effect.[13] While lidocaine may inhibit the cough reflex, compelling evidence of its efficacy as a pretreatment agent in the bronchospastic patient is similarly lacking, although it is probably not harmful. If attenuation of the pressor response to laryngoscopy and intubation is important, alternatives to IV lidocaine include an appropriate dose of induction sedative/hypnotic, together with pretreatment using a potent opioid or a short-acting beta-blocker such as esmolol.[54,55] Caution must be used with these latter approaches, to avoid hypotension in at-risk patients.

Lidocaine for Airway Anesthesia Applied Topically or by Regional Nerve Block

Lidocaine is the mainstay of topically-applied airway anesthesia for awake intubation in many institutions. Many formulations of lidocaine exist, including jelly, ointment, viscous, and liquid, in varying concentrations. Lidocaine can be applied topically to the airway by "gargle and swish" of the liquid and/or viscous formulations; tongue depressor application of the ointment or gel to the tongue; cotton pledgets held in forceps to access deeper structures such as the piriform recesses; atomizer or metered-dose sprayer; or direct injection through the cricothyroid membrane. The injectable formulation (e.g., 2%) can be used for regional percutaneous nerve blocks.

SUMMARY

Drug: Lidocaine.

Drug type: Local anesthetic.

Indication: Intravenous: Historically, attenuation of pressor response or cough reflex to intubation. **Applied topically, via cricothyroid injection or percutaneous nerve block:** Airway anesthesia for awake intubation.

Contraindications: Hypersensitivity to amide-type local anesthetics.

Dose—IV use: Dose is 1–1.5 mg/kg IV (average 75 kg = 100 mg).

Onset/Duration: Onset is 1–3 minutes. Duration is ~ 20 minutes.

Potential Complications: Symptoms of local anesthetic toxicity. Hypotension. Seizures.

Atropine

Atropine is an anticholinergic agent. More specifically, it is an antimuscarinic agent, meaning that it blocks the effects of acetylcholine at muscarinic receptors. These receptors are found in the heart, salivary glands, and the smooth muscle of the respiratory, gastrointestinal (GI), and genitourinary (GU) tracts. Clinically, atropine results in an increase in heart rate, decrease in secretions, and potential bronchodilation. In toxic doses, atropine can exert a central effect and cause sedation, amnesia, and confusion (i.e., central anticholinergic syndrome).

Historically, atropine was administered almost universally as a preinduction agent to protect against excessive vagal responses to induction and intubation. With currently available drugs, this is rarely necessary in adult patients. In fact, there is limited data to support this practice

even in pediatrics, and its routine use has been questioned.[57–60] In a study performed at a large pediatric ED, atropine pretreatment had no effect on the incidence of bradycardia post-RSI.[60] Although still widely used as a pretreatment agent in infant RSI, the lack of evidence documenting its efficacy in preventing laryngoscopy and intubation-related bradydysrhythmias, together with its potential adverse effects do not support its use outside the context of administration of a second dose of succinylcholine.[57,58] If used, the recommended dose in pediatric practice is 0.01–0.02 mg/kg, with a minimum dose of 0.1 mg and a maximum dose of 1 mg.

Regardless of whether a practitioner adheres to these guidelines, atropine should be immediately available in the event that the patient develops symptomatic bradycardia following intubation. It is also recommended that atropine be used in both adults and children prior to giving a second dose of succinylcholine (discussed in the next section).

SUMMARY

Drug: Atropine.

Drug type: Anticholinergic/antimuscarinic.

Indication: Bradycardia. Prophylaxis prior to repeated doses of succinylcholine or historically, pretreatment in pediatrics.

Contraindications: Glaucoma is a relative contraindication, as is any situation in which tachycardia may be undesirable.

Dose: Dose is .01–.02 mg/kg IV (average 75 kg = 0.5 –1 mg).

Onset/Duration: Onset is within 1 minute. Clinical duration is 20–30 minutes.

Potential Complications: Tachycardia. Central anticholinergic syndrome.

Defasciculating Agents

The issues surrounding the administration of small doses of nondepolarizing muscle relaxants to suppress muscle fasciculation associated with succinylcholine use are discussed in the upcoming section on succinylcholine.

► NEUROMUSCULAR BLOCKERS (MUSCLE RELAXANTS)

The use of muscle relaxants to facilitate RSI has become standard practice in most of the larger EDs throughout North America.[61] As discussed elsewhere in the text, there is now ample evidence to demonstrate the increased success and safety with this technique.[62] However, it remains critically important for practitioners who administer neuromuscular blockers as part of an RSI to be very knowledgeable in all their effects (intended and adverse) and to be skilled in the mechanics of airway management.

There are two classes of muscle relaxant: depolarizing and nondepolarizing. Succinylcholine remains the only depolarizing agent available for clinical use. While there are many non-depolarizing agents on the market, when given in conventional doses, only rocuronium is appropriate for RSI, due to its rapid onset.

Depolarizing Muscle Relaxants: Succinylcholine

Succinylcholine is a commonly used neuromuscular blocker for RSI in emergencies. It has multiple side effects, some of which, although extremely rare, are potentially serious. Notwithstanding, succinylcholine remains in widespread use, for three reasons: (a) it has a very rapid onset; (b) it usually has a very short duration of action, and (c) many clinicians are familiar with its use.

Succinylcholine works by mimicking the effects of acetylcholine on receptors at the neuromuscular junction, causing membrane depolarization. Unlike acetylcholine, succinylcholine remains bound to these receptors for a substantially longer time, thereby preventing normal repolarization of the muscle membrane. This results clinically in a short period of muscle fasciculation, followed by skeletal muscle relaxation. The succinylcholine molecules dissociate from the acetylcholine receptors after several minutes, whereupon they are rapidly metabolized by pseudocholinesterase in the blood stream. The duration of muscle relaxation following a single dose of 1–2 mg/kg is typically 5–10 minutes, although initial return of spontaneous respiration will often occur in less than 5 minutes.

Adequate intubating conditions are consistently achieved in less than 1 minute following an IV bolus 1–2 mg/kg of succinylcholine. When dosing succinylcholine, it is better to err on the side of giving a larger dose, as the majority of the adverse reactions are not dose dependent and the larger dose assures rapid onset and good skeletal muscle relaxation. The short duration of action is a potential benefit in the OR setting, where it may be possible to awaken the patient if intubation proves to be impossible. However, this is usually not an option for patients requiring intubation in emergencies, thus making the short duration of action less beneficial in this setting. In addition, it should be noted that following a dose of 1 mg/kg of succinylcholine, resumption of spontaneous ventilation will not necessarily occur quickly enough to prevent critical oxygen desaturation if a failed oxygenation ("can't intubate/can't oxygenate") situation develops.[63]

Some data suggests that smaller doses (e.g., 0.6 mg/kg) of succinylcholine can produce intubating conditions equivalent to those obtained with conventional doses, but with the advantage of an earlier return of spontaneous ventilation.[64,65] However, onset of paralysis may be delayed and, as mentioned, the clinical significance of an early return to spontaneous respirations in the emergency setting is not clear.

Succinylcholine administration can result in a transient rise (0.5–1 mEq/L) of serum potassium. This is of little consequence in most individuals. However, in patients presenting with preexisting hyperkalemia, this additional rise may be enough to cause electrocardiographic changes, or even result in asystole.

Damaged or denervated muscle may respond by developing new acetylcholine receptors that are located outside the neuromuscular junction. Stimulation of these extrajunctional receptors by succinylcholine may result in an exaggerated release of potassium from the muscle, and induce hyperkalemic cardiac arrest.[66] **Patients with major crush injuries, burns, stroke, or spinal cord injuries may exhibit this exaggerated release of potassium.** However, as it takes at least 24 hours for injured muscle to express new receptors, these patients are generally not at risk when they initially present as emergencies. The duration of the sensitivity is unclear and may in part depend on the extent of abnormal tissue.[66] Patients with certain genetic muscular disorders such as muscular dystrophy may also respond to succinylcholine administration with an exaggerated release of potassium. In clinical situations where this response may occur, or if an elevated potassium level may already exist (e.g., a patient with known history of renal failure requiring intubation before blood chemistry results are available), an alternative to succinylcholine should be used.

Succinylcholine may cause cardiac dysrhythmias. Bradydysrhythmias are most common and are more likely following a repeat dose of succinylcholine. In this regard, it is recommended that **atropine be administered prior to giving a second dose of succinylcholine**, even in a tachycardic patient.

Succinylcholine has been shown to increase intraocular pressure (IOP). However, in patients with open eye injuries, no adverse effects from succinylcholine administration have been reported, despite extensive use.[67] Coughing and straining during intubation will raise intraocular pressure significantly more than succinylcholine use alone. Rocuronium may be a better choice for patients with open-eye injuries, in that during RSI, compared to succinylcholine, it has been shown to significantly decrease the percentage of change from baseline IOP.[68]

Although published study results are contradictory, succinylcholine may cause an increase in ICP. Any rise in ICP does not appear to be related to muscle fasciculations, and is more likely due to an increase in afferent activity caused by muscle spindle firing. However, while succinylcholine may cause a transient rise in ICP in brain tumor patients, there is no direct evidence that succinylcholine similarly increases the ICP of brain-injured patients.[69] In brain tumor patients undergoing elective surgery, two studies have shown an attenuation of a succinylcholine-induced rise in ICP with nondepolarizing agent pretreatment.[70, 71] However, to date there is no similar data supporting the use of defasciculating agents prior to succinylcholine use in brain-injured patients. In practice, succinylcholine is commonly used to facilitate intubation in this population.[72]

Succinylcholine is a known trigger for **malignant hyperthermia** (MH). MH is an inherited metabolic disease of skeletal muscle. When susceptible individuals are exposed to succinylcholine and/or volatile anesthetics they may "trigger" this life-threatening condition. MH is characterized by generalized muscle contractions, tachycardia, hypercarbia, tachypnea, hypoxia, mixed respiratory and metabolic acidosis, arrhythmias, and (a late sign), hyperthermia. **Dantrolene** (starting at 2.5 mg/kg) is the definitive treatment and should be administered early when the diagnosis is suspected, in conjunction with supportive management. Fortunately, MH is rare, occurring in 1 in 50,000 adult anesthetics, although the susceptibility in the general population may be as high as 1 in 2000.[73]

Succinylcholine may result in **masseter muscle rigidity** (MMR). This is more common in children and occurs most often when used in conjunction with a volatile anesthetic, although it has also been described in the ED setting.[74] Generally, this rigidity can be overcome, and it usually subsides spontaneously in 2–3 minutes. MMR may be associated with MH.

The effects of succinylcholine will be prolonged in patients who have abnormal pseudocholinesterase. In the most severe form of pseudocholinesterase deficiency, the effects of succinylcholine may last 6–12 hours.

Other adverse effects possible with succinylcholine use include histamine release and the potential for allergic reactions. Succinylcholine has been associated with generalized myalgias after administration, although this phenomenon is usually not relevant in the patient requiring emergency intubation. These myalgias occur more frequently in young people with a large muscle mass. It may be related to fasciculations but is not reliably prevented by pretreatment with a nondepolarizing agent.[75]

The issue of pretreatment with a small dose (one-tenth of an intubating dose) of nondepolarizing muscle relaxant prior to succinylcholine administration remains unclear. Pretreatment in this fashion **does not protect** against MH, MMR, hyperkalemia, dysrhythmias, or prolonged muscle relaxation secondary to pseudocholinesterase deficiency. The effect on ICP is unknown but is likely of little clinical significance.[69] Pretreatment does necessitate a larger dose of succinylcholine (1.5 mg/kg) and may decrease the quality of muscle relaxation achieved.[72] Pretreatment also adds another step to the RSI process and adds the potential for premature muscle relaxation, especially if a larger dose is given in error.

Succinylcholine provides rapid onset of skeletal muscle relaxation allowing for excellent intubating conditions, with rapid offset. However, as outlined above, it is also a drug with a number of potentially serious side effects. Before using succinylcholine, the clinician must be familiar with contraindications to its use.

SUMMARY

Drug: Succinylcholine.

Drug type: Depolarizing muscle relaxant.

Indication: Skeletal muscle relaxation for RSI.

Contraindications: Predicted inability to either mask ventilate or intubate. Hyperkalemia. Malignant hyperthermia. Patients 24 hours or more postburn or denervation injury. Pseudocholinesterase deficiency is a relative contraindication.

Dose: Dose is 1–2 mg/kg IV (average 75 kg = 120 mg).

Onset/Duration: Onset is less than 1 minute. Clinical duration is 5–10 minutes.

Potential Complications: Hypoxia, hypercarbia, hyperkalemic arrest, malignant hyperthermia, prolonged paralysis, myalgias.

Nondepolarizing Muscle Relaxants

The nondepolarizing muscle relaxants act as competitive antagonists to acetylcholine at the neuromuscular junction. They do not stimulate acetylcholine receptors: rather, they block the binding of acetylcholine. Their effects may be antagonized by increasing the concentration of acetylcholine at the neuromuscular junction with agents that inhibit acetylcholine breakdown (see section on neuromuscular blocker reversal agents). Their side effect profile is fairly limited and the main differences between the agents relate to pharmacodynamics.

Rocuronium

Rocuronium is being used with increasing frequency in the emergency setting as part of RSI and when indicated, for post-intubation neuromuscular blockade. In larger doses (e.g., 1 mg/kg), it has a similar onset time and produces intubating conditions comparable to those achieved following a 1 mg/kg dose of succinylcholine.[76] However, this dose of rocuronium will produce clinical paralysis that may last up to 1 hour. While the extended duration of action may cause anxiety in some clinicians, others prefer this longer period of neuromuscular blockade as it produces good conditions for BMV and repeat intubation attempts, should difficulty be encountered (See Table 9–1, Chap. 9). In addition, the use of rocuronium avoids the need to consider the many contraindications and precautions associated with succinylcholine use. Smaller doses of rocuronium may be used to maintain relaxation in the postintubation period, if needed.

Rocuronium is devoid of cardiac effects. It is supplied as a 10 mg/mL solution in a 5 mL vial.

SUMMARY

Drug: Rocuronium.

Drug type: Nondepolarizing muscle relaxant.

Indication: Skeletal muscle relaxation for RSI, or post-intubation paralysis.

Contraindications: Predicted inability to either bag-mask ventilate or intubate.

Dose: Dose is 1 mg/kg IV (average 75 kg = 80 mg).

Onset/Duration: Onset is within 1–1.5 minutes. Clinical duration is 45–80 minutes, depending on dose administered.

Potential Complications: Hypoxia, hypercarbia. Pain on injection.

Vecuronium

Vecuronium is an intermediate-acting nondepolarizing muscle relaxant. An intubating dose of 0.1 mg/kg will produce adequate intubating conditions within 3 minutes, with effects lasting about 45 minutes. Larger doses of up to 0.3 mg/kg may decrease the onset time required to intubate to 1.5 minutes, however clinical relaxation may persist for up to 3 hours. Vecuronium has no cardiac effects and does not stimulate histamine release. Since the introduction of rocuronium, the role of vecuronium in airway management is limited largely to postintubation management.

Vecuronium is supplied as a powder and must be reconstituted with water or saline to produce a solution of either 1 or 2 mg/kg.

SUMMARY

Drug: Vecuronium.

Drug type: Nondepolarizing muscle relaxant.

Indication: Skeletal muscle relaxation post-intubation.

Contraindications: Predicted inability to either bag mask ventilate or intubate.

Dose: Intubating dose is 0.1–0.3 mg/kg IV (average 75 kg = 8 mg initially; 2–4 mg for maintenance of post-intubation paralysis).

Onset/Duration: Onset is within 1.5–3 minutes. Clinical duration is 45–90 minutes, depending on dose.

Potential complications: Hypoxia, hypercarbia.

Pancuronium

Pancuronium is a long-acting nondepolarizing muscle relaxant with a relatively slow onset of action. Clinical relaxation lasts at least an hour. Pancuronium has fallen out of favor with many clinicians due to concerns of residual subclinical paralysis that may increase post-operative respiratory complications when used in the OR setting.

Pancuronium consistently causes an increase in heart rate and rarely, may result in dysrhythmias. This effect may make pancuronium an undesirable agent for use in patients with coronary artery disease, as well as other patients in whom tachycardia is considered an important early warning of hemodynamic decompensation.

Pancuronium has no role to play in RSI because of its slow onset. It can be considered for post-intubation paralysis if the duration of paralysis is not of concern.

Pancuronium is supplied as a 2 mg/ml solution.

SUMMARY

Drug: Pancuronium

Drug type: Nondepolarizing muscle relaxant.

Indication: Pretreatment agent before succinylcholine administration. Skeletal muscle relaxation post-intubation.

Contraindications: Predicted inability to either bag-mask ventilate or intubate.

Dose: Intubating dose is 0.1 mg/kg IV (average 75 kg = 8 mg initially; 1–2 mg for maintenance of post-intubation paralysis). As a pretreatment agent before succinylcholine, .01 mg/kg (average = 0.5–1.0 mg).

Onset/Duration: Onset is within 5 minutes. Clinical duration is 60–90 minutes.

Potential Complications: Hypoxia, hypercarbia, tachycardia.

▶ OTHER AGENTS

Neuromuscular Blockade Reversal Agents

Residual effects of the nondepolarizing agents may be reversed by administration of an anticholinesterase agent. However, it must be appreciated that **a substantial amount of spontaneous recovery must already have occurred before these drugs can be used to reverse the residual paralyzing effects of a nondepolarizing agent.** Ideally, this is determined by use of a nerve stimulator monitor. The time required for this initial spontaneous recovery is dose-dependent and depends on the relaxant used, but tends to be at least 20–30 minutes. This is obviously too long to wait for return of spontaneous ventilation should intubation and oxygenation prove impossible.

Neuromuscular reversal agents are rarely used in the context of emergency airway management. Their one possible use may be to reverse residual neuromuscular blockade in the already intubated patient in order to facilitate a complete neurologic assessment.

These agents inhibit acetylcholinesterase throughout the body and therefore result in an accumulation of acetylcholine at both muscarinic and nicotinic receptors (at the neuromuscular junction). The effects on the muscarinic receptors cause a predictable decrease in heart rate, increased secretions and gut mobility, and pupillary constriction. Therefore, concurrent administration of an antimuscarinic agent such as atropine or glycopyrrolate should occur, which will help limit the clinical effects of these agents, as desired, to the neuromuscular junction.

A new compound not on the market at the time of publication of this text is **Sugammadex (Org 25969; modified gamma-cyclodextrin)**. This drug looks promising as a rapid-reversal agent for rocuronium, even from deep levels of neuromuscular blockade.[77–80]

The drug works by chemically "encapsulating" rocuronium molecules, thus dissociating them from the acetylcholine receptor and thereby reversing the neuromuscular blockade.[78, 81] Early studies suggest that it will be able to reverse profound rocuronium-induced neuromuscular blockade within 3 minutes.[79,80,82] This effect is confined to rocuronium and when tested has not worked with atracurium or mivacurium,[79] two other nondepolarizing neuromuscular blockers. The drug is hemodynamically inert,[78] and no concomitant use of an anticholinergic agent is needed.[81] The potential of this agent to rapidly reverse neuromuscular blockade induced by rocuronium in failed oxygenation (can't intubate/can't oxygenate) situations may add an additional layer of safety to RSI.

Neostigmine and Edrophonium

Neostigmine and edrophonium are two anticholinesterase agents commonly used by anesthesiologists to reverse residual muscle paralysis in surgical patients. Neostigmine is the more commonly used agent, combined with atropine or glycopyrrolate. Exceeding the recommended maximal dose may actually result in a more prolonged neuromuscular block. Edrophonium has a somewhat more rapid onset than neostigmine, and is used in a dose of 0.5–1.0 mg/kg, also with concomitant atropine or glycopyrrolate administration.

SUMMARY

Drug: Neostigmine.

Drug type: Anticholinesterase.

Indication: Reversal of residual nondepolarizing agent neuromuscular blockade.

Contraindications: Complete neuromuscular blockade without any spontaneous recovery.

Dose: Dose is 0.04–0.06 mg/kg IV (average 75 kg = 3–5 mg, used with concomitant atropine 1–2 mg or glycopyrrolate 0.6–1.0 mg).

Onset/Duration: Onset is within 1.5–3 minutes. Clinical duration is several hours.

Potential Complications: Bradycardia. Abdominal discomfort.

Vasopressors and Inotropes (Rescue Drugs)

A decrease in blood pressure is not uncommon following induction and intubation. Reasons for this include:

- Direct negative inotropic and peripherally vasodilating effects of pretreatment agents and/or induction sedative/hypnotics.
- Decreased venous return secondary to initiation of positive pressure ventilation, accentuated by the volume-depleted state of many patients requiring emergency intubation.
- Relief of high sympathetic tone from administration of anxiolytic/sedative medications.
- Less commonly, a tension pneumothorax, particularly in the setting of trauma, or in patients with lung disease.

The presence of preexisting hypovolemia will make any of the above effects more pronounced. **The initial response to hypotension of almost any cause should be volume expansion** (e.g., 10–20 mL/kg). This should be followed by a quick clinical assessment, looking for a correctable etiology. However, because of hypotension-associated morbidity/mortality (e.g., in the head-injured patient), administration of a temporizing corrective medication may be beneficial while a cause is sought. Examples include short-acting vasopressors such as ephedrine and phenylephrine. Many clinicians espouse having at least one of these two drugs diluted and ready for administration during *every* RSI.

Ephedrine

Ephedrine is a vasopressor which acts indirectly on alpha-1 receptors by causing noradrenaline release, and directly, through action on beta adrenergic receptors. It is commonly used in the OR, although its use in out-of-OR emergency intubations is less well established. It results in an increase in heart rate and blood pressure. In doses of 5–10 mg IV, it may be useful to temporarily support the blood pressure while the effects of the induction sedative/hypnotic wear off and any volume deficit is corrected. Ephedrine's effects generally last 5–10 minutes. This temporary support may be particularly important in head-injured patients, where even transient hypotension can lead to worsened outcome. If there is no improvement after 20–25 mg, then the etiology of the hypotension should be reexamined and the need for a more potent vasopressor or inotrope (e.g., phenylephrine, dopamine, or epinephrine) should be considered. Ephedrine is supplied as 50 mg in a 1 mL ampoule. It should be diluted before use to a concentration of 5 mg/mL, for example, by adding the contents of the vial to 9 mL of saline in a 10 cc syringe.

SUMMARY

Drug: Ephedrine.

Drug type: Vasopressor.

Indication: To attain a transient increase in blood pressure.

Contraindications: Elevated BP and/or heart rate. Contraindicated in the presence of monoamine oxidase (MAO) inhibitors.

Dose: Dose is 5–10 mg IV.

Onset/Duration: Onset is within 1 minute. Clinical duration is 5–10 minutes.

Potential Complications: Tachycardia. Hypertension. Aggravation of myocardial ischemia. Tachyphylaxis, that is, repeat doses will be less effective.

Phenylephrine

As a direct-acting alpha agonist, phenylephrine is **a potent peripheral vasoconstrictor. It causes an increase in blood pressure with no direct effect on heart rate**. However, a reflex slowing of heart rate is often seen due to baroreceptor stimulation by the increase in systemic blood pressure. Phenylephrine is a very potent vasopressor and is supplied in a highly concentrated form (10 mg in a 1-mL vial). **It must be diluted prior to use.** The 10 mg/1 mL vial can be diluted by injecting its contents into a 100 mL bag of saline to yield a 100 µg/mL solution, or the same vial injected into a 250 mL bag will yield a 40 µg/mL solution. It is typically administered in doses starting at 40–100 µg IV. Onset is within 1 minute, and the dose can be doubled every 1–2 minutes, titrating to effect. As with ephedrine, its effect lasts about 5–10 minutes. Both drugs are commonly used in the OR setting.

Phenylephrine as a vasopressor may be preferable for use in the patient in whom an increase in heart rate is undesirable (e.g., a patient with ischemic heart disease).

SUMMARY

Drug: Phenylephrine.

Drug type: Vasopressor.

Indication: To attain a transient increase in blood pressure.

Contraindications: Elevated BP.

Dose: 40–100 µg IV.

Onset/Duration: Onset is within 1 minute. Clinical duration is 5–10 minutes.

Potential Complications: Bradycardia. Hypertension. Aggravation of myocardial ischemia.

Dantrolene

Dantrolene is a direct-acting skeletal muscle relaxant, although it acts intracellularly and with no paralyzing effect at the neuromuscular junction. Dantrolene is the only therapeutic agent available for treatment of malignant hyperthermia (MH). If MH is suspected following succinylcholine use, dantrolene should be given, as if unrecognized and untreated, MH has a mortality of over 70%. Side effects of dantrolene are few—although it can cause some skeletal muscle weakness, no respiratory impairment was reported in one study of awake, spontaneously breathing volunteers receiving the drug.[83] The initial dose is 2.5 mg/kg. If MH is suspected, the initial dosage of dantrolene should be given and a consult obtained from Anesthesia for help with ongoing management. Dantrolene is supplied in vials of only 20 mg, and must be reconstituted with sterile water. Dantrolene should be stocked in any institution where succinylcholine is used.

SUMMARY

Drug: Dantrolene.

Drug type: Skeletal muscle relaxant.

Indication: To treat suspected malignant hyperthermia.

Contraindications: None, when used for an MH crisis.

Dose: 2.5 mg/kg IV (Average 75 kg = 200 mg, which is **10 vials**). Should be repeated, as needed, every 5 minutes to maximum 20 mg/kg or until hypermetabolic symptoms subside. If no clinical response, the diagnosis should be questioned.

Onset/Duration: Onset of action is within 5 minutes.

Potential Complications: Skeletal muscle weakness. Calcium channel blockers should be avoided if dantrolene has been used.

▶ SUMMARY AND FINAL WORDS OF CAUTION

Many factors affect the appropriate use of injectable medications, including patient weight, age, co-morbidities, volume status, and level of consciousness. Clinician experience is also invaluable in making drug choices and choosing dosages. The drug indications and dosages outlined in this text should therefore be used only as a guide.

Intravenously injected agents act quickly. The clinician using these drugs must have a solid knowledge of their indications, contraindications, dosing, and expected clinical effect. It is incumbent on the clinician to

read, seek the advice and experience of colleagues, and ideally observe the use of these medications in elective settings (e.g., the OR) prior to using them in critically ill patients.

REFERENCES

1. Kaplan JD, Schuster DP. Physiologic consequences of tracheal intubation. *Clin Chest Med*. 1991; 12(3):425–432.
2. Shribman AJ, Smith G, Achola KJ. Cardiovascular and catecholamine responses to laryngoscopy with and without tracheal intubation. *Br J Anaesth*. 1987;59(3):295–299.
3. Takahashi S, Mizutani T, Miyabe M, et al. Hemodynamic responses to tracheal intubation with laryngoscope versus lightwand intubating device (Trachlight) in adults with normal airway. *Anesth Analg*. 2002;95(2):480–484.
4. Laxton CH, Milner Q, Murphy PJ. Haemodynamic changes after tracheal intubation in cigarette smokers compared with non–smokers. *Br J Anaesth*. 1999;82(3):442–443.
5. Shafi S, Gentilello L. Hypotension does not increase mortality in brain-injured patients more than it does in non-brain-injured patients. *J Trauma*. 2005;59(4):830–834; discussion 834–835.
6. The Brain Trauma Foundation. The American Association of Neurological Surgeons. The Joint Section on Neurotrauma and Critical Care. Resuscitation of blood pressure and oxygenation. *J Neurotrauma*. 2000;17(6–7):471–478.
7. Sivilotti ML, Filbin MR, Murray HE, et al. Does the sedative agent facilitate emergency rapid sequence intubation? *Acad Emerg Med*. 2003;10(6):612–620.
8. Sivilotti ML, Ducharme J. Randomized, double-blind study on sedatives and hemodynamics during rapid-sequence intubation in the emergency department: the SHRED Study. *Ann Emerg Med*. 1998;31(3):313–324.
9. Casati A, Putzu M. Anesthesia in the obese patient: pharmacokinetic considerations. *J Clin Anesth*. 2005;17(2):134–145.
10. Franklin C, Samuel J, Hu TC. Life-threatening hypotension associated with emergency intubation and the initiation of mechanical ventilation. *Am J Emerg Med*. 1994;12(4):425–428.
11. Trapani G, Altomare C, Liso G, et al. Propofol in anesthesia. Mechanism of action, structure-activity relationships, and drug delivery. *Curr Med Chem*. 2000;7(2):249–271.
12. Vasile B, Rasulo F, Candiani A, et al. The pathophysiology of propofol infusion syndrome: a simple name for a complex syndrome. *Intensive Care Med*. 2003;29(9):1417–1425.
13. Hans P, Bonhomme V. Neuroprotection with anaesthetic agents. *Curr Opin Anaesthesiol*. 2001;14(5):491–496.
14. Proporol Injection 10 mg/ml Product Monograph. Montreal, QC, Canada: Hospira Healthcare Corporation.
15. Wheeler DS, Vaux KK, Ponaman ML, et al. The safe and effective use of propofol sedation in children undergoing diagnostic and therapeutic procedures: experience in a pediatric ICU and a review of the literature. *Pediatr Emerg Care*. 2003;19(6): 385–392.
16. Pentothal Product Monograph. Vaughan, ON, Canada: Abbot Laboratories Limited.
17. Grunberg G, Cohen JD, Keslin J, et al. Facilitation of mechanical ventilation in status asthmaticus with continuous intravenous thiopental. *Chest*. 1991;99(5):1216–1219.
18. Cromhout A. Ketamine: its use in the emergency department. *Emerg Med (Fremantle)*. 2003;15(2): 155–159.
19. Brown RH, Wagner EM. Mechanisms of bronchoprotection by anesthetic induction agents: propofol versus ketamine. *Anesthesiology*. 1999; 90(3):822–828.
20. Green SM, Krauss B. Clinical practice guideline for emergency department ketamine dissociative sedation in children. *Ann Emerg Med*. 2004;44(5): 460–471.
21. Sehdev RS, Symmons DA, Kindl K. Ketamine for rapid sequence induction in patients with head injury in the emergency department. *Emerg Med Australas*. 2006;18(1):37–44.
22. Himmelseher S, Durieux ME. Revising a dogma: ketamine for patients with neurological injury? *Anesth Analg*. 2005;101(2):524–534.
23. Albanese J, Arnaud S, Rey M, et al. Ketamine decreases intracranial pressure and electroencephalographic activity in traumatic brain injury patients during propofol sedation. *Anesthesiology*. 1997;87(6):1328–1334.
24. Sherwin TS, Green SM, Khan A, et al. Does adjunctive midazolam reduce recovery agitation after ketamine sedation for pediatric procedures? A

randomized, double-blind, placebo-controlled trial. *Ann Emerg Med.* 2000;35(3):229–238.

25. Wathen JE, Roback MG, Mackenzie T, et al. Does midazolam alter the clinical effects of intravenous ketamine sedation in children? A double-blind, randomized, controlled, emergency department trial. *Ann Emerg Med.* 2000;36(6):579–588.

26. Loh G, Dalen D. Low-dose ketamine in addition to propofol for procedural sedation and analgesia in the emergency department. *Ann Pharmacother.* 2007;41(3):485–492.

27. Willman EV, Andolfatto G. A prospective evaluation of "ketofol" (ketamine/propofol combination) for procedural sedation and analgesia in the emergency department. *Ann Emerg Med.* 2007;49(1):23–30.

28. Oglesby AJ. Should etomidate be the induction agent of choice for rapid sequence intubation in emergency department? *Emerg Med J.* 2004;21(6): 655–659.

29. Bramwell KJ, Haizlip J, Pribble C, et al. The effect of etomidate on intracranial pressure and systemic blood pressure in pediatric patients with severe traumatic brain injury. *Pediatr Emerg Care.* 2006;22(2):90–93.

30. Zed PJ, Abu-Laban RB, Harrison DW. Intubating conditions and hemodynamic effects of etomidate for rapid sequence intubation in the emergency department: an observational cohort study. *Acad Emerg Med.* 2006;13(4):378–383.

31. Choi YF, Wong TW, Lau CC. Midazolam is more likely to cause hypotension than etomidate in emergency department rapid sequence intubation. *Emerg Med J.* 2004;21(6):700–702.

32. Hoffman WE, Charbel FT, Edelman G, et al. Comparison of the effect of etomidate and desflurane on brain tissue gases and pH during prolonged middle cerebral artery occlusion. *Anesthesiology.* 1998;88(5):1188–1194.

33. Edelman GJ, Hoffman WE, Charbel FT. Cerebral hypoxia after etomidate administration and temporary cerebral artery occlusion. *Anesth Analg.* 1997;85(4):821–825.

34. Bergen JM, Smith DC. A review of etomidate for rapid sequence intubation in the emergency department. *J Emerg Med.* 1997;15(2):221–230.

35. Schenarts CL, Burton JH, Riker RR. Adrenocortical dysfunction following etomidate induction in emergency department patients. *Acad Emerg Med.* 2001;8(1):1–7.

36. Jackson WL, Jr. Should we use etomidate as an induction agent for endotracheal intubation in patients with septic shock?: a critical appraisal. *Chest.* 2005;127(3):1031–1038.

37. Murray H, Marik PE. Etomidate for endotracheal intubation in sepsis: acknowledging the good while accepting the bad. *Chest.* 2005;127(3):707–709.

38. Ray DC, McKeown DW. Effect of induction agent on vasopressor and steroid use, and outcome in patients with septic shock. *Crit Care.* 2007; 11(3):R56.

39. Annane D, Sebille V, Charpentier C, et al. Effect of treatment with low doses of hydrocortisone and fludrocortisone on mortality in patients with septic shock. *JAMA.* 2002;288(7):862–871.

40. Lipiner–Friedman D, Sprung CL, Laterre PF, et al. Adrenal function in sepsis: the retrospective Corticus cohort study. *Crit Care Med.* 2007;35(4): 1012–1018.

41. Zed PJ, Mabasa VH, Slavik RS, et al. Etomidate for rapid sequence intubation in the emergency department: Is adrenal suppression a concern? *Can J Emerg Med.* 2006;8(5):347–350.

42. Miner JR, Danahy M, Moch A, et al. Randomized clinical trial of etomidate versus propofol for procedural sedation in the emergency department. *Ann Emerg Med.* 2007;49(1):15–22.

43. Swanson ER, Fosnocht DE, Jensen SC. Comparison of etomidate and midazolam for prehospital rapid-sequence intubation. *Prehosp Emerg Care.* 2004;8(3):273–279.

44. Sagarin MJ, Barton ED, Sakles JC, et al. Underdosing of midazolam in emergency endotracheal intubation. *Acad Emerg Med.* 2003;10(4):329–338.

45. Reves JG, Fragen RJ, Vinik HR, et al. Midazolam: pharmacology and uses. *Anesthesiology.* 1985;62(3): 310–324.

46. Davis DP, Kimbro TA, Vilke GM. The use of midazolam for prehospital rapid-sequence intubation may be associated with a dose-related increase in hypotension. *Prehosp Emerg Care.* 2001;5(2): 163–168.

47. Avitsian R, Lin J, Lotto M, et al. Dexmedetomidine and awake fiberoptic intubation for possible cervical spine myelopathy: a clinical series. *J Neurosurg Anesthesiol.* 2005;17(2):97–99.

48. Bergese SD, Khabiri B, Roberts WD, et al. Dexmedetomidine for conscious sedation in difficult awake fiberoptic intubation cases. *J Clin Anesth.* 2007;19(2):141–144.

49. Kautto UM. Attenuation of the circulatory response to laryngoscopy and intubation by fentanyl. *Acta Anaesthesiol Scand*. 1982;26(3):217–221.

50. Murkin JM, Moldenhauer CC, Hug CC, Jr. High-dose fentanyl for rapid induction of anaesthesia in patients with coronary artery disease. *Can Anaesth Soc J*. 1985;32(4):320–325.

51. Adachi YU, Satomoto M, Higuchi H, et al. Fentanyl attenuates the hemodynamic response to endotracheal intubation more than the response to laryngoscopy. *Anesth Analg*. 2002;95(1):233–237.

52. Splinter WM, Cervenko F. Haemodynamic responses to laryngoscopy and tracheal intubation in geriatric patients: effects of fentanyl, lidocaine and thiopentone. *Can J Anaesth*. 1989;36(4):370–376.

53. Lev R, Rosen P. Prophylactic lidocaine use preintubation: a review. *J Emerg Med*. 1994;12(4):499–506.

54. Kindler CH, Schumacher PG, Schneider MC, et al. Effects of intravenous lidocaine and/or esmolol on hemodynamic responses to laryngoscopy and intubation: a double-blind, controlled clinical trial. *J Clin Anesth*. 1996;8(6):491–496.

55. Feng CK, Chan KH, Liu KN, et al. A comparison of lidocaine, fentanyl, and esmolol for attenuation of cardiovascular response to laryngoscopy and tracheal intubation. *Acta Anaesthesiol Sin*. 1996;34(2):61–67.

56. Robinson N, Clancy M. In patients with head injury undergoing rapid sequence intubation, does pretreatment with intravenous lignocaine/lidocaine lead to an improved neurological outcome? A review of the literature. *Emerg Med J*. 2001;18(6):453–457.

57. Rothrock SG, Pagane J. Pediatric rapid sequence intubation incidence of reflex bradycardia and effects of pretreatment with atropine. *Pediatr Emerg Care*. 2005;21(9):637–638.

58. Fleming B, McCollough M, Henderson HO. Myth: Atropine should be administered before succinylcholine for neonatal and pediatric intubation. *Cjem*. 2005;7(2):114–117.

59. McAuliffe G, Bissonnette B, Boutin C. Should the routine use of atropine before succinylcholine in children be reconsidered? *Can J Anaesth*. 1995;42(8):724–729.

60. Fastle RK, Roback MG. Pediatric rapid sequence intubation: incidence of reflex bradycardia and effects of pretreatment with atropine. *Pediatr Emerg Care*. 2004;20(10):651–655.

61. Sagarin MJ, Barton ED, Chng YM, et al. Airway management by US and Canadian emergency medicine residents: a multicenter analysis of more than 6,000 endotracheal intubation attempts. *Ann Emerg Med*. 2005;46(4):328–336.

62. Kovacs G, Law JA, Ross J, et al. Acute airway management in the emergency department by non–anesthesiologists. *Can J Anaesth*. 2004;51(2):174–180.

63. Benumof JL, Dagg R, Benumof R. Critical hemoglobin desaturation will occur before return to an unparalyzed state following 1 mg/kg intravenous succinylcholine. *Anesthesiology*. 1997;87(4):979–982.

64. El-Orbany MI, Joseph NJ, Salem MR, et al. The neuromuscular effects and tracheal intubation conditions after small doses of succinylcholine. *Anesth Analg*. 2004;98(6):1680–1685.

65. Naguib M, Samarkandi A, Riad W, et al. Optimal dose of succinylcholine revisited. *Anesthesiology*. 2003;99(5):1045–1049.

66. Martyn JA, Richtsfeld M. Succinylcholine-induced hyperkalemia in acquired pathologic states: etiologic factors and molecular mechanisms. *Anesthesiology*. 2006;104(1):158–169.

67. Libonati MM, Leahy JJ, Ellison N. The use of succinylcholine in open eye surgery. *Anesthesiology*. 1985;62(5):637–640.

68. Vinik HR. Intraocular pressure changes during rapid sequence induction and intubation: a comparison of rocuronium, atracurium, and succinylcholine. *J Clin Anesth*. 1999;11(2):95–100.

69. Clancy M, Halford S, Walls R, et al. In patients with head injuries who undergo rapid sequence intubation using succinylcholine, does pretreatment with a competitive neuromuscular blocking agent improve outcome? A literature review. *Emerg Med J*. 2001;18(5):373–375.

70. Stirt JA, Grosslight KR, Bedford RF, et al. "Defasciculation" with metocurine prevents succinylcholine-induced increases in intracranial pressure. *Anesthesiology*. 1987;67(1):50–53.

71. Minton MD, Grosslight K, Stirt JA, et al. Increases in intracranial pressure from succinylcholine: prevention by prior nondepolarizing blockade. *Anesthesiology*. 1986;65(2):165–169.

72. Silber SH. Rapid sequence intubation in adults with elevated intracranial pressure: a survey of emergency medicine residency programs. *Am J Emerg Med*. 1997;15(3):263–267.

73. Ali SZ, Taguchi A, Rosenberg H. Malignant hyperthermia. *Best Pract Res Clin Anaesthesiol.* 2003;17(4):519–533.

74. Gill M, Graeme K, Guenterberg K. Masseter spasm after succinylcholine administration. *J Emerg Med.* 2005;29(2):167–171.

75. Martin R, Carrier J, Pirlet M, et al. Rocuronium is the best non–depolarizing relaxant to prevent succinylcholine fasciculations and myalgia. *Can J Anaesth.* 1998;45(6):521–525.

76. McCourt KC, Salmela L, Mirakhur RK, et al. Comparison of rocuronium and suxamethonium for use during rapid sequence induction of anaesthesia. *Anaesthesia.* 1998;53(9):867–871.

77. Gijsenbergh F, Ramael S, Houwing N, et al. First human exposure of Org 25969, a novel agent to reverse the action of rocuronium bromide. *Anesthesiology.* 2005;103(4):695–703.

78. de Boer HD, van Egmond J, van de Pol F, et al. Reversal of profound rocuronium neuromuscular blockade by sugammadex in anesthetized rhesus monkeys. *Anesthesiology.* 2006;104(4):718–723.

79. de Boer HD, van Egmond J, van de Pol F, et al. Sugammadex, a new reversal agent for neuromuscular block induced by rocuronium in the anaesthetized Rhesus monkey. *Br J Anaesth.* 2006;96(4):473–479.

80. Shields M, Giovannelli M, Mirakhur RK, et al. Org 25969 (sugammadex), a selective relaxant binding agent for antagonism of prolonged rocuronium–induced neuromuscular block. *Br J Anaesth.* 2006;96(1):36–43.

81. Suzuki T. [Sugammadex (Org 25969, modified gamma-cyclodextrin)]. *Masui.* 2006;55(7):834–840.

82. Sparr HJ, Vermeyen KM, Beaufort AM, et al. Early reversal of profound rocuronium-induced neuromuscular blockade by sugammadex in a randomized multicenter study: efficacy, safety, and pharmacokinetics. *Anesthesiology.* 2007;106(5):935–943.

83. Krause T, Gerbershagen MU, Fiege M, et al. Dantrolene—a review of its pharmacology, therapeutic use and new developments. *Anaesthesia.* 2004;59(4):364–373.

CHAPTER 14

Central Nervous System Emergencies

▶ INTRODUCTION

Central nervous system emergencies may result from a wide variety of pathologies. To maximize the chances for a good outcome, the acute-care clinician should be knowledgeable about intracranial physiology, its response to resuscitative maneuvers, and how commonly used medications impact intracranial pressure dynamics.

▶ Case 14.1

A 24-year-old male went off the road while riding his bicycle during a triathlon. Despite wearing a helmet, he suffered a head injury and was brought into the emergency department (ED) actively seizing. His preseizure scene Glasgow Coma Scale (GCS) was reportedly 10. In the ED, the patient was on a backboard, with a cervical collar in place. There was a significant amount of blood present around the mouth and he had an obvious nasal injury. The seizures had begun 10 minutes prior to arrival, and the patient's teeth were clenched. The paramedics, who were a Basic Life Support (BLS) crew, had given him diazepam 10 mg without effect. In the ED, the patient's GCS was now 8. His heart rate was 120, BP 175/95, and SaO$_2$ was 94% on a non-rebreathing mask.

Traumatic brain injury remains the primary cause of death in trauma and contributes significantly to the overall burden of injury to society, in both human and economic terms.[1,2] The major priority in assessing the head-injured patient is to identify any surgically correctable focal neurological deficits. However, it is also clear that relatively basic resuscitative interventions, including optimal oxygenation and preservation of cerebral perfusion pressure (CPP) help prevent significant secondary brain injury, and decrease mortality.[3–6]

- *It has been clearly demonstrated that even transient hypoxia or hypotension in the severely head-injured patient may as much as double mortality.*[6–8]
- *In perhaps no other injury is the end-organ (brain) more adversely affected by compromise of the basic elements of resuscitative care.*

The patient presenting with neurologic impairment or blunt trauma to the torso must also be suspected of spinal cord injury until proven otherwise. The probability of associated cervical spine injury triples if the patient has a craniofacial injury[9] and/or a GCS of 8 or less.[10,11] To avoid secondary cervical spinal cord injury, cervical immobilization should be maintained during airway management.

► PHYSIOLOGIC CONSIDERATIONS

Historically, management of the patient with increased intracranial pressure (ICP) has focused on the principle that the cranium has a fixed volume that must accommodate brain, blood, and cerebrospinal fluid (CSF). With an increase in volume in one component (e.g., tumor, or extravascular blood clot), some compensation will occur initially, for example, by shifting CSF to the spinal canal, and blood away from venous sinuses. However, once compensatory mechanisms become exhausted, ICP will rise. Raised ICP eventually causes reduced local tissue blood flow, and ultimately, brain herniation and death.

The normal brain is able to protect against compromised cerebral blood flow (CBF) by autoregulation, whereby CBF remains constant over a wide range of mean arterial pressures (MAPs). However, in the injured brain, this capacity to autoregulate is at least somewhat diminished, so that a lowered MAP may significantly lower cerebral blood flow, leading to secondary brain injury. Conversely, if autoregulation remains intact, a lowered MAP may lead to compensatory cerebral vasodilation in the effort to maintain CBF, which in turn can increase ICP from the resulting raised cerebral blood volume. Thus, a lowered MAP is probably always detrimental in the patient with traumatic brain injury (TBI).[12]

The importance of MAP in maintaining CBF is such that CPP has become the target clinical variable to monitor and manage in the TBI patient.[3–5,6,13,14] CPP is defined as the difference between MAP and the ICP (i.e., CPP = MAP − ICP). As a normal ICP is around 10 mm Hg, and a normal MAP* is 90, a normal CPP is approximately 80 mm Hg. In the brain-injured patient, inadequate CPP is considered to be less than 60–70 mm Hg.[15,16] ICP is often increased in the patient with TBI, so that if accompanied by a low MAP, significant compromise of CPP will occur.

*MAP = diastolic blood pressure + 1/3(systolic − diastolic blood pressure). Thus, a blood pressure of 120/80 = 80 + 1/3(40) = MAP of 92

- *A clinical approximation of ICP in a (nonsedated) patient with TBI can be estimated, as follows:*
  - *A drowsy and confused (GCS 13–15) patient, ICP = 20 mm Hg.*
  - *An unconscious (GCS <8) patient, ICP = 30 mm Hg.[17]*

Other major determinants of CBF and cerebral blood volume are the arterial tensions of oxygen and carbon dioxide. When the PaO_2 drops below 50 mm Hg, CBF and cerebral blood volume increase rapidly, with the potential for increased ICP. CBF also reacts to $PaCO_2$, with raised levels causing cerebral vasodilation, while conversely, hyperventilation-induced hypocapnia will cause cerebral vasoconstriction, which can in turn lead to cerebral ischemia.

- *Once used automatically for the patient with TBI, routine hyperventilation is no longer espoused, as worse patient outcomes have been noted with its indiscriminant use.[18]*

These poor outcomes are most likely related to several physiologic factors. CBF is already significantly decreased in the TBI patient for the first day following injury, and there is a risk that further, hyperventilation-induced cerebral vasoconstriction could lead to cerebral ischemia. In addition, ventilatory dynamics required to achieve hyperventilation can have adverse effects on venous return, cardiac output, and in turn, MAP. Finally, with hypocapnia, the oxyhemoglobin dissociation curve shifts to the left, making oxygen less available to tissues.

- *In contemporary practice, the patient with TBI should be ventilated to target the lower levels of normocapnia (i.e., 35 mm Hg), with short-term hyperventilation reserved for signs of acute neurological deterioration such as cerebral herniation with posturing and asymmetrically or bilaterally dilated pupils.[19]*

► PHARMACOLOGIC CONSIDERATIONS

The goal of rapid sequence intubation (RSI) in the critically ill patient is to facilitate intubation as a means of maintaining or improving gas exchange in a manner that does not further compromise end-organ perfusion. Unless contraindicated, RSI is generally the preferred route for intubation of the patient with TBI, as drugs used during RSI may have a beneficial effect on ICP, and a lack of cooperation generally precludes an awake approach.

"Pretreatment" agents

Pretreatment medications have been espoused during RSI of the patient with TBI to help attenuate a further rise in ICP due to (a) laryngoscopy and intubation or (b) other administered medications.

- *Pretreatment with agents (e.g., narcotics or lidocaine) to prevent the "pressor" response to laryngoscopy and intubation, including a rise in ICP, is of questionable clinical value and not without the risk of contributing to postintubation hypotension.[20–22]*
- *Pretreatment with small doses of nondepolarizing neuromuscular blockers to prevent a possible ICP rise associated with succinylcholine use is also falling out of favor.[22,23] Indeed, a number of studies have failed to demonstrate any increase in ICP with succinylcholine use in the TBI patient.[24,25]*

Induction Sedative/Hypnotics

The most important clinically relevant factors in pharmacologic decision making in the patient with traumatic brain injury relate to the need to avoid hypoxia and hypotension. Although the etiology of postintubation hypotension is multifactorial, the choice and dosage of induction sedative/hypnotic is often a major contributing factor.

- *In this seizing, hypertensive patient, propofol (1–2 mg/kg) or thiopental (3–4 mg/kg) could be considered for induction.*
- *The use of etomidate (0.2–0.3 mg/kg) can be considered, as it has been shown to decrease ICP while maintaining MAP.[26–28] However, as discussed in Chap. 13, its use may render the at-risk brain less tolerant of ischemia.*
- *In the head-injured patient with **concomitant hypotension**, ketamine may also be considered as an induction agent for RSI.[29,30]*

Ketamine use in the patient with increased ICP remains somewhat controversial.[31] In general, it may be appropriate to avoid its use in the hypertensive head-injured patient. However, its ability to preserve, or increase blood pressure and offer some neuroprotective effects (currently being studied), may be useful in the trauma patient.

Neuromuscular Blockers

Both succinylcholine and rocuronium are appropriate agents to use for RSI in the TBI patient.

Rescue Vasopressors

For RSI of the patient with TBI, it is particularly important to have a short-acting vasopressor such as ephedrine or phenylephrine drawn up, to treat any postintubation hypotension.

► TECHNICAL CONSIDERATIONS

Airway Management Decisions

The patient described in Case 14–1 has probable intracranial pathology and a declining level of consciousness. Tracheal intubation is indicated for predicted clinical course, and for airway protection.

- *Although often used for the purpose, a GCS of 8 or less does not always correlate with an absence of protective airway reflexes,[32–35] and on its own should rarely be used to dictate the need to intubate.*

The GCS was developed and subsequently validated primarily as a tool for predicting outcomes in head-injured patients.[36,37] Interrater agreement is relatively poor and its use as a prospective decision tool to intubate is even less grounded in science.[38] However, this does not negate the value of monitoring the level of consciousness by GCS, or other method, as an important contributory factor in the decision to intubate the trachea.

The blunt trauma patient should always be assumed to have a cervical spine injury and will require immobilization until this is ruled out. The true incidence of secondary spinal cord injury caused by emergent airway management is unknown, however reported cases are extremely rare.[39–41] An inappropriate fear of causing a cord injury may lead to a delay in airway management, which is likely to pose a more significant risk to the head-injured patient.

- *A cervical collar will predictably make direct laryngoscopy difficult by limiting range of motion of both the neck and mandible.[39,40,42–44]*

The incidence of Cormack-Lehane Grade 3 (epiglottis only) views encountered at direct laryngoscopy has been reported to be up to 60% when a cervical collar is in place.[43–45] Before an intubation proceeds, the anterior portion of the collar should be removed, and replaced with manual in-line neck stabilization (MILNS). In addition to facilitating laryngoscopy, this will provide for easier access to the thyroid cartilage for external laryngeal manipulation (ELM) and the cricoid cartilage for the Sellick maneuver.

- *With the substitution of MILNS for the cervical collar, the incidence of grade 3 views at laryngoscopy drops to 20%–25% of cases.[43,44]*

- *The presence of a cervical collar can increase ICP in the TBI patient.[46–48]*

As always, the decision to perform an RSI should be based on predicted difficulty, patient cooperation, and clinician skill and knowledge. RSI is safe and is generally the preferred method of facilitating intubation in the trauma patient.[39,49–52] RSI is not contraindicated in cases of suspected or known c-spine injury.[41,53]

Intubation and Postintubation Considerations

During preparations for intubation of the patient presented in Case 14–1, the stretcher may be tilted somewhat head-up, to promote cerebral venous drainage. A fluid bolus should be considered, to help avoid a drop in blood pressure peri-intubation, and the patient should be well preoxygenated. Assistants should be coached in anticipation of their tasks, including application of MILNS, and cricoid pressure. If only because of the MILNS, difficulty should be anticipated, and preparations should include immediate availability of a bougie, and an alternative intubation technique, such as an LMA Fastrach, Trachlight, fiberoptic stylet, or videolaryngoscope. RSI medications should be drawn up, as should vasopressors to treat transient postintubation hypotension. As close monitoring of blood pressure will be needed during and after intubation, a noninvasive cuff should be set to cycle at 1–3 minute intervals.

- *If located at the patient's head, the assistant applying MILNS should be positioned out of the laryngoscopist's way, to the left.*
- *MILNS must be maintained even during BMV, as this can cause as much movement of the cervical spine as laryngoscopy.*
- *Apnea times should be limited in the head-injured patient during intubation attempts to avoid the adverse effects of hypercarbia.*
- *ELM and/or a bougie should be used early (i.e., on the first attempt), if difficult laryngoscopy is encountered.*

- *Very often, a view of only the interarytenoid notch or posterior cartilages is obtained during laryngoscopy in the presence of MILNS. The bougie can be passed above the notch, and the endotracheal tube advanced over the bougie.*
- *A change to a straight or levering tip blade can be considered if the initial "best look" laryngoscopy fails.*[54–57]

Following intubation, tube position should be objectively confirmed, cricoid pressure released, and the cervical collar replaced. **The blood pressure should be rechecked,** and additional fluid and vasopressor given, if low. However, if the blood pressure is intact, or once it recovers, a head-up (reverse Trendelenberg) position should be resumed, or considered, to promote venous drainage. The endotracheal tube (ETT) should be affixed to the patient, although tightly encircling ties around the neck should be avoided. The clinician should ensure that the patient is not being inadvertently hyperventilated: this is best accomplished with quantitative end tidal CO_2 monitoring, or the judicious utilization of blood gases.

▶ SUMMARY

The patient with known or suspected CNS injury must be treated with particular attention to maintenance of cerebral perfusion pressure, and the avoidance of hypoxemia. Manual in-line stabilization should be maintained after removal of the cervical collar, and extra preparations should be made for an anticipated difficult laryngoscopy.

REFERENCES

1. Thurman DJ, Alverson C, Dunn KA, et al. Traumatic brain injury in the United States: a public health perspective. *J Head Trauma Rehabil.* 1999;14(6):602–615.
2. Langlois JA, Rutland-Brown W, Thomas KE. *Traumatic Brain Injury in the United States: Emergency Department Visits, Hospitalizations, and Deaths.* Atlanta GA Centers for Diseae Control and Prevention, National Center for Injury Prevention and Control; 2004.
3. Balestreri M, Czosnyka M, Hutchinson P, et al. Impact of intracranial pressure and cerebral perfusion pressure on severe disability and mortality after head injury. *Neurocrit. Care.* 2006;4(1): 8–13.
4. The Brain Trauma F. The American Association of Neurological Surgeons. The Joint Section on Neurotrauma and Critical Care. Guidelines for cerebral perfusion pressure. *J Neurotrauma.* 2000;17(6–7): 507–511.
5. Ling GS, Neal CJ. Maintaining cerebral perfusion pressure is a worthy clinical goal. *Neurocrit. Care.* 2005;2(1):75–81.
6. The Brain Trauma F. The American Association of Neurological Surgeons. The American Association of Neurological Surgeons. The Joint Section on Neurotrauma and Critical Care. Resuscitation of blood pressure and oxygenation. *J Neurotrauma.* 2000;17(6–7):471–478.
7. Chestnut RM, Marshall LF, Klauber MR, et al. The role of secondary brain injury in determining outcome from severe head injury. *J. Trauma.* 1993;34(2): 216–222.
8. Dunford JV, Davis DP, Ochs M, et al. Incidence of transient hypoxia and pulse rate reactivity during paramedic rapid sequence intubation. *Ann Emerg Med.* 2003;42(6):721–728.
9. Hackl W, Hausberger K, Sailer R, et al. Prevalence of cervical spine injuries in patients with facial trauma. *Oral Surg Oral Med Oral Pathol Oral Radiol Endod.* 2001;92(4):370–376.
10. Holly LT, Kelly DF, Counelis GJ, et al. Cervical spine trauma associated with moderate and severe head injury: incidence, risk factors, and injury characteristics. *J Neurosurg.* 2002;96(3 Suppl):285–291.
11. Demetriades D, Charalambides K, Chahwan S, et al. Nonskeletal cervical spine injuries: epidemiology and diagnostic pitfalls. *J Trauma.* 2000;48(4): 724–727.
12. Bouma GJ, Muizelaar JP, Bandoh K, et al. Blood pressure and intracranial pressure-volume dynamics in severe head injury: relationship with cerebral blood flow. *J Neurosurg.* 1992;77(1):15–19.
13. Rose JC, Mayer SA. Optimizing blood pressure in neurological emergencies. *Neurocrit. Care.* 2004;1(3): 287–299.
14. Myburgh JA. Driving cerebral perfusion pressure with pressors: how, which, when? *Crit Care Resusc.* 2005;7(3):200–205.
15. Chan KH, Miller JD, Dearden NM, et al. The effect of changes in cerebral perfusion pressure upon middle cerebral artery blood flow velocity and

jugular bulb venous oxygen saturation after severe brain injury. *J Neurosurg*. 1992;77(1):55–61.

16. The Brain Trauma Foundation. The American Association of Neurological Surgeons. The Joint Section on Neurotrauma and Critical Care. Guidelines for cerebral perfusion pressure. *J Neurotrauma*. 2000;17(6–7):507–511.

17. Walters FJM. Intracranial pressure and cerebral blood blow. *Update in Anaesthesia: Physiology*; 1998.

18. Muizelaar JP, Marmarou A, Ward JD, et al. Adverse effects of prolonged hyperventilation in patients with severe head injury: a randomized clinical trial. *J Neurosurg*. 1991;75(5):731–739.

19. The Brain Trauma F. The American Association of Neurological Surgeons. The Joint Section on Neurotrauma and Critical Care. Initial Management. *J Neurotrauma*. 2000;17(6–7):463–469.

20. Feng CK, Chan KH, Liu KN, et al. A comparison of lidocaine, fentanyl, and esmolol for attenuation of cardiovascular response to laryngoscopy and tracheal intubation. *Acta Anaesthesiol. Sin.* 1996;34(2):61–67.

21. Robinson N, Clancy M. In patients with head injury undergoing rapid sequence intubation, does pretreatment with intravenous lignocaine/lidocaine lead to an improved neurological outcome? A review of the literature. *Emerg Med J*. 2001;18(6):453–457.

22. Bozeman WP, Idris AH. Intracranial pressure changes during rapid sequence intubation: a swine model. *J Trauma*. 2005;58(2):278–283.

23. Clancy M, Halford S, Walls R, et al. In patients with head injuries who undergo rapid sequence intubation using succinylcholine, does pretreatment with a competitive neuromuscular blocking agent improve outcome? A literature review. *Emerg Med J*. 2001;18(5):373–375.

24. Brown MM, Parr MJ, Manara AR. The effect of suxamethonium on intracranial pressure and cerebral perfusion pressure in patients with severe head injuries following blunt trauma. *Eur J Anaesthesiol*. 1996;13(5):474–477.

25. Kovarik WD, Mayberg TS, Lam AM, et al. Succinylcholine does not change intracranial pressure, cerebral blood flow velocity, or the electroencephalogram in patients with neurologic injury. *Anesth Analg*. 1994;78(3):469–473.

26. Bramwell KJ, Haizlip J, Pribble C, et al. The effect of etomidate on intracranial pressure and systemic blood pressure in pediatric patients with severe traumatic brain injury. *Pediatr Emerg Care*. 2006;22(2):90–93.

27. Modica PA, Tempelhoff R. Intracranial pressure during induction of anaesthesia and tracheal intubation with etomidate–induced EEG burst suppression. *Can J Anaesth*. 1992;39(3):236–241.

28. Moss E, Powell D, Gibson RM, et al. Effect of etomidate on intracranial pressure and cerebral perfusion pressure. *Br J Anaesth*. 1979;51(4):347–352.

29. Sehdev RS, Symmons DA, Kindl K. Ketamine for rapid sequence induction in patients with head injury in the emergency department. *Emerg Med Australas*. 2006;18(1):37–44.

30. Himmelseher S, Durieux ME. Revising a dogma: ketamine for patients with neurological injury? *Anesth Analg*. 2005;101(2):524–534, table.

31. Sehdev RS, Symmons DA, Kindl K. Ketamine for rapid sequence induction in patients with head injury in the emergency department. *Emerg Med Australas*. 2006;18(1):37–44.

32. Moulton C, Pennycook AG. Relation between Glasgow coma score and cough reflex. *Lancet*. 1994;343(8908):1261–1262.

33. Kolb JC, Galli RL. No gag rule for intubation. *Ann Emerg Med*. 1995;26(4):529–530.

34. Moulton C, Pennycook A, Makower R. Relation between Glasgow coma scale and the gag reflex. *Bmj*. 1991;303(6812):1240–1241.

35. Davies AE, Stone SP, Kidd D, et al. Pharyngeal sensation and gag reflex in healthy subjects. *The Lancet*. 1995;345(8948):487–488.

36. Teasdale G, Jennett B. Assessment of coma and impaired consciousness. A practical scale. *Lancet*. 1974;2(7872):81–84.

37. Teasdale GM, Pettigrew LE, Wilson JT, et al. Analyzing outcome of treatment of severe head injury: a review and update on advancing the use of the Glasgow Outcome Scale. *J Neurotrauma*. 1998;15(8):587–597.

38. Gill MR, Reiley DG, Green SM. Interrater reliability of Glasgow Coma Scale scores in the emergency department. *Ann Emerg Med*. 2004;43(2):215–223.

39. Crosby E. Airway management after upper cervical spine injury: what have we learned? *Can J Anaesth*. 2002;49(7):733–744.

40. Crosby ET. Airway management in adults after cervical spine trauma. *Anesthesiology*. 104(6):1293–1318.

41. Manoach S, Paladino L. Manual In-Line Stabilization for Acute Airway Management of Suspected Cervical Spine Injury: Historical Review and Current Questions. *Ann Emerg Med*. 2007.

42. Ollerton JE, Parr MJ, Harrison K, et al. Potential cervical spine injury and difficult airway management for emergency intubation of trauma adults in the emergency department—a systematic review. *Emerg Med J*. 2006;23(1):3–11.

43. Heath KJ. The effect of laryngoscopy of different cervical spine immobilisation techniques. *Anaesthesia*. 1994;49(10):843–845.

44. Nolan JP, Wilson ME. Orotracheal intubation in patients with potential cervical spine injuries. An indication for the gum elastic bougie. *Anaesthesia*. 1993;48(7):630–633.

45. MacQuarrie K, Hung OR, Law JA. Tracheal intubation using Bullard laryngoscope for patients with a simulated difficult airway. *Can J Anaesth*. 1999;46(8):760–765.

46. Davies G, Deakin C, Wilson A. The effect of a rigid collar on intracranial pressure. *Injury*. 1996;27(9): 647–649.

47. Kolb JC, Summers RL, Galli RL. Cervical collar-induced changes in intracranial pressure. *Am J Emerg Med*. 1999;17(2):135–137.

48. Mobbs RJ, Stoodley MA, Fuller J. Effect of cervical hard collar on intracranial pressure after head injury. *ANZ J Surg*. 2002;72(6):389–391.

49. Bushra JS, McNeil B, Wald DA, et al. A comparison of trauma intubations managed by anesthesiologists and emergency physicians. *Acad Emerg Med*. 2004;11(1):66–70.

50. Levitan RM, Rosenblatt B, Meiner EM, et al. Alternating day emergency medicine and anesthesia resident responsibility for management of the trauma airway: a study of laryngoscopy performance and intubation success. *Ann Emerg Med*. 2004;43(1):48–53.

51. Sagarin MJ, Barton ED, Chng YM, et al. Airway Management by US and Canadian Emergency Medicine Residents: A Multicenter Analysis of More Than 6,000 Endotracheal Intubation Attempts. *Ann Emerg Med*. 2005;46(4):328–336.

52. Graham CA, Beard D, Henry JM, et al. Rapid sequence intubation of trauma patients in Scotland. *J Trauma*. 2004;56(5):1123–1126.

53. Ghafoor AU, Martin TW, Gopalakrishnan S, et al. Caring for the patients with cervical spine injuries: what have we learned? *J Clin Anesth*. 2005;17(8):640–649.

54. Gerling MC, Davis DP, Hamilton RS, et al. Effects of cervical spine immobilization technique and laryngoscope blade selection on an unstable cervical spine in a cadaver model of intubation. *Ann Emerg Med*. 2000;36(4):293–300.

55. Gabbott DA. Laryngoscopy using the McCoy laryngoscope after application of a cervical collar. *Anaesthesia*. 1996;51(9):812–814.

56. Laurent SC, de Melo AE, Alexander–Williams JM. The use of the McCoy laryngoscope in patients with simulated cervical spine injuries. *Anaesthesia*. 1996;51(1):74–75.

57. Uchida T, Hikawa Y, Saito Y, et al. The McCoy levering laryngoscope in patients with limited neck extension. *Can J Anaesth*. 1997;44(6):674–676.

CHAPTER 15
Cardiovascular Emergencies

► INTRODUCTION

The critically ill patient is dependent on the integrity of the cardiovascular system to maintain perfusion and deliver oxygen to vital tissue beds. Many patients requiring emergency airway intervention will have a degree of coronary artery disease. In the patient with suspected or known ischemic heart disease (IHD), including an acute coronary syndrome (ACS), the general principle of management is to retain a favorable balance between myocardial oxygen supply and demand.

► ISCHEMIC HEART DISEASE

► **Case 15.1**

An intoxicated and confused 64-year-old man presented after a low-velocity single vehicle crash resulting from an unexplained "blackout." In the emergency department (ED), his blood pressure (BP) was 140/90, heart rate (HR) 100, respiratory rate (RR) 18, and his oxygen saturation (SaO₂) was 99% on a nonrebreathing facemask. Due to a depressed level of consciousness, the question of tracheal intubation for "airway protection" arose, especially in the context of examination within a computed tomography (CT) suite. His spouse mentioned that he had suffered two heart attacks and still experienced frequent angina. Blood glucose was normal.

Physiologic Considerations

The patient presented in Case 15–1 may be placed at risk of myocardial ischemia related to the stress of laryngoscopy and intubation. This physiologic stress is mediated primarily through sympathetic nervous system stimulation and can include an increase in HR and BP. Both responses can increase myocardial oxygen demand, potentially causing or worsening myocardial ischemia. Conversely, significant hypotension (as can happen with the use of rapid-sequence intubation [RSI] sedative/hypnotics) can compromise coronary perfusion pressure and also potentially exacerbate myocardial ischemia. With reference to the cardiovascular system, physiologic goals in managing this patient's airway include the following:

- *Attenuation or control of patient hemodynamics with judicious pharmacological intervention, seeking:*
  - *Minimal increase in heart rate.*
  - *Minimal variation in blood pressure.*

- *Optimization of cardiac function in the presence of possible hypovolemia or compromised ventricular function.*

Pharmacologic Considerations

Many publications in the anesthesiology literature have described methods of blunting the sympathetic response to laryngoscopy and intubation with the use of pretreatment agents.[1–4] However, it is important to realize that the majority of this data has been gathered in the setting of stable patients in a non-emergent setting. Both narcotics and beta blockers have been used as pretreatment agents in the patient with ischemic heart disease:

- *Fentanyl will reliably attenuate the HR and BP response to laryngoscopy and intubation, although at doses higher than those traditionally used for analgesia.*
- *At lower pretreatment doses (e.g., 1–3 µg/kg), fentanyl will usually, but less consistently attenuate the BP, but not necessarily the HR response to intubation.*
- *Esmolol can be effective in blunting both the HR and BP response to laryngoscopy and intubation.[3,4]*
- *The benefits of using these agents must be balanced against their risk of compromising coronary perfusion pressure, or precipitating a general state of hemodynamic decompensation.*
- *Post-intubation hypotension is best treated with small boluses (e.g., 40–100 µg) of phenylephrine, to avoid any increase in HR (as may happen with ephedrine).*

Technical Considerations

The patient with known or suspected ischemic heart disease should be well monitored, and intubated gently, yet expeditiously. As prolonged efforts at intubation are associated with a more pronounced hemodynamic response, equipment preparation and patient positioning should be optimized for "first-pass" success.

- *Vital signs should be closely monitored during and after tracheal intubation, with a noninvasive cuff cycling at 3-minute intervals.*
- *An intravenous fluid bolus of 10–20 mL/kg is not contraindicated in the patient with myocardial ischemia, and should usually be given, to help avoid post-intubation hypotension.*
- *Hypotension following tracheal intubation should be aggressively treated with additional fluid and vasopressors. Unexpected tachycardia can be treated with esmolol.*
- *Hypertension, while undesirable if excessively high, will usually settle on its own.*

▶ CONGESTIVE HEART FAILURE

▶ Case 15.2

A 79-year-old female arrived in the ED in acute respiratory distress. She was unable to speak more than two words at a time, and her coarse, rasping breath sounds could be heard from the foot of the bed. Her spouse reported that she had been complaining of chest pain for 2 hours, and that she had begun coughing up pink, frothy sputum just before leaving for the hospital. She had a history of Type 2 diabetes and hypertension. Her electrocardiogram (ECG) showed new ST segment depression in the precordial leads. A trial of noninvasive positive pressure ventilation had failed. Her BP was 100/60, HR 138, RR 34, and her SaO_2 was 83% on a nonrebreathing facemask.

Physiologic Considerations

The patient in Case 15–2 presented in pulmonary edema secondary to an acute coronary syndrome. She required tracheal intubation primarily to correct gas exchange by improving oxygen delivery. Several considerations should be addressed:

- *This patient is in part dependent on sympathetic nervous system tone to compensate for left ventricular (LV) dysfunction.*

- *Tachycardia and low normal BP in a patient with congestive heart failure and a history of hypertension is a harbinger of cardiovascular collapse.*
- *As always, the goal is to facilitate tracheal intubation without further compromising the patient's hemodynamic status.*

Pharmacologic Considerations

With or without a pretreatment agent, use of an induction sedative/hypnotic as part of an RSI in the patient with compromised ventricular function will negatively affect both myocardial contractility and peripheral vascular tone. Circulatory collapse may ensue. If the patient is not actively uncooperative, an awake intubation may present an attractive strategic option. However, if an RSI is chosen, great care must be taken in choice and dosage of sedative/hypnotic.[5] A number of considerations apply:

- *Although ketamine is intrinsically a negative inotrope, its administration results in additional sympathetic nervous system (SNS) stimulation and an increase myocardial oxygen demand. It is therefore potentially problematic in patients with evolving myocardial ischemia.*
- *Etomidate will not affect myocardial contractility at usual doses.[6] However, a reduced dose (e.g., 0.15–0.20 mg/kg) should still be considered, based on the patient's age and presenting vital signs.*
- *Unless used in very modest doses, both thiopental and propofol could potentially cause catastrophic hypotension in this patient by further depressing myocardial contractility and causing peripheral vasodilation.[7]*
- *Propofol and ketamine can be blended ("off-label") in a 50/50 mix, with greater stability than either agent alone, but caution must still occur, with use of judicious doses (e.g. 0.1 cc/kg of the mixture).*

- *These patients are at significant risk for post-intubation hypotension, as relief of the work of breathing, relative hypocarbia, and decrease in venous return results in loss of sympathetic tone.*
- *Reliable vascular access should be in place, and a short-acting vasopressor such as phenylephrine diluted and available for immediate use.*

In the patient with compromised ventricular function, a slow circulation time will delay the clinical onset of administered sedative-hypnotics. The clinician must not fall into the trap of giving more drug to hasten the onset time, as a profound drop in BP may result.

Technical Considerations

If intubating with an RSI, the patient should be left in a position of comfort (often sitting, if dyspneic) until loss of consciousness, if the BP allows. Immediately upon loss of consciousness, the stretcher can be lowered to the supine position. An awake intubation can be done in the semisitting position, to maximize patient comfort and cooperation during the procedure.

- *Pulmonary edema may result in difficult mask ventilation. An oral airway and two-person technique should be employed early.*
- *If possible, a large endotracheal tube should be used, in order to facilitate suctioning of pulmonary edema fluid.*
- *End-tidal CO_2 (ETCO$_2$) detection may be impaired in patients with cardiogenic shock and pulmonary edema.[8]*
- *PEEP (positive end-expiratory pressure) may be beneficial, but patients in congestive heart failure are very sensitive to its adverse effects on venous return.*

▶ CARDIAC ARREST

▶ Case 15.3

A 53-year-old male sustained a cardiac arrest in the intensive care unit (ICU). The day before, he had undergone an abdominal-perineal resection of the colon for neoplastic disease. He had exhibited ST-depression in the operating room (OR), and in the recovery room had ECG changes suggestive of inferolateral ischemia. Troponin rise was suggestive of myocardial infarction. He had been sent to the ICU, unintubated, for overnight monitoring. The next morning, while talking to his nurse, he suddenly became unresponsive. The monitor tracing was suggestive of ventricular fibrillation, and pulse oximeter and arterial line tracings had become flat. The patient, of average body habitus, had a history of treated hypertension, and Type-2 diabetes mellitus.

Physiologic Considerations

Following a sudden ventricular fibrillation cardiac arrest, blood oxygen levels will remain in a near-normal range for the first few minutes. However, with myocardial and cerebral oxygen delivery limited by absent cardiac output, chest compressions should ideally begin without delay. As the cardiac arrest continues beyond the first few minutes, both compressions and oxygenation/ventilation are important, as is the case for patients hypoxic at the time of arrest.

During cardiopulmonary resuscitation (CPR), cardiac output is only 25%–33% of normal,[9] so an adequate ventilation-perfusion ratio can be maintained with much lower tidal volumes and respiratory rates than usual. The lower required minute ventilation has the advantage of minimizing intrathoracic pressure, which could otherwise interfere with venous return and cardiac output. In addition, small tidal volumes will help minimize gastric insufflation during bag-mask ventilation (BMV).

Unlike other clinical scenarios, airway management efforts in the cardiac arrest situation do not take precedence over attempts to establish a return of circulation. Chest compressions are essential for providing blood flow during CPR, and will increase the likelihood of successful defibrillation.

- *To minimize interruption of compressions, intubation can be deferred until the patient has failed to respond to initial CPR and defibrillation attempts.*
- *If tracheal intubation is undertaken during CPR, each attempt should be as brief as possible, occurring only after full preparations have been made.*

Cricoid pressure application during airway management in the cardiac arrest patient may help prevent passive regurgitation and aspiration of gastric contents, all the more likely as lower esophageal sphincter tone relaxes in the arrested patient,[10] as well as during the pre-arrest phase.[11] Cricoid pressure may also help minimize gastric insufflation during bag-mask ventilation.

Pharmacologic Considerations

The arrested patient usually offers little resistance to BMV, laryngoscopic intubation, or extraglottic device (EGD) insertion. However, if the patient were to retain sufficient muscle tone to have a clenched jaw, a skeletal muscle relaxant such as succinylcholine can be given. Succinylcholine should be avoided if the arrest may have been caused by hyperkalemia.

Technical Considerations

For the patient presented in Case 15–3, adult basic life support recommendations call for establishing unresponsiveness, performing an airway opening maneuver, and assessing the patient's breathing.

- *For the clinician inexperienced in the use of EGDs or laryngoscopic intubation, BMV can be used for intermittent ventilation throughout a cardiac arrest.*
- *When performing BMV during breaks in chest compressions, two positive pressure ventilations are provided during a brief (3–4 seconds) pause after every 30 compressions.[12] Inspiratory time should be limited to 1 second and should seek simply to achieve a visible chest rise (using a volume of 6–7 mL/kg).*
- *EGDs (e.g., Combitube and the LMA) have also been successfully used and studied in the setting of cardiac arrest.[12] No interruption of chest compressions is required during EGD placement or subsequent ventilation.*
- *In skilled hands, laryngoscopic intubation is often easily performed in cardiac arrest. Interruptions to chest compressions should be minimized during any one attempt.*
- *Correct tracheal placement of the ETT in the cardiac arrest situation should, as always, make use of objective confirmatory methods. End-tidal CO_2 may be unreliable in non-perfusing states.*

In addition to visualization of the tube going between cords, an $ETCO_2$ detector or an esophageal detector device (EDD) can be used. False negative $ETCO_2$ readings (i.e., no CO_2 detected despite the ETT being in trachea) may occur in the setting of cardiac arrest for one of a number of reasons: low blood flow and CO_2 delivery to the lungs; pulmonary embolus; device contamination with drug or acidic gastric contents; systemic epinephrine bolus; or severe lower airway obstruction (e.g., pulmonary edema or *status asthmaticus*).[12] Unless the arrest was witnessed, or a return to circulation has occurred, an EDD is the preferred method for confirming correct ETT placement.

Following tracheal intubation or placement of an extraglottic device, chest compressions should no longer be paused for delivery of positive pressure ventilation (PPV)—compressions now continue uninterrupted at a rate of 100 per minute, with PPV at 8–10 breaths per minute, using a volume of 500–600 mL in the adult. PPV at this rate and tidal volume will help avoid excessive intrathoracic positive pressure, which could otherwise interfere with venous return.[12] Following the return of a perfusing rhythm, 10–12 breaths per minute can be delivered, although the patient at risk of air-trapping ("auto-PEEP") should be ventilated at the lower rate of 6–8 breaths per minute.[12]

▶ SUMMARY

Intubation of the patient with ischemic heart disease and its sequellae can be challenging. A significant increase in HR or BP can be detrimental by increasing myocardial oxygen demands, while conversely, hypotension must also be avoided in order to maintain coronary perfusion pressure. The clinician must walk this tightrope by choosing the best method of proceeding with the intubation, and, if RSI is chosen, the correct dosage of an appropriate sedative/hypnotic.

REFERENCES

1. Wiest D. Esmolol. A review of its therapeutic efficacy and pharmacokinetic characteristics. *Clin Pharmacokinet.* 1995;28(3):190–202.
2. Yuan L, Chia YY, Jan KT, et al. The effect of single bolus dose of esmolol for controlling the tachycardia and hypertension during laryngoscopy and tracheal intubation. *Acta Anaesthesiol Sin.* 1994;32(3):147–152.
3. Feng CK, Chan KH, Liu KN, et al. A comparison of lidocaine, fentanyl, and esmolol for attenuation of cardiovascular response to laryngoscopy and tracheal intubation. *Acta Anaesthesiol Sin.* 1996;34(2):61–67.

4. Helfman SM, Gold MI, DeLisser EA, et al. Which drug prevents tachycardia and hypertension associated with tracheal intubation: lidocaine, fentanyl, or esmolol? *Anesth Analg.* 1991;72(4):482–486.

5. Horak J, Weiss S. Emergent management of the airway. New pharmacology and the control of comorbidities in cardiac disease, ischemia, and valvular heart disease. *Crit Care Clin.* 2000;16(3):411–427.

6. Sprung J, Ogletree-Hughes ML, Moravec CS. The effects of etomidate on the contractility of failing and nonfailing human heart muscle. *Anesth Analg.* 2000;91(1):68–75.

7. Rouby JJ, Andreev A, Leger P, et al. Peripheral vascular effects of thiopental and propofol in humans with artificial hearts. *Anesthesiology.* 1991;75(1):32–42.

8. Bozeman WP, Hexter D, Liang HK, Kelen GD. Esophageal detector device versus detection of end-tidal carbon dioxide level in emergency intubation. *Ann Emerg Med.* 1996;27(5):595–599.

9. Part 4: Adult Basic Life Support. *Circulation.* 2005;112(24):19–34.

10. Bowman FP, Menegazzi JJ, Check BD, et al. Lower esophageal sphincter pressure during prolonged cardiac arrest and resuscitation. *Ann Emerg Med.* 1995;26(2):216–219.

11. Gabrielli A, Wenzel V, Layon AJ, et al. Lower esophageal sphincter pressure measurement during cardiac arrest in humans: potential implications for ventilation of the unprotected airway. *Anesthesiology.* 2005;103(4):897–899.

12. Part 7.1: Adjuncts for Airway Control and Ventilation. *Circulation.* 2005;112(24):51–57.

CHAPTER 16
Respiratory Emergencies

▶ INTRODUCTION

Management of a patient presenting with either upper or lower airway pathology can be challenging for any clinician, regardless of experience. Understanding the etiology of, and having an approach to the patient in respiratory distress is critical to ensuring a good clinical outcome.

▶ OBSTRUCTING UPPER AIRWAY PATHOLOGY

The causes of pathologic upper airway obstruction are listed in Table 16–1. While the etiology of obstruction is often self-evident (e.g., trauma or thermal injury), occasionally the cause may be more subtle (e.g., previously undiagnosed laryngeal tumor).

While the likely diagnosis of adult epiglottitis is not difficult in the patient presented in Case 16–1, the management of such a patient can be either smooth and life-saving, or fraught with complications, up to and including death. The need for early control of this patient's airway must be recognized. Delay may result in loss of airway patency due to worsening inflammation and edema.

Securing the airway of a patient with obstructing pathology can be difficult and anxiety-provoking, even for expert airway managers. The adage "take early control of the airway" can compete with a strong instinct to "first do no harm." Early, preemptive airway management

▶ Case 16.1

A 48-year-old man presented to a rural emergency department (ED) with a 3-day history of a severe sore throat. Two days before, he had been seen at an urgent-care clinic and started on amoxicillin. That morning, the patient and his spouse were concerned because he could not "swallow his own spit" and was making a "funny noise" when he breathed. The patient was conscious, but looked anxious; he was sitting upright, protruding his jaw, and drooling. His temperature was 38.8°C; heart rate (HR) 130; respiratory rate (RR) 26; blood pressure (BP) 110/90; and his oxygen saturation (Sao$_2$) was 96% on room air. His oral exam showed no pathology. He had inspiratory stridor.

requires a clinician with the appropriate skills. An early call for help should be placed—often the best setting for managing this type of patient is the operating room (OR), with the presence of both an anesthesiologist and surgeon. However, acuity and clinician availability will often dictate where and by whom the patient is managed.

Physiologic Considerations

The patient with obstructing airway pathology bears special consideration for a number of reasons. Substantial narrowing of the airway can

▶ **TABLE 16–1** CLASSIFICATION OF OBSTRUCTING CONDITIONS OF THE UPPER AIRWAY

Class of Obstruction	Etiology
INFECTIOUS	Acute epiglottitis/ supraglottitis
	Croup
	Retropharyngeal abscess
	Ludwig's angina
INFLAMMATORY	Anaphylaxis
	Angioedema
MECHANICAL	Inhaled foreign body
	Tumor (hemorrhage, swelling, infection)
	Posttraumatic strictures
TRAUMATIC	Blunt or penetrating anterior neck trauma
	Postoperative swelling or hematoma
	Thermal or chemical injury

occur before signs (e.g., stridor) or symptoms (e.g., dyspnea) occur.[1] Unfortunately, this means that on presentation, the patient may be close to respiratory *extremis* or even complete obstruction. Especially with advanced stages of pathologic airway obstruction, airway patency is sometimes maintained only with patient effort. Interfering with this effort by the administration of sedatives, or proceeding with rapid-sequence intubation (RSI), can precipitate complete obstruction.

- *Regardless of the etiology, inspiratory stridor is a hallmark of the patient with obstructing pathology at or just above the level of the laryngeal inlet. Stridor on expiration suggests obstructing pathology below the cords.*
- *A change in voice (often described as "muffled," or "hot potato") and odynophagia, with a normal oral exam, should also raise concern of pathology in or around the laryngeal inlet.*

- *Voice changes and stridor apart, the external airway examination may look otherwise normal in the patient with obstructing airway pathology. In such a patient, additional information on the state of the laryngeal inlet can be obtained by performing nasopharyngoscopy with a small flexible endoscope.*
- *Once present, stridor should be looked upon as a sign of impending complete airway obstruction.*
- *Patients with obstructing upper airway pathology are usually anxious, and often present sitting upright or leaning forward, in an attempt to maintain an open airway and better manage secretions.*
- *Obstruction may be relatively fixed (e.g., tumor or foreign bodies) or dynamic and progressive (e.g., infection; burns; hemorrhage).*

Pharmacologic Considerations

Generally, an awake approach is preferred for intubation of the patient with obstructing airway pathology. Application of topical airway anesthesia can proceed as usual. Systemic sedation should ideally be completely avoided, or if used, should be minimized. If sedation is employed, a number of options are available, with caveats:

- *If used, benzodiazepines, such as midazolam (e.g., 0.5–1.0 mg in an average adult) must be employed very judiciously.*
- *Ketamine (e.g., 0.25–0.5 mg/kg) can be titrated to effect if needed. Although ketamine has the theoretic advantage of minimizing respiratory depression in otherwise healthy patients, little data exists on its use in patients with obstructing airway pathology.[2]*
- *Ketamine has been associated with laryngospasm (more frequently described in pediatric patients with concurrent respiratory disease)[3, 4] and increased respiratory secretions, both of which would be very unwelcome in the obstructing patient.*

- *In an uncooperative patient, other sedative medications potentially useful to assist an awake intubation may include haloperidol or dexmedetomidine.*

Technical Considerations

Airway Management Decisions

Obstructing airway pathology has the potential to create **difficulty with all "dimensions" of airway management**: bag-mask ventilation (BMV), laryngoscopy and intubation, and rescue oxygenation with an extraglottic device (Fig. 11–1).

- *As such, in general, the presence of pathological airway obstruction is a **relative contraindication to RSI.***

A patient in the early stages of upper airway obstruction will often be cooperative, allowing the option of an awake approach to intubation (see *Approach to Tracheal Intubation* algorithm, Chapter 11, Fig. 11–3, **track 3**). The awake approach will allow the patient to maintain a tenuous airway and, if landmarks are indistinct during the intubation attempt, movement of laryngeal structures (i.e., abduction of edematous cords/false cords during inspiration) may afford the clinician an additional and valuable landmark. In contrast, apnea from significant sedation or RSI with paralysis may cause static edematous structures to obscure all landmarks and further constrict the airway. In addition to making direct laryngoscopy difficult or impossible, this will also compromise the efficacy of BMV or an extraglottic device (EGD). Even small amounts of sedation in the patient with advanced obstruction can interfere with the muscle tone related patency of a tenuous airway.[5]

With advanced degrees of obstruction, tracheal intubation from above will always be risky, and even with an awake approach, complete obstruction can occur during the attempt.[5] Because of this, for some patients with an advanced degree of obstructing pathology, a primary awake tracheostomy using local anesthesia may be the method of choice. However, if an attempt at intubation from above is made in the patient with obstructing pathology, it should proceed only with a **double set-up**, whereby the cricothyroid membrane has been identified, and the needed equipment is available for immediate cricothyrotomy.

- *Performed with skill on selected, cooperative patients, an awake technique is generally safe, usually successful and in the opinion of many authors, the preferred route when significant airway obstruction is present.[2,6,7]*
- *For the uncooperative patient, (see Approach to Tracheal Intubation algorithm, Chapter 11, Fig. 11–3, **track 5**), options include a trial of a sedative such as ketamine; intubation following an inhalational induction of anesthesia in the operating room (OR); or awake tracheostomy or cricothyrotomy. Rarely, in a high acuity situation with an actively uncooperative patient, **RSI with a double setup** may be needed, with the expectation to proceed to cricothyrotomy without delay, if failed oxygenation ensues.*
- *Although extraglottic devices would generally not be expected to work for failed oxygenation with pathologic obstruction at or below the cords, there are sporadic case reports of their successful use in this situation.[8,9]*

Temporizing Measures

The following temporizing measures may allow time for arrival of additional expertise and equipment, or transfer of the patient with obstructing pathology to another location:

- *To promote venous drainage, the head of the bed should be elevated (if the patient has not naturally assumed the sitting position).*
- *Heliox (a helium:oxygen mixture in 80:20, 70:30 or 60:40 proportions) can be used.[10,11] Heliox eases the work of breathing in upper airway obstruction by reducing the obstruction-related turbulent flow. The*

more laminar flow thus afforded can symptomatically improve the patient, but comes at the cost of a reduced inspired concentration of oxygen.

- *For certain inflammatory obstructing conditions, a nebulized epinephrine aerosol may help temporarily shrink the edematous component.[12,13]*

- *In certain cases of angioedema, a conservative approach including the use of epinephrine may reverse the obstruction, thereby averting the need for intubation.*

- *Well applied BMV may be effective as a temporizing measure in the face of upper airway pathology.[14]*

Intubation and Postintubation Considerations

Intubation of the patient with obstructing airway pathology should proceed with the patient in a position of comfort (usually sitting).

- *Preoxygenation should be undertaken, even for an awake intubation.*

- *As stated, in most cases, preparations should include a "double setup" for urgent cricothyrotomy, in case the patient completely obstructs during intubation attempts.*

- *Equipment preparation should include the availability of small endotracheal tubes and a bougie. While direct laryngoscopy can be used for awake intubation, an indirect visualization technique, using a rigid or flexible fiberoptic or video-based device, will be particularly useful if availability and clinician expertise permit.*

- *"Blind" alternatives to direct laryngoscopy, such as the LMA Fastrach or Trachlight, are relatively contraindicated with distorted airway anatomy.*

- *Topical airway anesthesia and precision direct laryngoscopy, if used, should be performed as described in Chapter 8.*

- *Distorted laryngeal inlet anatomy can be difficult to interpret: sometimes the only fea-ture identifying the glottic opening in the awake patient is a suggestion of movement on inspiration, or the appearance of bubbles on expiration. A small tube or a bougie can be aimed through the hole. Prior passage of a bougie has the advantage of providing tactile feedback to confirm tracheal entry, although in the awake patient it should not be advanced to or beyond the carina.*

- *In an unconscious, apneic patient with unidentifiable anatomy at laryngoscopy, having an assistant perform a single chest compression may sometimes produce a bubble at the laryngeal inlet, through which a bougie can be passed.*

Surgical Considerations

The presence of a surgeon at the bedside of an obstructing patient should always be a welcome sight. If acuity permits, primary awake tracheostomy using local anesthesia, performed by a skilled clinician is a safe and well-tolerated option in the patient with advanced airway obstruction.[15]

- *Emergent surgical access should be via the cricothyroid membrane. Tracheostomy, although quickly performed by some surgeons, can take time and should generally be reserved for more controlled scenarios.*

▶ PENETRATING NECK TRAUMA

Penetrating trauma to the neck can involve the upper or lower airway, and bears special mention. Case series reporting experience with penetrating neck injuries have reported very high success rates with the use of RSI.[7, 16] RSI is, in fact, probably safe in penetrating neck injuries involving no direct or indirect (e.g., distortion of the airway by an adjacent neck hematoma) trauma to the airway. However, clinically identifying these particular injuries before airway management is commenced is not always possible or reliable. Although reports of poor outcomes attributable to RSI use in penetrating neck trauma (and for that matter, all upper airway pathology) are relatively rare, this may in part be explained by publication bias. It is a well-known phenomenon that "success stories" are more commonly submitted to and accepted in peer-reviewed journals.[17] Caution should be exercised before performing RSI in any patient with a penetrating neck injury, and full preparations should be made for encountering a very difficult situation.

▶ LOWER AIRWAY DISEASE

Lower airway disease of sufficient severity to require intubation may stem from processes involving large (e.g., acute exacerbation of chronic obstructive pulmonary disease [COPD]) or small (e.g., bronchospasm) conducting airways, or lung parenchyma and alveoli (e.g., pneumonia, pulmonary contusion, or pulmonary edema). Many conditions of the lower airway requiring correction of gas exchange can be managed conservatively, for example, with use of noninvasive positive pressure ventilation. Often, the patient requiring intubation for lower airway pathology is experiencing fatigue and a marked deterioration of gas exchange.

▶ Case 16.2

A 19-year-old known asthmatic male presented by ambulance, in extreme respiratory distress. Despite continuous treatment with inhaled beta agonists en route to the ED, the patient was now drowsy and unable to speak in complete sentences. His breath sounds were diminished bilaterally and he had paradoxical abdominal respirations. His SaO_2 was 82% on oxygen via a nonrebreathing face mask; he had a RR of 30, HR of 150, and BP of 150/100.

Physiologic Considerations

Practically speaking, patients with recurrent reactive airways disease can be distinguished on the basis of age as having either asthma (in the younger patient), or COPD (in the older patient). Although they share the common pathophysiology of lower airway obstruction, their responses to therapies are different.

* *Noninvasive positive pressure ventilation (NPPV) has proven benefit in the COPD patient and may avert the need for endotracheal intubation when employed early.[18–20] The evidence for the use of NPPV in the asthmatic patient is less clear.[21, 22]*

The patient presented in Case 16–2 is in extreme distress, and any delay in definitive management may be fatal. In addition to treatment with B-agonists and corticosteroids, other agents such as ketamine and magnesium have been advocated as adjunctive therapy in cases of acute severe asthma.[23,24] However, these therapies are unlikely to be effective in the late stages of respiratory failure. As respiratory muscle fatigue ensues, tracheal intubation is indicated for predicted further clinical deterioration and correction of progressive hypoxemia, hypercarbia, and the resultant mixed respiratory and metabolic acidosis.

Pharmacologic Considerations

Tracheal intubation of the patient with lower airway disease can proceed with an awake approach or RSI. Generally, RSI is the preferred route, as placement of an endotracheal tube (ETT) in a deeply anesthetized patient is less likely to stimulate further bronchospasm. Any induction sedative/hypnotic can be used for induction, although ketamine is the only agent that may also provide some bronchodilation.

- *Although commonly recommended, there is little evidence to support the use of intravenous lidocaine as a pretreatment agent during RSI in the asthmatic patient.*[25]
- *As it bronchodilates in higher doses, ketamine is the ideal agent for induction of the patient in* status asthmaticus. *However, it should be noted that most evidence supporting its use comes from experience in pediatrics, as an adjunctive therapy in either the pre- or post-intubation phase.*[26-29]
- *The deep level of anesthesia needed to prevent further bronchospasm in response to laryngoscopy and intubation can be achieved with a large dose of induction sedative/ hypnotic, with or without pretreatment with a narcotic such as fentanyl.*
- *A rapid-onset neuromuscular blocker (succinylcholine or rocuronium) should be used during RSI. Although there is theoretic concern related to histamine release with some agents (e.g., thiopental; succinylcholine), there is no clinical evidence precluding the use of these medications to facilitate intubation of the asthmatic.*

Technical Considerations

As always, an airway assessment should be performed. The decision to intubate should ideally be made before hypoxia, or patient obtundation by hypercarbia precludes patient cooperation.

Airway Management Decisions

Direct laryngoscopy with endotracheal intubation is a potent stimulus for bronchospasm. The least traumatic, most effective means of achieving endotracheal intubation in the asthmatic *in extremis* is RSI with a deep plane of anesthesia.

- *However, in approaching an asthmatic requiring endotracheal intubation, it is also important to recognize that "tight" lungs may pose an obstacle to both mask ventilation and extraglottic rescue device use.*

- *Extraglottic devices with higher "pop-off" pressures would be appropriate to have available for the patient with poor lung compliance. Examples include the LMA ProSeal, LMA Supreme, and Combitube.*

Intubation and Postintubation Considerations

Airway management considerations in this population include the following:

- *No matter what the cause, the patient in respiratory distress often chooses to assume an upright position. BP permitting, this position should be retained until the patient undergoing RSI is rendered unconscious.*
- *If an awake intubation is performed on the patient in respiratory distress, it should be done with the patient in a sitting position. As long as the patient is not confused, awake intubations are often well tolerated in this population.*
- *In contrast to the patient with obstructing upper airway pathology, a larger sized endotracheal tube should be used for the patient with lower airway pathology: this will decrease airflow resistance and facilitate suctioning of secretions.*
- *Preoxygenation may be difficult but should be attempted, including patients known to be functioning on the basis of hypoxic drive.*
- *If RSI is chosen, rapid oxygen desaturation will occur (and should be anticipated) once apnea occurs. Bag-mask ventilation is essential, as soon as the patient stops breathing.*
- *Postintubation hypotension is not uncommon from a combination of hypovolemia from insensible losses, loss of sympathetic drive, and the effects of dynamic lung hyperinflation on venous return. A fluid bolus may be beneficial before proceeding with the tracheal intubation.*

Particularly in the patient with lower airway diseases, successful placement of an endotracheal tube is only the beginning of effective management. Postintubation challenges include decreased compliance, copious secretions, and hypotension.

- *Stimulation of the carina may cause worsening of bronchospasm, and should be avoided by ensuring appropriate location of the ETT tip.*
- *Ongoing sedation with neuromuscular blockade will prevent ventilator asynchrony, minimize the risk of barotrauma, reduce oxygen consumption and diminish CO_2 production.[27]*
- *"Breath stacking," or dynamic hyperinflation due to inadequate expiratory time, can significantly raise mean intrathoracic pressure ("auto-PEEP"). This can interfere with venous return, potentially causing cardiovascular collapse or barotrauma.*
- *The patient intubated for respiratory failure from pulmonary edema, pneumonia, or COPD may require frequent suctioning.*

Ventilator strategies to minimize complications include the use of permissive hypercapnia (i.e., controlled hypoventilation) whereby CO_2 levels of under 90 mm Hg may be accepted,[30] and attention to the expiratory phase of the ventilatory cycle. Recommended pressure-control ventilator settings[27] in *status asthmaticus* appear in Table 16–2.

▶ **TABLE 16–2** RECOMMENDED INITIAL VENTILATOR SETTINGS FOR STATUS ASTHMATICUS

Rate: 10–15 breaths/min
Tidal volume: 6–10 mL/kg
Minute ventilation: 8–10 L/min
PEEP: none
Inspiratory/expiratory ratio: (1:3
Inspiratory flow: (100 L/min
Maintain SaO_2 >90%
Pplat (end-inspiratory plateau pressure) <35 cm H_2O
V_{EI} (end-inspired volume above apneic FRC) <1.4 L

Adapted from Papiris.[27]

▶ SUMMARY

Patients presenting with acute respiratory disease require careful assessment and management choices, specific to the location and nature of the disease process. With upper airway obstruction, the most complex decisions revolve around the choices made during the preintubation phase, and the technical challenges of proceeding with an awake approach to the intubation. In contrast, in the patient with disease of the lower airway, (e.g., bronchospasm), management challenges continue and can be even greater after tracheal intubation.

REFERENCES

1. Mason RA, Fielder CP. The obstructed airway in head and neck surgery. *Anaesthesia.* 1999;54(7): 625–628.
2. Cload B, Howes D, Sivilotti M, et al. Where is the ET tube? *CJEM.* 2006;8 (6):436.
3. Green SM, Krauss B. Clinical practice guideline for emergency department ketamine dissociative sedation in children. *Ann Emerg Med.* 2004;44(5): 460–471.
4. Cohen VG, Krauss B. Recurrent episodes of intractable laryngospasm during dissociative sedation with intramuscular ketamine. *Pediatr Emerg Care.* 2006;22(4):247–249.
5. McGuire G, el-Beheiry H. Complete upper airway obstruction during awake fibreoptic intubation in patients with unstable cervical spine fractures. *Can J Anaesth.* 1999;46(2):176–178.
6. Kovacs G, Law JA, Petrie D. Awake fiberoptic intubation using an optical stylet in an anticipated difficult airway. *Ann Emerg Med.* 2007;49(1): 81–83.
7. Tallon JM, Ahmed JM, Sealy B. Airway management in penetrating trauma of the neck in a Canadian tertiary trauma centre. *Can J Emerg Med, in press.* 2007.
8. Martin R, Girouard Y, Cote DJ. Use of a laryngeal mask in acute airway obstruction after carotid endarterectomy. *Can J Anaesth.* 2002;49(8):890.
9. King CJ, Davey AJ, Chandradeva K. Emergency use of the laryngeal mask airway in severe upper airway obstruction caused by supraglottic oedema. *Br J Anaesth.* 1995;75(6):785–786.

10. Ho AM, Dion PW, Karmakar MK, et al. Use of heliox in critical upper airway obstruction.: Physical and physiologic considerations in choosing the optimal helium:oxygen mix. *Resuscitation.* 2002;52(3):297–300.

11. Smith SW, Biros M. Relief of imminent respiratory failure from upper airway obstruction by use of helium-oxygen: a case series and brief review. *Acad Emerg Med.* 1999;6(9):953–956.

12. MacDonnell SP, Timmins AC, Watson JD. Adrenaline administered via a nebulizer in adult patients with upper airway obstruction. *Anaesthesia.* 1995;50(1):35–36.

13. Nutman J, Brooks LJ, Deakins KM, et al. Racemic versus l-epinephrine aerosol in the treatment of postextubation laryngeal edema: results from a prospective, randomized, double-blind study. *Crit Care Med.* 1994;22(10):1591–1594.

14. Ghirga G, Ghirga P, Palazzi C, et al. Bag-mask ventilation as a temporizing measure in acute infectious upper-airway obstruction: does it really work? *Pediatr Emerg Care.* 2001;17(6):444–446.

15. Goldberg D, Bhatti N, Cummings Charles W. *Management of the impaired airway in the adult, Otolaryngology, Head and Neck Surgery.* Philadelphia Mosby;2005.

16. Mandavia DP, Qualls S, Rokos I. Emergency airway management in penetrating neck injury. *Ann Emerg Med.* 2000;35(3):221–225.

17. Moscati R, Jehle D, Ellis D, et al. Positive-outcome bias: comparison of emergency medicine and general medicine literatures. *Acad Emerg Med.* 1994;1(3):267–271.

18. Majid A, Hill NS. Noninvasive ventilation for acute respiratory failure. *Curr. Opin. Crit Care.* 2005;11(1):77–81.

19. Crummy F, Buchan C, Miller B, et al. The use of noninvasive mechanical ventilation in COPD with severe hypercapnic acidosis. *Respir. Med.* 2006.

20. Phua J, Kong K, Lee KH, et al. Noninvasive ventilation in hypercapnic acute respiratory failure due to chronic obstructive pulmonary disease vs. other conditions: effectiveness and predictors of failure. *Intensive Care Med.* 2005;31(4):533–539.

21. Ram FS, Wellington S, Rowe B, et al. Non-invasive positive pressure ventilation for treatment of respiratory failure due to severe acute exacerbations of asthma. *Cochrane. Database. Syst. Rev.* 2005(3):CD004360.

22. Agarwal R, Malhotra P, Gupta D. Failure of NIV in acute asthma: case report and a word of caution. *Emerg. Med. J.* 2006;23(2):e9.

23. Silverman RA, Osborn H, Runge J, et al. IV magnesium sulfate in the treatment of acute severe asthma: a multicenter randomized controlled trial. *Chest.* 2002;122(2):489–497.

24. Rowe BH, Bretzlaff JA, Bourdon C, et al. Intravenous magnesium sulfate treatment for acute asthma in the emergency department: a systematic review of the literature. *Ann Emerg Med.* 2000;36(3):181–190.

25. Butler J, Jackson R. Best evidence topic report. Lignocaine as a pretreatment to rapid sequence intubation in patients with status asthmaticus. *Emerg. Med. J.* 2005;22(10):732.

26. Cromhout A. Ketamine: its use in the emergency department. *Emerg. Med. (Fremantle).* 2003;15(2):155–159.

27. Papiris S, Kotanidou A, Malagari K, et al. Clinical review: severe asthma. *Crit Care.* 2002;6(1):30–44.

28. Denmark TK, Crane HA, Brown L. Ketamine to avoid mechanical ventilation in severe pediatric asthma. *J. Emerg. Med.* 2006;30(2):163–166.

29. Allen JY, Macias CG. The efficacy of ketamine in pediatric emergency department patients who present with acute severe asthma. *Ann Emerg Med.* 2005;46(1):43–50.

30. Oddo M, Feihl F, Schaller MD, et al. Management of mechanical ventilation in acute severe asthma: practical aspects. *Intensive Care Med.* 2006;32(4):501–510.

CHAPTER 17

The Critically Ill Patient

▶ INTRODUCTION

By definition, virtually all patients requiring emergency airway management are critically ill. Although the circumstances, challenges, and outcomes of these cases will always be patient-specific, certain generalizations can be made. In all cases, the goal should be to predict technical, anatomic, and physiologic barriers to safe airway management, and then take appropriate steps to meet the identified challenges.

▶ Case 17.1

A 60-year-old male was brought by ambulance to the emergency department (ED), complaining of shortness of breath. Earlier in the day, he had been begun on an oral antibiotic for a chest infection. He had a past history of coronary artery disease, hypertension and chronic bronchitis. In the ED, the patient was observed to be an anxious, overweight male, in marked respiratory distress. His vital signs were as follows: temperature 39.5°C; heart rate 120 (sinus tachycardia); blood pressure 106/60 mm Hg; respiratory rate 28/minute and SaO$_2$ of 88% on a nonrebreathing face mask (NRFM). A portable chest x-ray showed diffuse bilateral pulmonary infiltrates, consistent with a diagnosis of pneumonia.

▶ PHYSIOLOGIC CONSIDERATIONS

The physiologic goal of airway management in the critically ill patient is to maximize oxygen delivery and minimize injury at the cellular level. In the attempt to preserve oxygen delivery to the brain and heart in such patients, physiologic compensation occurs with vasoconstriction and catecholamine release. However, once such reserves are exceeded, the patient decompensates, and cellular injury occurs. Injured and ischemic cells swell, in turn compromising the microcirculation and preventing clearance of local toxins. This decompensated state may become irreversible and lead to multisystem organ failure, despite normalization of the patient's vital signs.

The patient who is, or may become critically ill must be recognized early. Appropriate treatment, including aggressive airway management, should be begun without delay, before irreversible changes occur. The clinician should anticipate the potential for physiologic decompensation and attempt to minimize procedurally related hypotension and worsened hypoxemia.

- *Due to his underlying chronic illnesses, the patient described in Case 17–1 has a significantly reduced physiologic reserve.*
- *Without appropriate action, his condition may quickly deteriorate to a decompensated state.*
- *Given his history of chronic hypertension, the patient's blood pressure is inappropriately*

low, quite possibly indicating a state of partially compensated septic shock.

• *Definitive emergent airway management is needed in this patient to facilitate end-organ oxygen delivery.*

▶ AIRWAY DECISIONS IN THE CRITICALLY ILL

Appropriate airway management in the critically ill patient requires consideration of three major decision nodes, each of which may be represented as part of a continuum (Fig. 17–1). The three nodes relate to patient **acuity, predicted difficulty,** and patient **cooperation.**

Patient Acuity

Acuity defines how much time is available to manage the patient's airway. An arrested, or rapidly deteriorating ("crashing"), hypoxic patient will present fewer airway management options than a more stable one. Help is often not available, difficult airway equipment may be some distance away, and trained assistants scarce. Although the basic principles of airway management should still be observed (e.g., pre-oxygenation), typically, the patient who is rapidly deteriorating will need intervention before optimal conditions are obtained. In very high acuity situations (e.g., the arrested patient),

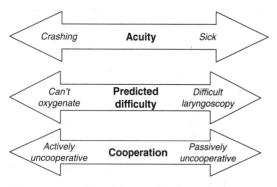

Figure 17–1. Decision nodes in the critically ill.

this may equate to simply proceeding with laryngoscopy and intubation there and then—very often, the patient will offer little resistance. On occasion, high-acuity situations may also lead to the need for RSI in scenarios where an awake intubation would have been chosen had time allowed.

• *Although the patient presented in Case 17–1 requires urgent airway management, his acuity is such that an airway assessment can be performed, and appropriate preparations for intubation made, prior to proceeding.*

The Predicted Difficult Airway

The second decision node considers the **predicted difficult airway**, a topic discussed in more detail in previous chapters. As always, if time permits, an assessment of the patient for predicted difficulty with bag-mask ventilation (BMV), laryngoscopy and intubation, and rescue oxygenation via extraglottic device (EGD) or cricothyrotomy should occur. However, in the critically ill patient, two additional considerations apply:

A. **Limited oxygen reserves**

The critically ill patient often has decreased oxygen reserves and increased consumption. If the patient is rendered apneic, any difficulty with subsequent oxygen delivery during the transition to positive pressure ventilation (e.g., by BMV, or via an endotracheal tube) will generally be very poorly tolerated, with rapid oxygen desaturation.

This propensity for rapid desaturation in the critically ill patient should prompt one of two responses: (a) an "awake" approach to tracheal intubation, whereby the patient helps maintain oxygenation with spontaneous respirations; or (b) if rapid-sequence intubation (RSI) is undertaken, full preparations for a difficult situation should occur

before proceeding, including the presence of an extra assistant for two-person BMV; fully prepared primary and alternative intubation devices, and a rescue EGD.

- *The patient in Case 17–1, with his suspected pulmonary pathology, is likely to have an increased shunt fraction. Obesity and his shallow breathing will limit his functional residual capacity (FRC). The effectiveness of preoxygenation will thus be limited, and he will desaturate quickly if rendered apneic.*
- *In the critically ill patient, assisted BMV may be needed during the preoxygenation phase, to improve oxygenation.*
- *If an RSI is undertaken, BMV should occur with the onset of apnea (if not already being assisted), anticipating rapid oxygen desaturation.*
- *Even without anticipated difficulty, in the critically ill patient, time available for intubation attempts will be shortened before reoxygenation by BMV is needed. Here again, the critically ill patient is poorly forgiving of difficulty.*

B. **Difficult physiology**

The critically ill patient is almost always significantly volume depleted, and may be hypotensive. A patient who is predicted to be poorly tolerant of induction sedative/hypnotic medications is sometimes best intubated using an "awake" approach.

- *Especially in the critically ill patient who is dyspneic and tachypneic, it is easy to overlook volume status. The patient in Case 17–1 (and most critically ill patients) should receive a fluid bolus via large-bore IV access prior to intubation, if acuity permits.*
- *For all emergency intubations, but especially those in the critically ill, rescue vasopressors such as ephedrine and phenylephrine should be drawn up and ready for administration.*

Patient Cooperation

The third decision node in the critically ill patient addresses the practical issue of **patient cooperation**. The critically ill patient may be **passively uncooperative** on the basis of hypoxemia, hypercarbia (as with the patient in respiratory failure) or simply hypotension. Although drowsy, the patient may not actively resist management interventions. This passive state may allow for an "awake" (i.e., non-RSI) approach to intubation, with application of topical airway anesthesia. In contrast, an **actively uncooperative** patient, who is agitated, or has clenched teeth, will almost always require pharmacologic relaxation as part of an RSI.

- *The assessment of patient cooperation requires bedside judgment.*
- *Many experienced clinicians with an appropriate skill set would choose to use an RSI for the patient presented in Case 17–1.*

Theoretically, for appropriate decision-making at each of the foregoing decision nodes, the clinician's skill set should also be considered. However, as discussed above, situation acuity in the critically ill patient often mandates proceeding before more expert assistance can be summoned. It is important to recognize that a delay in appropriate airway management in this patient population may lead to an irreversible clinical state, and ultimately, death.

- *With predictors of at least difficult BMV, the patient in Case 17–1 should have full preparations and a planned response for difficulty, including 2-person BMV with an OPA during ventilation between laryngoscopy attempts.*
- *Obese patients will desaturate quickly in the supine position, as will patients with respiratory failure.[1]*
- *Once supine, a "ramped" position (see Chap.5, figure 5–6) will facilitate airway management in the morbidly obese, including laryngoscopy.[2]*

• *Following successful tracheal intubation in this patient with COPD, during manual ventilation, adequate time must be allowed for expiration, to avoid further cardiovascular collapse from air-trapping and "auto-PEEP."*

▶ SHOCK STATES

▶ Case 17.2

A 22-year-old man was ejected from his vehicle in a high speed motor vehicle collision. He arrived in the ED on a spine board, with a cervical collar in place. He had a GCS of 9, an open fracture of the right femur, a visible contusion on the right side of his chest, and abdominal distension. His jaw was clenched shut. Blood pressure was 70/54, heart rate 134, respiratory rate 34, and SaO$_2$ 89% on a NRFM.

Shock defines a state of inadequate tissue perfusion and oxygen delivery. There are a variety of classifications used to describe the severity and causes of shock, based on physiologic parameters.

• *Clinically, shock is most commonly, although not exclusively, recognized by hypotension.*
• *In terms of severity, shock may be compensated (with preserved blood pressure) or uncompensated (low blood pressure).*
• *Pathology causing shock may arise from problems with the pump (i.e., cardiac), vessels (i.e., sepsis) or fluid (i.e., hemorrhage).*
• *Diminished venous return, loss of sympathetic tone and drugs given during airway management may all contribute to the development of an uncompensated shock state.*

Management of shock must always involve fluid resuscitation, regardless of etiology. Severely hypotensive patients will be obtunded, and a non-RSI approach (i.e., proceeding with direct laryngoscopy after applying some topical airway anesthesia) may be easily performed. If RSI is chosen in a more uncooperative patient with profound shock, the clinician must be aware that even very small doses of sedative/ hypnotic medications can have profoundly adverse hemodynamic effects. As discussed in the next section, if RSI is undertaken, induction doses must be reduced.

Pharmacologic Considerations in Shock States

Patients in shock are very sensitive to sedative/ hypnotic agents. Animal studies suggest that in hemorrhagic shock, alterations occur to pharmacokinetics and pharmacodynamics of both narcotics and sedative/hypnotics.[3–9] Changes in volumes of distribution and clearances for propofol,[3–5] etomidate,[6] fentanyl,[7] and remifentanil[8] in hemorrhagic shock result in higher brain drug concentrations, more rapid onset, and more profound effect.[9] In addition, for propofol, the brain sensitivity to the drug increases.[3–5,9] This translates to decreased dose requirements of at least 50% for narcotics, and even more (up to an 80%–90% decrease in dosage) for propofol in the setting of unresuscitated hemorrhagic shock.[9] For propofol, these effects appear to be partially, but not completely reversed after crystalloid resuscitation.[5]

In contrast to propofol, etomidate has performed well in animal studies of hemorrhagic shock, with little requirement for dosing adjustment.[6,9] This is in keeping with etomidate's reputation for maintenance of stable hemodynamics during RSI, and accounts for its widespread usage in North American EDs. As discussed in Chapter 13, etomidate will cause adrenocortical suppression with a resultant reduced circulating cortisol level.[10] This has led to calls by some for restriction of its use in the setting of a critically ill patient in whom having adequate levels of circulating cortisol is thought to be a determinant of outcome.[11,12]

▶ **TABLE 17–1** SUGGESTED DOSE RANGES FOR RSI SEDATIVE/HYPNOTIC AGENTS IN THE HYPOTENSIVE PATIENT

Systolic Blood Pressure	Etomidate (mg/kg)	Ketamine (mg/kg)	Propofol (mg/kg)
100	0.2–0.3	1–1.5	1–2
80–100	0.2	1.0	0.5–1
<80	0.15–0.2	0.5–1.0	0.25–0.5

Ketamine has traditionally been viewed as an agent of choice for RSI in the presence of hypotension, as blood pressure is often maintained, or indirectly raised by sympathetic nervous system stimulation. However, ketamine is intrinsically a negative inotrope, and may therefore further lower the blood pressure in the critically ill, hypotensive patient who is already using maximum compensatory sympathetic drive.[13]

Ketamine is usually avoided in head-injured patients, unless also suspected to be hypovolemic or known to be hypotensive. In the profoundly hypotensive, sympathetically driven head-injured patient, ketamine dosage should be reduced.[14] Approximate dosage reductions for sedative/hypnotic agent use in the hypotensive patient appear in Table 17–1.

Unfortunately, despite best efforts, postintubation hypotension may still ensue in the critically ill patient. The use of bolus doses of vasopressors as "rescue agents" in the postintubation phase should be considered to treat transient drops in blood pressure, but should never be considered a replacement for volume resuscitation.

▶ SUMMARY

The critically ill patient should ideally be identified prior to decompensation. Early airway management is indicated to ensure effective gas exchange. For safe clinical outcomes to occur, tracheal intubation decisions must consider patient acuity, cooperation, and predicted difficulty. Irrespective of the approach chosen for intubation, the critically ill patient will always require attention to fluid resuscitation, and careful choice and dosing of adjuvant medications.

REFERENCES

1. Dixon BJ, Dixon JB, Carden JR, et al. Preoxygenation is more effective in the 25 degrees head-up position than in the supine position in severely obese patients: a randomized controlled study. *Anesthesiology.* 2005;102(6):1110–1115.

2. Collins JS, Lemmens HJ, Brodsky JB, et al. Laryngoscopy and morbid obesity: a comparison of the "sniff" and "ramped" positions. *Obes Surg.* 2004;14(9):1171–1175.

3. De Paepe P, Belpaire FM, Rosseel MT, et al. Influence of hypovolemia on the pharmacokinetics and the electroencephalographic effect of propofol in the rat. *Anesthesiology.* 2000;93(6):1482–1490.

4. Johnson KB, Egan TD, Kern SE, et al. The influence of hemorrhagic shock on propofol: a pharmacokinetic and pharmacodynamic analysis. *Anesthesiology.* 2003;99(2):409–420.

5. Johnson KB, Egan TD, Kern SE, et al. Influence of hemorrhagic shock followed by crystalloid resuscitation on propofol: a pharmacokinetic and pharmacodynamic analysis. *Anesthesiology.* 2004;101(3):647–659.

6. Johnson KB, Egan TD, Layman J, et al. The influence of hemorrhagic shock on etomidate: a pharmacokinetic and pharmacodynamic analysis. *Anesth Analg.* 2003;96(5):1360–1368.

7. Egan TD, Kuramkote S, Gong G, et al. Fentanyl pharmacokinetics in hemorrhagic shock: a porcine model. *Anesthesiology.* 1999;91(1):156–166.

8. Johnson KB, Kern SE, Hamber EA, et al. Influence of hemorrhagic shock on remifentanil: a pharmacokinetic and pharmacodynamic analysis. *Anesthesiology.* 2001;94(2):322–332.

9. Shafer SL. Shock values. *Anesthesiology.* 2004;101(3):567–568.

10. Schenarts CL, Burton JH, Riker RR. Adrenocortical dysfunction following etomidate induction in emergency department patients. *Acad Emerg Med.* 2001;8(1):1–7.

11. Jackson WL Jr. Should we use etomidate as an induction agent for endotracheal intubation in patients with septic shock?: a critical appraisal. *Chest.* 2005;127(3):1031–1038.

12. den Brinker M, Joosten KF, Liem O, et al. Adrenal insufficiency in meningococcal sepsis: bioavailable cortisol levels and impact of interleukin-6 levels and intubation with etomidate on adrenal function and mortality. *J Clin Endocrinol Metab.* 2005;90(9):5110–5117.

13. Weiskopf RB, Bogetz MS, Roizen MF, et al. Cardiovascular and metabolic sequelae of inducing anesthesia with ketamine or thiopental in hypovolemic swine. *Anesthesiology.* 1984;60(3): 214–219.

14. Sehdev RS, Symmons DA, Kindl K. Ketamine for rapid sequence induction in patients with head injury in the emergency department. *Emerg Med Australas.* 2006;18(1):37–44.

CHAPTER 18

The Very Young and the Very Old Patient

▶ INTRODUCTION

People at the extremes of age often present with emergencies that require airway intervention. Patients in these age cohorts can present significant airway management challenges to clinicians with acute-care responsibilities.

▶ THE VERY YOUNG

The challenges encountered during airway management in infants are psychological, physiologic, and anatomic. The presentation of a "sick" infant, accompanied by distraught parents, can produce significant and potentially debilitating anxiety for many clinicians. Proportionately, far fewer children than adults present critically ill to the emergency department (ED). This fact may limit clinician comfort and familiarity with the "when and how" to perform acute airway management. Critically

▶ Case 18.1

A 9-day-old male infant, born at term following an uneventful pregnancy, had been discharged from hospital within 48 hours of birth. His 4-year-old brother was recovering from an upper respiratory tract infection. Within days, the baby had developed a runny nose and cough. The mother set out to return the infant to the hospital, but during the car ride, he became apneic and turned blue. On arrival, the baby was breathing again but had severe indrawing, head bobbing, eye rolling, hypotonia, and visible cyanosis. The triage nurse started oxygen by facemask and rushed the baby into the resuscitation area.

Sao_2 was 88% on high-flow oxygen by face mask. Respirations were irregular and at times gasping. A decision was made to immediately intubate the trachea. However, the attempt at emergency awake intubation was abandoned due to patient resistance, and an alarming drop in oxygen saturation.

Having failed to establish an airway by emergent awake intubation, the decision was made to proceed with an RSI. Prior to induction, using good bag-mask ventilation (BMV) technique synchronized to the baby's efforts, the Sao_2 rose to 94%, although the work of breathing remained extreme.

ill children, and in particular infants, may rapidly physiologically decompensate ("crump"), mandating immediate attention. Furthermore, size- and age-related anatomic variations may make recognition and management of this decompensated state challenging.

Physiologic Challenges

A number of physiologic challenges directly impact airway management of the infant. These include the following:

- **High oxygen consumption:** Infants have a relatively high cardiac output, minute volume of ventilation, and oxygen consumption, to match their high metabolic rate. This equates to rapid arterial desaturation when delivered oxygen or ventilation is reduced.[1,2]
- **Small oxygen reservoir:** Infants have relatively low-volume lungs, with functional residual capacities that overlap closing capacity. This results in a small oxygen reservoir and a tendency to ventilation/perfusion (V/Q) mismatch, which may in turn reduce the effectiveness of preoxygenation.[2]
- **Drug dosing:** Infants have higher extracellular fluid compartments than older children or adults. This expands the volume of distribution for water-soluble drugs such as succinylcholine. When combined with a high cardiac output, this translates to rapid onset and short duration of action of these drugs, together with the need for higher initial doses.[3]
- **High risk of regurgitation on induction:** The gastroesophageal junction is often incompetent in infants. The injection of succinylcholine can rapidly be followed by regurgitation of large volumes of formula or breast milk. Despite this, the occurrence of significant aspiration pneumonitis seems relatively uncommon. However, the use of cricoid pressure is still recommended (as part of a rapid-sequence intubation [RSI]) in an attempt to minimize this complication.[4,5]

For these reasons, it is important to appreciate that an RSI in infants is **really rapid**. Preoxygenation can usually be accomplished in less than 3 minutes. Although the pace following drug injection should be swift, the agents must still be allowed time to work. If assisted BMV is required to maintain oxygenation, applied cricoid pressure may reduce gastric insufflation, which, in the infant population, can otherwise cause clinically significant impairment of chest expansion.[6] This may also mandate gastric decompression by naso- or orogastric tube following tracheal intubation.[5]

Anatomic Challenges

Although infants can generally be intubated quite easily by direct laryngoscopy, there are clinically significant anatomic differences that must be recognized. Specific techniques may be required to overcome these challenges.

- **Acute airway axes:** Infants have large heads compared to their bodies. When lying flat on a stretcher, both their necks and atlanto-occipital (A-O) joints tend to be flexed. This positioning, combined with a relatively larger tongue, means that (in the supine infant) the trachea lies more anteriorly, and at an acute angle (less than 90°) relative to the axis of the oral cavity—far from the 180° ultimately needed for direct vision! Alignment of airway axes in the infant can be achieved in part simply by extending the head, as the lower neck is already flexed. Historically, it has been suggested that a rolled towel is needed under the shoulders of the small infant, as the proportionally larger head can otherwise cause excessive flexion at the A-O junction.
- **Large tongue, small jaw:** Infants naturally have a degree of glossoptosis—the "large tongue, small jaw" conundrum. The tongue is hypertrophied and muscular to facilitate suckling, and cannot be fully displaced into the relatively small submental space by the

laryngoscope blade. The laryngoscopist experiences this as an "anterior larynx."

- **Prominent preglottic structures:** The laryngeal inlet structures—epiglottis, false cords, and aryepiglottic folds—are prominent, redundant, soft, and highly mobile. To the uninitiated, they look "strange" and can interfere with visualization of the cords, or passage of the endotracheal tube (ETT). The epiglottis is "retroverted" i.e. angled toward the posterior pharyngeal wall, increasing the probability of a Grade 3 view at laryngoscopy. These anatomic variations in part contribute to the fact that children are more prone to airway obstruction, be it secondary to apposition of normal tissues during sedation, or from an underlying pathologic process.[7]

- **The "pseudo-larynx" deception:** The cricopharyngeal ring, at the esophageal inlet, when distorted by the anterior lift of a laryngoscope blade, can become a triangular structure with white side-walls (due to stretch-induced mucosal devascularization). This can mimic the appearance of an adult larynx quite convincingly. As a result, inadvertent esophageal intubation is a common complication for the inexperienced clinician.[8]

Technical Challenges

Many of the alternative intubation tools used in adults are not available in infant sizes. For those tools that are available, there is less supporting literature, compared to their adult congeners.

- **Bougie limitations:** Pediatric bougies are rarely used in infants, although they are available, with a distal coudé tip and in a size small enough to accept an ETT with internal diameter (ID) of 3 mm (Cook Medical Inc, Bloomington, IN). However, many clinicians experienced in infant intubation preferentially use a styletted ETT, angled as needed.

- **Few alternatives:** As previously mentioned in Chap. 6, the choices of proven alternative intubation tools available in infant sizes are limited. For example, the LMA Fastrach is not available for use in patients under 30 kg. The Bullard laryngoscope, the Glidescope and flexible fiberoptic bronchoscope are available in sizes consistent with use in the infant. However, few of these devices have significant supporting published literature on pediatric use. Pediatric fiberoptic stylets are available (e.g., the Shikani Seeing Optical Stylet [SOS] and the Brambrinck), accepting ETTs as small as 2.5 mm ID. The Shikani SOS is supported by some published accounts of success in the pediatric difficult airway.[9,10] The Trachlight, while available in child and infant sizes, has not produced results in this population as favorable as those experienced in the adults.[11] Traversing the laryngeal inlet with the Trachlight is challenging in the pediatric patient, and the light transmitted from the trachea is often indistinguishable from that obtained with esophageal placement.

- **Rescue oxygenation devices:** Fortunately, LMAs and other extraglottic devices are available in sizes to fit even a small premature baby (see Chap.7, Table 7–1). They are easily inserted and highly effective. They remain the only proven rescue technique for the failed infant airway.[12,13] The Combitube is not available in a pediatric size.

- **Surgical Airways:** The cricothyroid membrane is not developed at this age, so transtracheal access would occur below the cricoid cartilage in the infant. Specialized equipment for emergency transtracheal access is very limited for the infant: the smallest Melker needle-guided percutaneous cricothyrotomy cannula has an ID of 3.5 mm, while the Pedia-Trake Pediatric Emergency Cricothyrotomy Kit (Smiths Medical MD Inc., St. Paul MN) contains uncuffed cannulae of 3, 4, and 5 mm ID. For the failed oxygenation situation in an infant, unrelieved by EGD placement, many clinicians would proceed with percutaneous tracheal placement of a 20G (or larger) intravenous (IV) cannula connected to a self-inflating bag (See Chap. 7).

Awake Intubation in Infants

Awake intubation in infants was once popular: fear of failure to intubate led to a reluctance to use muscle relaxants. There is a rather perverse logic in the belief that awake intubation in infants is a reasonable option because infants have less muscular power than adults. Apart from the obvious ethical issues behind this logic, it is also the case that awake intubation in infants is generally more difficult, because cooperation is lacking. The current view among pediatric emergency physicians and anesthesiologists is that in general, RSI is the technique of choice for intubation of infants, unless a contraindication (such as known glottic pathology) exists.

RSI in Infants

The indications for and contraindications to RSI in infants do not differ from those in adults, but the technique does require modification, as described in the following sections:

A. **Preparation for infant RSI:** The standard "STOP IC BARS" mnemonic, previously presented in Chap. 5, can also be used in preparing equipment for infant intubation. Some special considerations apply:

- **Suction:** The suction catheter should be of a large size—nothing is more frustrating than attempting to clear thick secretions through a miniscule suction catheter. Nothing smaller than a 10 French catheter should be considered, and many clinicians recommend using the full size adult Yankauer suction tip.

- **Tubes:** Tracheal tubes should be marked with cord markers (one or more transverse lines on the tube that should be aligned with the vocal cords) to reduce the risk of right mainstem intubation. #3.0, 3.5 and 4.0 ID tubes should be ready. Most term infants will accept a 3.5 tube. The tubes should be styletted and bent to the appropriate shape. For infants beyond the newborn period, cuffed tubes

are probably as safe as uncuffed, provided that tube size, position and cuff pressures are optimized.[5]

- **Oxygen and positive pressure:** A range of suitable pediatric masks should be readied and test-fitted to the patient during preoxygenation. An oropharyngeal airway, sized by the "corner of mouth to angle of mandible" technique (usually 5–6 cm or 00–0 size), should be ready. Pediatric-sized manual resuscitators are available: to help avoid barotrauma, most have incorporated "pop-off" valves which can be adjusted to limit applied positive pressure.

- **Pharmacology:** Ketamine 2.5 mg/kg, succinylcholine 2.0 mg/kg, rocuronium 1 mg/kg, atropine 0.1 mg, and ephedrine 5 mg diluted to 1mg/mL should be drawn up.

- **Intravenous Access:** Intravenous access using a #22G IV catheter should be obtained. Failing this, an intraosseous needle should be inserted. Vascular access by intravascular or intraosseous routes is critical to successful pediatric airway management, as drugs delivered by the intramuscular (IM) route are of marginal value at best.

- **Connect to Monitors and Confirmation:** At a minimum, a pulse oximeter and automatic blood pressure (BP) cuff set to 3-minute measurement intervals must be applied. Optimally, ECG leads should also be applied. A pediatric $ETCO_2$ detection device, or quantitative CO_2 monitoring should be available.

- **Blades:** Recommended laryngoscope blades for infant intubation are #0 and #1 straight blades, preferably of the Wisconsin or Flagg design, as these provide more room inside the cross-sectional arc of the blade than the classic Miller blade. A lightweight, small laryngoscope handle is preferred, but the adult handle can also be used.

- **Alternative intubation, rescue oxygenation, and surgical airway** options have been discussed above. A size 0 and 1 LMA (or other infant-sized EGD) should be prepared for rescue oxygenation, and the difficult airway cart should be on hand.

B. **Infant RSI: the procedure**
  - With the monitors applied and the IV dripping, preoxygenation is carried out for 3 minutes. The technique of holding a mask on the face of a frightened child may be difficult, but is not impossible. Bundling the infant to restrain the arms and legs and using a "cradling technique" (the operator's arms prevent head movement while applying the mask with a two-hand grip) is usually successful.
  - A rapid fluid bolus of 10–20 mL/kg is desirable, and mandatory if there is any suspicion of dehydration or shock. An assistant can push this in during preoxygenation.
  - Optimal positioning for laryngoscopy should be undertaken, as discussed earlier in this chapter.
  - After 3 minutes of preoxygenation, ketamine 2 mg/kg and succinylcholine 2 mg/kg, for example, are injected by an assistant, using rapid IV push. Many clinicians have historically also used atropine pretreatment in this context, although, as discussed in more detail in Chap.13, evidence is lacking for this practice.
  - If the lungs are reasonably healthy, and preoxygenation has been successful, the RSI can often be completed without performing BMV. However, as discussed, rapid desaturation is common. This should be prevented or rapidly remedied with BMV, with an oropharyngeal airway in place.
  - Infants do not always fasciculate—they may simply go limp following administration of succinylcholine. Laryngoscopy should start once "relaxation" is achieved

(usually earlier than the adult, that is, in about 20–30 seconds).
  - The right hand should extend the atlanto-occipital joint and open the mouth. The left hand inserts the blade into the right paraglossal gutter and follows the edge of the tongue until the epiglottis is seen. The epiglottis is then everted, either directly, by placing the blade beneath the epiglottis and lifting, or indirectly, with blade advancement into the vallecula and engaging the hyoepiglottic ligament. The blade should now be moved towards the middle of the oral cavity to displace the tongue to the patient's left, thereby creating more room for tube insertion on the right.
  - Once the cords are visualized, the endotracheal tube is inserted, preferably from the right corner of the mouth, so as not to occlude the view down the blade. The transverse cord marker printed on the distal ETT is placed at the level of the vocal cords, and the position of the tube relative to the upper lip is noted.
  - If difficulty is encountered in attaining a view of the larynx with DL, consideration should be given to easing or releasing cricoid pressure, performing external laryngeal manipulation (ELM), or adjusting the blade tip location.
  - The tube is held firmly in place while the self-inflating bag and ETCO$_2$ confirmation device are attached, manual ventilation is commenced, and correct tracheal placement confirmed.
  - Several (relatively) large breaths are administered to permit assessment of chest expansion and auscultation for equal air entry.
  - If oxygen saturation is difficult to maintain, if air entry appears unequal, or if the chest feels "stiff," the most likely problem is right main-stem bronchial intubation. Laryngoscopy should be repeated, and the ETT withdrawn until the cord marker

sits at the appropriate level, prior to re-taping the tube in place.

C. **Failed intubation in the infant**

- Laryngoscopy should be discontinued when the SaO_2 falls below 90%, or an intubation attempt approaches 30 seconds.
- After a failed attempt at intubation, BMV should be reestablished, using an oropharyngeal airway if necessary.
- If the airway can be maintained and BMV is successful, a second dose of succinylcholine 2 mg/kg may be administered, or rocuronium 1 mg/kg. Before giving a second dose of succinylcholine, atropine 0.1 mg should be given.
- For a second or third attempt at intubation, a blade change can be considered, as can the use of an alternative intubation device, if availability and clinician skill permit.
- Following three unsuccessful attempts at intubation, an EGD such as an LMA should be inserted, the cuff inflated and ventilation maintained. Alternatively, one may revert to BMV with applied cricoid pressure, until definitive care can be arranged.

D. **Postintubation care in the infant**

- Once the tube is confirmed to be correctly positioned, it should be secured with obsessive attention to detail. Skin preparation with Friar's Balsam or alcohol is recommended to maximize tape adherence. The maxilla is a more stable fixation point than the mandible. Many pediatric clinicians fix the tube to both the maxilla and mandible and cover the tape with a second layer of waterproof tape. Alternatively, if available, a commercial fixation device may be used to secure the tube.
- Succinylcholine will wear off in a very short time (i.e., less than 5 minutes) after administration. A longer acting muscle relaxant such as rocuronium 1 mg/kg is usually required, if paralysis is to be maintained.

- Postintubation hypotension should be treated with fluid boluses and pressor administration.
- Gastric distension due to BMV is common— following tracheal intubation, a gastric tube should be inserted to aid decompression.[5]
- A chest x-ray should be obtained to confirm ETT positioning above the carina.
- Suctioning the tube until free of secretions is essential.
- Sedation can be achieved with agents such as midazolam or propofol. Although rare, propofol infusion syndrome has been described, most commonly associated with prolonged pediatric use in the intensive care unit (ICU) setting.[14] Analgesia and further sedation may occur using morphine 0.1 mg/kg/h, or fentanyl 1 µg/kg/h.

▶ THE VERY OLD

▶ Case 18.2

An 82-year-old man arrived in the ED with fever, cough, and confusion. On examination, he had scattered crackles in both lung fields and was in severe respiratory distress. He had a history of stable angina, arthritis, and hypertension. He had a mild stroke 2 years before. His temperature was 38.8°C, pulse 120, respiratory rate 32/minute, BP 170/90, and his Sao_2 was 82% on a nonrebreathing face mask. His chest x-ray showed bilateral pulmonary infiltrates. With a presumptive diagnosis of pneumonia, antibiotic therapy was begun, and a decision was made to proceed with tracheal intubation.

As with the infant in the first case, the elderly patient poses age-related physiologic and anatomic challenges, and is at increased risk for conditions that will require airway management. It is sobering to realize that many elderly patients suffer permanent reduction in cerebration even after well-managed general anesthesia. This is attributed, at least in part, to regional cerebral blood flow problems, related to cerebrovascular disease.

End-of-life issues may complicate tracheal intubation decisions in the elderly. However, age alone should never be the sole determinant of whether or not to initiate resuscitation. Withholding acute care in the emergency setting is generally less common than subsequent withdrawal of therapy, simply because the information needed to make these decisions is often not yet available.[15] Understandably, physicians and families are frequently uncomfortable in addressing these issues in the acute setting. However, while the decision to intubate should consider patient and family wishes, a judgment should also be made as to whether the intervention represents futile care.

Physiologic Challenges

- **Pulmonary limitations:** As with infants, octogenarians have a relatively low ratio of functional residual capacity (FRC) to total lung capacity, with closing volumes that may encroach on normal tidal breathing.[16] In addition, they may have ongoing conditions such as chronic obstructive pulmonary disease (COPD) or restrictive lung disease. These diseases may increase shunt fraction, airway closure, air trapping, and dead space. This will limit the effectiveness of preoxygenation, and places the elderly patient at increased risk of hypoxia and hypercarbia.
- **Circulatory limitations:** The elderly are prone to cerebrovascular, coronary, and large-vessel atherosclerotic disease. The physiologic consequence is a reduction in effective organ blood flow, autoregulation, and pressure-dependant organ perfusion. Changes in BP can lead to hypoperfusion, with devastating effects such as stroke or myocardial infarction.
- **Pharmacologic intolerance:** For less well-understood reasons, but perhaps linked to reduced myocardial performance and low vascular compliance, the aged are prone to swings in BP with physiologic stress. Moderate stress may cause severe BP spikes. Conversely, small doses of benzodiazepines, narcotics, and sedative/hypnotics may cause unexpected unconsciousness and severe hypotension. The hypotension, especially in combination with reflex tachycardia, may lead to coronary insufficiency, arrhythmias, cardiac arrest, stroke, and other organ damage.[17,18]

Anatomic Challenges

- **Bag-mask ventilation:** Loss of subcutaneous fat in the face, presence of facial hair, and limited dentition may make mask fit difficult. Dentures, if secure, may be left in place during BMV, while beards can be slathered with water-soluble lubricant to facilitate mask seal.
- **Laryngoscopy:** Limited mouth opening and prominent or asymmetric dentition can make laryngoscope blade insertion difficult. Tooth loss is always a risk and can be a serious complication where single teeth anchors dental prostheses. Dentures should normally be removed for laryngoscopy. Reduced atlantooccipital and neck mobility due to degenerative joint disease may fix the oral-tracheal angle near 90°, interfering with laryngeal visualization.

In contrast to the situation for the very young, a wide variety of alternatives to direct laryngoscopy exist for the adult patient. Devices previously described such as the LMA Fastrach, Trachlight, and various rigid fiberoptic or video-based instruments can be extremely helpful in the patient with reduced jaw or neck mobility.

Technical Challenges

In general, indications for, and contraindications to RSI and awake intubation in the elderly are the same as those for younger adults. Successful awake intubation requires skill and appropriate patient selection. While an awake approach avoids the hemodynamic consequences of induction agents, the unabated pressor response to laryngoscopy and intubation also has the potential to cause harm in certain patients. Execution of the RSI procedure does require modification.

A. **Preparation for RSI in the elderly**
   - **Airway assessment**: Recognition of the age-related anatomic challenges previously presented requires preparation for both difficult BMV and difficult laryngoscopy.
   - **Equipment should be prepared**. The edentulous patient will require a face mask one or two sizes smaller. A bougie should be within reach for use as an adjunct to direct laryngoscopy.
   - **Intravenous access** and cautious volume loading with 10–20 mL/kg of crystalloid is still appropriate, in an attempt to mitigate the hypotensive effect of RSI drugs.
   - **Preoxygenation** should occur, including assisted BMV, if needed to raise the SaO_2. The conservative use of oxygen for fear of adversely affecting the "hypoxic drive to breathe" in the COPD patient is not appropriate in the preintubation phase.
   - **Drug doses** for RSI sedative/hypnotics should be adjusted downward for the elderly patient, often by 50% or more. Muscle relaxant doses do not require adjustment. Pressor drugs such as ephedrine or phenylephrine should always be drawn up for use in maintaining the BP close to the patient's baseline. It is probably better to err on the side of hypertension, although tachycardia and profound elevation of BP should be avoided.
   - **Adjuncts, alternative intubation, and rescue devices.** The airway cart should be on stand-by, and the alternative intubation device (e.g., LMA Fastrach) with which the clinician is most familiar should be sized and prepared for use. A rescue oxygenation device, such as a Combitube or other EGD should also be chosen and sized before proceeding with an RSI.

B. **RSI in the elderly: the procedure**
   - RSI in the elderly requires a light touch. The goal throughout the intubation process is to maintain an unchanged pulse and BP, while maintaining adequate oxygenation and ventilation.
   - Because of its hemodynamic stability, etomidate is an attractive choice for RSI in the elderly. However, as previously discussed, etomidate will cause adrenal suppression. Although the clinical significance of this effect is unclear, in general, etomidate should be avoided in the septic patient when an appropriate alternative agent is available. Propofol often produces hypotension, especially if doses are not appropriately adjusted downward for the elderly, while the sympathetic stimulation caused by ketamine may produce unwanted hypertension and tachycardia. The mixture of propofol and ketamine (widely used off-label in pediatrics) may be of value in the elderly, but published experience is limited.
   - It is critical to remain aware of vital signs throughout the RSI sequence—this can be difficult. Prolonged efforts at intubation, with attendant vital sign changes, must be avoided. The laryngoscopist should abandon the intubation attempt before the patient becomes hypoxemic, hypercarbic, tachycardic, or hypo- or hypertensive.

C. **Failed intubation in the elderly**
   - Again, persistent laryngoscopy is hazardous to the patient: reoxygenation should precede any further attempts.

- An alternative intubation technique should be considered, if "best look" laryngoscopy and the use of an adjunct such as a bougie or fiberoptic stylet has failed. A change to a longer, or differently shaped (e.g., straight or levering tip) blade may be of use in selected patients. Alternative device use should consider operator experience and the likelihood of success. It may be more appropriate to temporize by proceeding to a rescue EGD in lieu of using an unfamiliar alternative technique, when "best look" laryngoscopy has failed after two or three attempts.

D. **Postintubation care in the elderly**

- Successful airway management should not detract from the recognition that even with a secured airway, the elderly patient remains fragile and prone to cerebrovascular and cardiac catastrophe. Airway management is only the first step in providing the critically ill elderly patient an opportunity to return to meaningful life. The aging heart, brain, and kidney need optimal oxygenation and perfusion if they are to survive.

▶ SUMMARY

Most aspects of airway management at the extremes of life are similar to those needed for the older child and non-elderly adult. However, the clinician must be cognizant of the anatomic and physiologic differences which may be encountered, with the resultant need to prepare for difficulty and adjust drug dosing appropriately.

REFERENCES

1. Patel R, Lenczyk M, Hannallah RS, et al. Age and the onset of desaturation in apnoeic children. *Can. J. Anaesth.* 1994;41(9):771–774.

2. Morrison JE, Jr., Collier E, Friesen RH, et al. Pre-oxygenation before laryngoscopy in children: how long is enough? *Paediatr. Anaesth.* 1998;8(4):293–298.

3. Meretoja OA, Bissonnette B, Dalens B. *Muscle relaxants in Children in Pediatric Anesthesia: Principles and Practice.* New York: McGraw-Hill 2002.

4. Zelicof-Paul A, Smith-Lockridge A, Schnadower D, et al. Controversies in rapid sequence intubation in children. *Curr. Opin. Pediatr.* 2005;17(3):355–362.

5. 2005 AHA Guidelines for CPR and ECC. Part 12. Pediatric Advanced Life Support. *Circulation.* 2005;112(24 Supplement):167–187.

6. Moynihan RJ, Brock-Utne JG, Archer JH, et al. The effect of cricoid pressure on preventing gastric insufflation in infants and children. *Anesthesiology.* 1993;78(4):652–656.

7. Goldmann K. Recent developments in airway management of the paediatric patient. *Curr. Opin. Anaesthesiol.* 2006;19(3):278–284.

8. O'Donnell CP, Kamlin CO, Davis PG, et al. Endotracheal intubation attempts during neonatal resuscitation: success rates, duration, and adverse effects. *Pediatrics.* 2006;117(1):e16–e21.

9. Pfitzner L, Cooper MG, Ho D. The Shikani Seeing Stylet for difficult intubation in children: initial experience. *Anaesth Intensive Care.* 2002;30(4):462–466.

10. Shukry M, Hanson RD, Koveleskie JR, et al. Management of the difficult pediatric airway with Shikani Optical Stylet. *Paediatr. Anaesth.* 2005;15(4):342–345.

11. Fisher QA, Tunkel DE. Lightwand intubation of infants and children. *J. Clin. Anesth.* 1997;9(4):275–279.

12. Bortone L, Ingelmo PM, De Ninno G, et al. Randomized controlled trial comparing the laryngeal tube and the laryngeal mask in pediatric patients. *Paediatr. Anaesth.* 2006;16(3):251–257.

13. Grein AJ, Weiner GM. Laryngeal mask airway versus bag–mask ventilation or endotracheal intubation for neonatal resuscitation. *Cochrane. Database. Syst. Rev.* 2005(2):CD003314.

14. Fudickar A, Bein B, Tonner PH. Propofol infusion syndrome in anaesthesia and intensive care medicine. *Curr Opin Anaesthesiol.* 2006;19(4):404–410.

15. Iserson KV. Withholding and withdrawing medical treatment: an emergency medicine perspective. *Ann. Emerg. Med.* 1996;28(1):51–54.

16. Birnbaumer D, Marx JA, Hockberger RS, et al. The Elder Patient. *Rosen's Emergency Medicine: Concepts and Clinical Practice.* Vol 5th: CV Mosby; 2002:2485.

17. John AD, Sieber FE. Age associated issues: geriatrics. *Anesthesiol. Clin. North America.* 2004;22(1): 45–58.

18. Burton DA, Nicholson G, Hall GM. Anaesthesia in elderly patients with neurodegenerative disorders: special considerations. *Drugs Aging.* 2004;21(4): 229–242.

CHAPTER 19

Prehospital Airway Management Considerations

► GENERAL CONSIDERATIONS

Emergency airway management should be performed by a skilled clinician. In this book, the term "clinician" has included both physician and nonphysician health-care providers. Depending on the setting, paramedics, nurse practitioners, and respiratory technicians may be expected to independently manage patients with acute airway emergencies. As long as they possess the appropriate knowledge base and procedural skills, this is entirely appropriate. The practice of airway management should be defined by educational and competency-based

► Case 19.1

A 20-year-old male was ejected as the result of a high-speed rollover motor vehicle crash (MVC), on a rural highway. When the paramedics arrived on the scene, they were faced with a hypotensive patient who was breathing spontaneously, but with a Glasgow Coma Scale (GCS) of 8, and a clenched jaw. The crew had given a "ten minute head's up" prior to their arrival at the local emergency department. At that time, they reported vital signs of BP 90/75, HR 100, RR 20, and SaO₂ 98% on a nonrebreathing face mask.

criteria, and not limited by departmental or discipline-related turf battles.

Prehospital care of the patient in case 19-1 will include the following:

- Ensuring scene safety.
- Attention to oxygenation, ventilation, and blood pressure.
- Recognizing the potential for cervical spine injury, and taking appropriate precautions.
- Being ready for the unexpected, such as vomiting or seizure.
- Ruling out reversible causes of coma, such as hypoglycemia or drug toxicity.
- Making decisions about appropriate on-scene interventions prior to transport.

Without doubt, airway management skills are necessary in the prehospital setting, with early support of oxygenation and ventilation for the acutely ill. However, whether this is achieved by bag-mask ventilation (BMV) or tracheal intubation depends on a number of factors, including, most immediately, anticipated time and type of transport. Local Emergency Medical Services (EMS) jurisdictions may also have established algorithms or protocols.

The general approach to airway management in the prehospital environment should follow the **same principles** already espoused in this text. Appropriate airway management decisions require consideration of:

- Clinician factors (knowledge base, psychomotor skills, equipment, and the availability of trained assistants).
- Higher acuity (obtain/maintain an airway, and/or correction of gas exchange) versus lower acuity (airway protection and/or predicted clinical deterioration) indications for tracheal intubation.
- Patient assessment (anatomy, physiology, cooperation, and **time**).

▶ CLINICIAN FACTORS

Prehospital care providers with acute airway management responsibilities should have a cognitive level of understanding comparable to that of clinicians staffing the emergency department (ED). They must understand the indications and contraindications for advanced airway management, including tracheal intubation. Providers should be comfortable in performing an airway assessment and predicting difficulty. They should be able to choose a safe and effective method to manage the patient's airway, have the procedural skills to competently perform it, and have an approach to difficult situations.

The education of prehospital providers must also be realistic and should reflect their practice mandate. For example, knowledge of rapid-sequence intubation (RSI) drug pharmacology should be included only if it is within their scope of practice. Their procedural skill set will be similarly guided. In an ideal world, training objectives for attaining and maintaining procedural skills in BMV or endotracheal intubation would be identical for all individuals, regardless of their professional designation. In practice, for the prehospital provider, the logistics of attaining and maintaining these competencies are often difficult, with the practical pressures of equipment availability, cost, and the sheer volume of trainees posing a problem. Medical directors must understand these limitations when designing educational and continuous quality improvement (CQI) programs, or when

designing protocols for prehospital airway management providers. Pragmatically, North American standards of prehospital care often include a higher level of cognitive and skills training in airway management if the providers work in an air ambulance program, or as part of a dedicated ground-based critical care transport team.

▶ PREHOSPITAL INDICATIONS FOR ADVANCED AIRWAY MANAGEMENT

"Advanced" airway management in the context of prehospital practice refers primarily to tracheal intubation. However, in some EMS settings, advanced airway management involves the use of an extraglottic device (EGD) such as the Combitube or Laryngeal Mask Airway (LMA). In general, however, the indications for tracheal intubation are as previously discussed in this text: to obtain or maintain an airway; correct gas exchange, protect the airway against aspiration of gastric contents, or for predicted clinical deterioration. However, it is important to understand that each of these indications represents a very different scenario. The high acuity, apneic (e.g., cardiac arrest) patient requires an immediate, "crash" airway. A patient hypoxic from respiratory failure due to congestive heart failure (CHF) may also be higher acuity and require tracheal intubation, but can often be safely temporized during transport. A head injured patient with a GCS of 8 and an SaO_2 of 98% may well require intubation for airway protection, but with less urgency for the intervention. Predicted clinical deterioration is a similarly lower acuity indication for intubation.

▶ PATIENT ASSESSMENT

The three components of patient assessment discussed in Chap. 11—that is, airway anatomy, system physiology, and patient cooperation are very relevant to the prehospital provider.

However, a fourth variable must be emphasized in the assessment of the patient in a prehospital setting, and this is **time**. Simply put, when is it better to attempt definitive airway management on the scene, and when is it better to wait?

- *The patient described in* **Case 19–1** *clearly represents a critically ill, head-injured trauma patient who is hemodynamically compromised.*
- *He will be immobilized in a cervical collar and has clenched teeth, which may make direct laryngoscopy difficult. Conversely, his patent airway and stable SaO₂ create a lower acuity need for immediate tracheal intubation.*
- *If this patient is relatively close to the trauma center, then it may be advisable to transport while monitoring the patient's spontaneous ventilations and oxygenation status.*
- *If transport with assisted BMV is required, attention to good technique is important, to avoid gastric insufflation. Otherwise, regurgitation could occur, potentially leading to aspiration and a difficult mask ventilation scenario.*
- *In contrast, if the same patient did not have clenched teeth, had marginal oxygen saturation ($SaO_2<90\%$) despite assisted BMV, and was 40 minutes from a trauma center, then an intubation attempt could be considered, if provider skills and protocols allowed.*

In either scenario, both "airway protection" and "predicted clinical deterioration" are legitimate but lower acuity indications for intubation. However, the chosen approach in the prehospital setting will also be based on the added issue of transport time. A short transport time, combined with a predicted difficult airway and a lower acuity indication for intubation, favors skillful BMV *en route* to the ED, where definitive airway management can occur. Training of prehospital personnel must thus emphasize that optimal airway management does not always equate to tracheal intubation. In other words, the **technical imperative** of "getting the tube" should not overshadow the **outcome imperative** of maintaining adequate gas exchange.

► CHOOSING A METHOD OF TRACHEAL INTUBATION

In general, the choices to facilitate tracheal intubation (RSI; non-RSI [i.e., "awake" or deep sedation] and 1° surgical) in the prehospital setting are similar to those used in-hospital. Realistically, most ground EMS systems are limited by training and maintenance of competence issues to non-RSI intubation choices and/or EGDs such as the LMA or Combitube.[1] Non-RSI choices for tracheal intubation span the spectrum from truly "awake" to an intubation facilitated by deep sedation. The dangers of deep sedation to facilitate intubation are just as relevant in the prehospital arena as they are in-hospital. In fact, the use of sedative agents to facilitate airway management in the prehospital setting parallels the history of their use in the ED. Rightly or wrongly in the prehospital arena, familiarity with using drugs such as diazepam and morphine in the context of symptom relief has allowed for a gradual acceptance of their use to facilitate intubation using deep sedation.

Cardiac arrest is the clinical context for up to two-thirds of all tracheal intubations in a typical ground EMS system.[2] For these patients, there is generally no requirement for pharmacologic adjuncts to facilitate intubation. The remainder of the EMS patient cohort requiring airway management tends to be evenly split among respiratory failure, nontraumatic central nervous system (CNS) conditions, trauma, and shock states. In general, helicopter Emergency Medical Services (HEMS) operations do not respond to primary cardiac arrest victims and, therefore, deal with a patient population of similar complexity to that in the ED. With this clearly different patient population, and more manageable provider numbers, educational

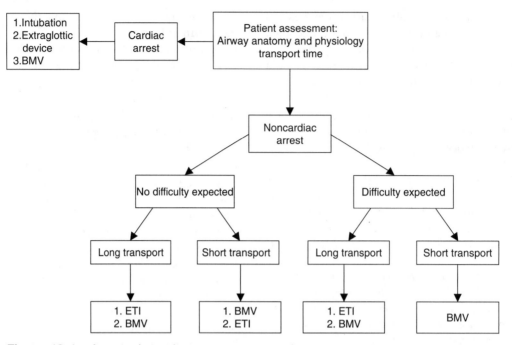

Figure 19–1. Approach to airway management for prehospital ground systems.

support is more feasible, which in turn has allowed many HEMS programs to introduce RSI as a safe management option for use by their crews.

The evidence in the EMS literature supporting the use of RSI is scant,[3,4] save for some very specific circumstances. For ground EMS systems, several well-conducted studies have consistently shown worsened, or insignificant differences in outcome in traumatic brain injury patients when prehospital RSI is used to facilitate endotracheal intubation.[5–8] Head injury was deliberately chosen in these studies, as previous studies had suggested that optimal and timely oxygenation of these patients improved outcomes.[9] However, despite the lack of efficacy of RSI demonstrated in ground-based EMS systems, a distinct pattern of improved outcomes has in fact emerged in the subpopulation of those patients where air medical transport had been utilized.[8,10–13] It would thus appear that the key to improved outcomes lies in the initial training and maintenance

of competence programs (addressing both cognitive and procedural skills components) for prehospital providers, with particular attention to the avoidance of transient hypoxia and/or hyperventilation.[14–16]

Given this evidence, a well-prepared HEMS program could use an approach to tracheal intubation algorithm similar to that previously presented (see Chap.11, Fig. 11–3) in this text. However, a prehospital ground system *not* using RSI may require a different approach, as shown in Fig. 19–1.

► EQUIPMENT OPTIONS AND THE DIFFICULT AIRWAY

The procedural skills required for successful BMV and laryngoscopy and intubation are the same for all providers. However, the environmental context of the prehospital setting adds an additional layer of complexity to airway management.

Issues of lighting, weather, scene safety and location, and the presence of distraught family members often create unique challenges to the prehospital care provider.

Direct laryngoscopy (DL) remains the most appropriate approach to tracheal intubation in the prehospital setting, despite its significant learning curve. Unlike the blind or indirect visualization intubation techniques, DL retains the advantage of enabling the provider to assess the oral cavity for presence of foreign material during the intubation attempt.

The approach to the difficult airway in the prehospital setting is similar to that previously outlined in this text. Difficult tracheal intubation, once encountered, requires an approach that employs first attempt "best look" laryngoscopy, including the use of external laryngeal manipulation (ELM) and a bougie. A change in the blade type or length may be useful depending on the encountered problem. The benefit of repeated attempts at intubation should always be weighed against the risk of prolonging the scene time. The advisability of proceeding to an alternative intubation device such as the LMA Fastrach if laryngoscopic intubation fails is less clear in the prehospital setting. Indeed, failed intubation in this context might be defined by two unsuccessful attempts (as opposed to three) and would usually mean reverting to BMV or an EGD such as the Combitube or LMA. A falling oxygen saturation after an initial attempt at laryngoscopy should preclude further attempts at intubation until the patient's oxygenation has been corrected by BMV, EGD or ultimately, cricothyrotomy.

For the paramedic, although the principles of airway management are the same, the spectrum of available equipment may not be as wide. However, prehospital systems considering an RSI program should have several difficult airway devices available:

- The **bougie** is simple, inexpensive, and proven in the prehospital arena;[17] **blade change** options should also be available.

- **Alternative intubating devices:** the LMA Fastrach is simple and may provide a reasonable prehospital option;[18] the Trachlight is a less realistic option because of skill maintenance issues and the inability to control environmental lighting. Fiberoptic- or video-based devices may be useful, but, especially for ground EMS systems, cost often precludes outfitting of entire fleets.

- **Rescue oxygenation devices:** the Combitube has a long track record in prehospital care, used as a rescue oxygenation device[19] or as a primary airway, especially in the setting of cardiac arrest.[20] An LMA can also be used as a primary or rescue device in this setting.[20,21] Newer EGDs such as the King LTS-D and the LMA ProSeal and Supreme look promising for the prehospital setting due to their esophageal drainage tubes and design features enabling higher ventilating pressures, if needed. However, scientific validation of their use in the field is still required.

- **Surgical airway:** many EMS systems now stock needle-guided percutaneous cricothyrotomy devices (e.g., the Melker or the Portex PCK), which are relatively simple to use.[22]

Finally, confirmation of correct endotracheal tube (ETT) placement, initially and continuously, is vitally important in the chaotic prehospital environment, as the consequences of an unrecognized misplaced endotracheal tube are always devastating. The exact number of unrecognized esophageal intubations in the prehospital setting is uncertain, as many EMS systems do not systematically gather this data. Very low rates are found in systems with specific tube verification protocols, including end-tidal CO_2 (ETCO$_2$) monitoring, and ongoing quality improvement programs to ensure compliance.[23] Conversely, unacceptably high rates of esophageal intubation are found when no such protocols are in place.[24]

Prehospital care providers can objectively confirm correct placement of the ETT in the same ways previously discussed in this text: by visualization of tube going between cords;

use of an ETCO$_2$ detector and/or by using a mechanical esophageal detector device (EDD). ETCO$_2$ verification of correct ETT placement has become the standard of care in the EMS arena.[25] The limitations of each of these techniques have been previously discussed.

▶ SUMMARY

Despite the provider's quiet sigh of relief following ETCO$_2$ detection, it is what has happened up to the point of successful tracheal intubation that will determine patient outcome. Tracheal intubation alone will almost never save a life, unless it has been done without further compromising the patient's condition. Irrespective of the setting in which airway management occurs, attention must be directed throughout towards the basics of maintaining oxygenation, ventilation and perfusion.

REFERENCES

1. Wang HE, Davis DP, Wayne MA, et al. Prehospital rapid-sequence intubation—what does the evidence show? Proceedings from the 2004 National Association of EMS Physicians annual meeting. *Prehosp. Emerg. Care.* 2004;8(4):366–377.

2. Wang HE, Kupas DF, Paris PM, et al. Preliminary experience with a prospective, multi-centered evaluation of out-of-hospital endotracheal intubation. *Resuscitation.* 2003;58(1): 49–58.

3. Gausche M, Lewis RJ, Stratton SJ, et al. Effect of out-of-hospital pediatric endotracheal intubation on survival and neurological outcome: a controlled clinical trial. *JAMA.* 2000;283(6):783–790.

4. Wang HE, Yealy DM. Out-of-hospital rapid sequence intubation: is this really the "success" we envisioned? *Ann. Emerg. Med.* 2002;40(2):168–171.

5. Bochicchio GV, Ilahi O, Joshi M, et al. Endotracheal intubation in the field does not improve outcome in trauma patients who present without an acutely lethal traumatic brain injury. *J. Trauma.* 2003;54(2):307–311.

6. Davis DP, Hoyt DB, Ochs M, et al. The effect of paramedic rapid sequence intubation on outcome in patients with severe traumatic brain injury. *J. Trauma.* 2003;54(3):444–453.

7. Dunford JV, Davis DP, Ochs M, et al. Incidence of transient hypoxia and pulse rate reactivity during paramedic rapid sequence intubation. *Ann. Emerg. Med.* 2003;42(6):721–728.

8. Wang HE, Peitzman AB, Cassidy LD, et al. Out-of-hospital endotracheal intubation and outcome after traumatic brain injury. *Ann. Emerg. Med.* 2004;44(5): 439–450.

9. Chesnut RM, Marshall LF, Klauber MR, et al. The role of secondary brain injury in determining outcome from severe head injury. *J. Trauma.* 1993;34(2): 216–222.

10. Ma OJ, Atchley RB, Hatley T, et al. Intubation success rates improve for an air medical program after implementing the use of neuromuscular blocking agents. *Am. J. Emerg. Med.* 1998;16(2):125–127.

11. Murphy-Macabobby M, Marshall WJ, Schneider C, et al. Neuromuscular blockade in aeromedical airway management. *Ann. Emerg. Med.* 1992;21(6): 664–668.

12. Sing RF, Rotondo MF, Zonies DH, et al. Rapid sequence induction for intubation by an aeromedical transport team: a critical analysis. *Am. J. Emerg. Med.* 1998;16(6):598–602.

13. Slater EA, Weiss SJ, Ernst AA, et al. Preflight versus en route success and complications of rapid sequence intubation in an air medical service. *J. Trauma.* 1998;45(3):588–592.

14. Davis DP, Douglas DJ, Koenig W, et al. Hyperventilation following aero-medical rapid sequence intubation may be a deliberate response to hypoxemia. *Resuscitation.* 2007;73(3):354–361.

15. Davis DP, Stern J, Sise MJ, et al. A follow-up analysis of factors associated with head-injury mortality after paramedic rapid sequence intubation. *J Trauma.* 2005;59(2):486–490.

16. Davis DP, Fakhry SM, Wang HE, et al. Paramedic rapid sequence intubation for severe traumatic brain injury: perspectives from an expert panel. *Prehosp Emerg Care.* 2007;11(1):1–8.

17. Phelan MP, Moscati R, D'Aprix T, et al. Paramedic use of the endotracheal tube introducer in a difficult airway model. *Prehosp. Emerg. Care.* 2003;7(2):244–246.

18. Swanson ER, Fosnocht DE, Matthews K, et al. Comparison of the intubating laryngeal mask airway versus laryngoscopy in the Bell 206–L3 EMS helicopter. *Air Med. J.* 2004;23(1):36–39.

19. Davis DP, Valentine C, Ochs M, et al. The Combitube as a salvage airway device for paramedic rapid sequence intubation. *Ann. Emerg. Med.* 2003;42(5):697–704.

20. Rumball CJ, MacDonald D. The PTL, Combitube, laryngeal mask, and oral airway: a randomized prehospital comparative study of ventilatory device effectiveness and cost-effectiveness in 470 cases of cardiorespiratory arrest. *Prehosp. Emerg. Care.* 1997;1(1):1–10.

21. Hulme J, Perkins GD. Critically injured patients, inaccessible airways, and laryngeal mask airways. *Emerg. Med. J.* 2005;22(10):742–744.

22. Keane MF, Brinsfield KH, Dyer KS, et al. A laboratory comparison of emergency percutaneous and surgical cricothyrotomy by prehospital personnel. *Prehosp. Emerg. Care.* 2004;8(4):424–426.

23. Bozeman WP, Hexter D, Liang HK, et al. Esophageal detector device versus detection of end-tidal carbon dioxide level in emergency intubation. *Ann. Emerg. Med.* 1996;27(5):595–599.

24. Katz SH, Falk JL. Misplaced endotracheal tubes by paramedics in an urban emergency medical services system. *Ann. Emerg. Med.* 2001;37(1):32–37.

25. O'Connor RE, Swor RA. Verification of endotracheal tube placement following intubation. National Association of EMS Physicians Standards and Clinical Practice Committee. *Prehosp. Emerg. Care.* 1999;3(3):248–250.

CHAPTER 20

Human Factors in Airway Management

▶ INTRODUCTION TO HUMAN FACTORS

From a patient safety standpoint, airway management is a key determinant of patient outcome. In this book, the emphasis has inevitably fallen on two main areas: procedural skills, and the knowledge required to safely secure an airway. Prepared with a comprehensive knowledge of anatomy, physiology, equipment options, and pharmacology, tracheal intubation proceeds as a complex integration of visual, motor, and haptic (i.e., touch feedback) skills.

For the patient, a successful intubation will be one during which the clinician has avoided significant error. However, for the clinician (as long as it is recognized), error is a necessary component of learning any procedure.[1] Failure and adversity have the potential to make behavior more robust and adaptive. Indeed, recognizing that errorless practice is an unrealistic goal, the term "quality assurance" has been replaced by "continuous quality improvement" (CQI).

In an unpublished study, investigators queried novice paramedics on their self-perceived competence in laryngoscopic intubation. The paramedics had performed 5, 10, or 20 tracheal intubations as part of another study seeking

*Personal communication, Orlando Hung, 2006

to define the learning curve for the procedure.[2] Interestingly, the group who had performed only five intubations perceived themselves as most competent in the skill.* Presumably, their limited exposure had not provided them the opportunity to encounter difficulty and fully engage the three principal domains of human performance: psychomotor, cognitive, and affective.[3]

▶ PSYCHOMOTOR PERFORMANCE

Historically, the maxim of skills acquisition in medicine has been "see one, do one, and teach one,"[1] often on compromised and vulnerable patients. The shortcomings of this approach are immediately obvious, and include adverse effects on patient safety. In an attempt to address this problem, training using human patient simulators is becoming increasingly common. Indeed, most trainees in airway management techniques will begin their skills acquisition on a manikin or airway simulator of some sort.

Unfortunately, psychomotor skills transfer from simulator to human is hampered by issues of tissue fidelity. Although simulators may be anatomically correct, their "tissues" don't respond to manipulation in the same way human tissue does. Thus, while psychomotor skills acquisition in airway management can begin in the simulation environment, it must then be augmented and reinforced in real patients. This in turn presents logistical (where and when to get the experience) and ethical (whether elective surgical patients should bear the brunt of such training) dilemmas. Going forward, there is a significant need for training programs using airway management simulators[4] of increased fidelity, coupled with multimedia presentations[5] and expert instructors.

Having said this, good psychomotor skills may not necessarily translate to improved patient outcomes. Although success in airway management has historically been measured by whether "they got the tube," the occurrence of process-related adverse events, such as hypotension, hypoxia, or aspiration, are much more likely to influence patient outcome. Fortunately, simulation can also provide a valuable venue for improving cognitive decision making and addressing contextual issues.

▶ COGNITIVE PERFORMANCE

Spinal reflexes in a transected cord apart, no behavioral act can be performed without cognitive input from the brain. The cognitive components required during the acquisition of procedural skills are those needed for basic learning processes: intelligence, alertness, attention, and concentration. However, once the skills have been acquired and are being maintained, a second cognitive imperative comes into play—that associated with clinical decision-making. These skills are vital in deciding when (or when not) to apply specific airway management strategies. Good decision-making embraces all aspects of the clinical milieu, and involves reasoning that minimizes the potential for harm to the patient.[6] The mode of clinical reasoning is important: it may be intuitive, rapid, heuristic, and recognition primed ("System 1"); or more analytical, deliberate, reasoned, and deductive ("System 2").[7] Sometimes, the situation might call for a blend of the two. It is important to be aware of the strengths and limitations of each mode.[8]

"System 1" reasoning will typically impel the decision maker reflexively toward what is familiar and comfortable; it is the rapid cognitive style described in the book *Blink* as "thinking without thinking."[9] It is often algorithmic in nature and may be achieved through deliberate preparation and rehearsal, in a specific attempt to achieve a stage of "reflexive responsiveness." Thus, faced with a Cormack-Lehane Grade 3 view, the clinician might "automatically" perform a head lift (if not contraindicated), external laryngeal manipulation (ELM) or reach for a bougie. However, without rehearsal and preprogramming, this "System 1" type of response may not be cognitively accessible during times of stress, and the clinician may simply revert to a lower pattern of untrained behavior: repeated attempts at direct laryngoscopy.

In contrast, stepping back from the immediate pull of the situation to reflect on the wider picture, engage in more analytical thinking, and consider less obvious consequents is reflective of "System 2," and when there is greater uncertainty, or less predictability, this might be the preferred course.[10] Why did head lift, ELM and the bougie fail? Was it a problem with managing the tongue? Would a blade change

▶ Case 20.1

Consider a complex patient with a head injury and a Glasgow Coma Score of 8, in a community emergency department. The patient was obese, immobilized on a spine board and had significant facial injuries. He was hemodynamically stable, with an oxygen saturation of 97%. Prior to transfer, the attending physician had spoken to a resident at the referral trauma center and had been advised to intubate the patient. The attending clinician was a family physician, working alone, whose last tracheal intubation had been performed during a cardiac arrest over a year previously.

be helpful? System 2 decision-making may still involve reference to an algorithm or decision-tree, but is less prescribed, requires some degree of reflection, and the greater use of judgment. Obtaining a colleague for help in a difficult situation will allow the primary clinician to emotionally and physically "step back" and engage in this type of thought process.

"System 1" thinking ("Glasgow 8, intubate") applied to Case 20-1 would not take into account the complexities of the decisions at hand. More analytical consideration of the risk/benefit ratio of a relatively inexperienced clinician managing this patient's potentially difficult airway, with no back-up, represents a "System 2" process.

Similar considerations apply widely. Being trained to perform a complex act is not an indication to proceed with it, simply because the opportunity has arisen. In the interest of patient safety, the benefit of the intervention should always outweigh the risk of proceeding. Sometimes, there is great virtue in reflection, and recognition of when **not** to do something: therein lies the stuff of clinical acumen.

▶ AFFECTIVE PERFORMANCE

The affective state of a clinician refers to his or her internal emotional milieu. Rarely are we in an affect-neutral state—usually there is a greater or lesser degree of ongoing confidence, energy, positivity, hesitation, fear, anger, and negativity. The affective state is highly relevant to both learning, and subsequent performance in the clinical arena.

• **Learning.** Learning can no sooner proceed without an appropriate affective state than it could without cognition. With a negative affect (e.g., that caused by excessive anxiety), or without the desire and motivation to learn, the learning process is clearly impoverished and will be adversely impacted. Thus, emotional and cognitive processes are inextricably related.[11]

Simulation training has the potential to remove the negative impact of the affective state from the learning process. Some performance anxiety may still occur in a peer-observed situation, or when learning is being evaluated, but for the most part the undesirable anxieties of learning on a real patient have been neutralized. The implied "permission to fail" enables learning to proceed under more optimal conditions.

• **Clinical Performance.** The intrinsic contribution of the affective state to the execution of a psychomotor skill is reflected in the Yerkes-Dodson law, which describes the inverted-U relationship between level of arousal and performance.[12] Arousal is a physiological and psychological state in which emotion is crucial. It raises the level of alertness and readiness to act, although too little or too much can adversely affect performance (Fig. 20–1). The corollary of the law is that there must exist an optimal level of arousal for any given task.

In the real-life situation, clinician anxiety may result in excessive arousal and compromised performance. For example, during a rapid-sequence intubation (RSI), a progressively dropping oxygen saturation that is audibly broadcast to all resuscitation team

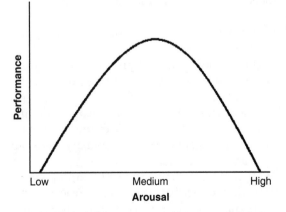

Figure 20–1. The Yerkes-Dodson law. The relationship between level of arousal and performance.[12]

members by a well-meaning helper may contribute to clinician anxiety, and compromise performance. At its worst, "paralysis" of cognition and action can occur. In contrast, it is well recognized that a second clinician *of equal skills or experience*, summoned for help, will often successfully intubate a patient within seconds of arriving, after an anxious primary clinician had failed. Not being emotionally invested in the situation empowers the second clinician to optimally perform a basic technique! Other strategies to help allay clinician anxiety are presented in the following sections.

▶ HUMAN FACTORS: TIPS AND PEARLS

A number of human factors tactics found useful over the years by the authors are presented below. Although little scientific validation exists for these tips, most are simply common sense!

The Importance of Helpers

The clinician undertaking airway management needs at least one helper. The helper may be needed for a gamut of facilitating activity:

- Drawing up, and possibly administering drugs.
- Application of cricoid pressure.
- Application of external laryngeal manipulation (ELM).
- Maintaining a head lift with a hand under the patient's head, if the view of the larynx was initially obtained by the primary clinician using a head lift.
- Handing the clinician the ETT in the correct orientation, so that direct visual contact with the laryngeal inlet can be maintained, once seen.
- Loading a tube over a bougie, then stabilizing the proximal end of the bougie as the clinician passes the tube.

- Obtaining, opening, and lubricating equipment needed unexpectedly, for example, a smaller tube for an encountered subglottic stenosis.
- Changing bags of intravenous (IV) fluid.
- Making phones calls for help, if needed.

A **second assistant** should be obtained for the patient with an anticipated difficult airway, specifically for the purpose of contributing to a two-person bag-mask ventilation (BMV) technique. The original helper will still be needed for all of the foregoing needs.

Less obvious to some clinicians is the need for the presence of a qualified colleague for **cognitive and moral support**, especially if difficulty is anticipated. In particular, the colleague can provide one or more of the following:

- Being a "sounding board" off whom to bounce the plan for intubation, and any concerns about anticipated difficulty.
- Being a very knowledgeable helper who will know without explanation what is wanted or needed by the primary clinician.
- Ensuring a confident and supportive environment. This is vitally important, and is one strategy that can be used to allay potentially counterproductive anxiety. The presence of a colleague allows the primary clinician to in effect "offload" some anxiety onto that individual.
- Facilitating the opportunity for "System 2" reflection.
- As an individual less emotionally invested in, and thus less anxious about the situation, the colleague may be in a better position to make suggestions and optimally perform skills.

For many clinicians, a colleague may not always be available. However, in the difficult situation, the importance of the presence of qualified help is such that it is worth "thinking outside the box" for where such help could be obtained—even calling in a colleague from home.

Even if patient acuity demands proceeding with a tracheal intubation before the colleague has arrived, simply knowing that help is on the way may contribute to relieving anxiety.

A corollary to the foregoing is the need for willingness, empathy and enthusiasm on the part of those who are called for help. Frequently, it is only the experienced clinician who can "say it like it is" (e.g., *"I think I have a tough one here—he looks really scary, and I could use a hand, as soon as you can get here"*). Even having initiated the call, some clinicians still hesitate to directly request help (e.g., *"I'm just calling to give you a "heads-up" that I may need you if this one turns out to be tough. . ."*). When receiving such a call, one should always read between the lines—for most clinicians, just initiating the call means, "please come now," regardless of what's actually said!

The "Visual Roadmap"

Particularly for the patient in whom difficulty is anticipated, although the clinician will have thought through the approach being planned, these additional preparations will also help:

- **Laying out a "visual roadmap" for the anticipated difficult situation.** Equipment should be prepared for both the initial attempt at tracheal intubation (including the bougie!), as well as the chosen alternative intubation method (e.g., an LMA Fastrach, optical stylet, or videolaryngoscope) *and* rescue EGD such as an LMA or Combitube. These devices should be correctly sized for the patient, out of the packaging, lubricated and ready for use. Furthermore, the devices should all be physically laid out, in order of anticipated usage, on a nearby work surface. This way, in the potentially stressful situation of a failed intubation attempt, no thought will be needed: the go-to device is already sitting there, ready for use, and prompting the clinician what to do next. It just needs to be picked up and used.

- **Team Briefing.** Before proceeding, a verbal briefing of the assembled helpers about the planned intubation and the transition to alternative intubation and rescue oxygenation devices can be useful, thus: *"O.K., folks, we're doing an RSI (rapid-sequence intubation) here. If I get in there and have trouble seeing where I'm going, I'm going to need the bougie, which is sitting right here on the patient's chest. If that doesn't work, I'm going to back out and bag-mask ventilate the patient. If I have trouble with that, I'll tell you, [Joan], to ease up on the cricoid pressure, and if that doesn't help, I'll proceed to a two-person technique, with you, [Bob], squeezing the bag. For a second attempt after that, I'm to going use a longer blade. If that doesn't do it, for the third attempt I'm going to use the Fastrach LMA, which is the thing with the metal handle right here. The Fastrach tube is over there, in a bottle of warm water. If for whatever reason the patient still isn't intubated after that third attempt, we're going to call a halt, ventilate through the Fastrach, and re-think things."*

Apart from the obvious benefit of letting the team know what to expect, the verbal briefing is even more beneficial for the primary clinician, as it helps solidify the plan in his or her mind; and more importantly, it ensures that a plan really exists!

Handling Anxiety During the Event

An intubation attempt can be very anxiety provoking. In an arrested patient, interventional airway management is a nonnegotiable part of a resuscitation. Conversely, in the patient who is conscious and breathing, undertaking an RSI (thereby rendering the patient apneic, unconscious and with an unprotected airway) places the onus on the clinician to effectively assume all of these vital functions—a substantially anxiety invoking paradigm. A good strategy in this situation is to concentrate on the ease and success of **BMV**. Even with a failed intubation, as long as oxygenation can occur with successful BMV, really, no problem exists! Other strategies for reassurance include obtaining help, employment of an accepted management paradigm, and simply having confidence in one's skills and knowledge, including a good approach to difficult BMV (Chap. 4).

The Ego, and When to Park It

The clinician should never be concerned that initiating a call for help to a colleague will be perceived by assistants as a sign of insecurity or incompetence. Experienced healthcare staff recognize a call for help as just the opposite—the sign of an effective clinician who knows his or her limitations and has recognized the challenges inherent in the situation. It is the inexperienced or dangerous clinician who fails to call for help out of concern that he or she will "look bad," and the assisting staff know it!

Overcoming Psychological Barriers

So-called psychological barriers exist for all. In the airway management arena, one of the most significant of these barriers may be proceeding with a cricothyrotomy. The very words *failed* oxygenation and *can't* intubate or oxygenate can connote personal failure. However, when indicated, the procedure itself is really no more complex than placing a chest tube or obtaining central venous access. Most cricothyrotomies are inappropriately delayed until a patient is no longer viable and the requirement for timely intervention is absolute (see Chap. 12). One should practice the technique regularly (see Chap. 7), so that there is minimal anxiety about not knowing the steps. With regular practice on part-task simulators and/or cadaveric specimens, if available, the technique can easily become familiar, and performed in under a minute. In addition, it can be beneficial to

mentally rehearse failed oxygenation situations where cricothyrotomy may be needed.

Making the Effort

As with cricothyrotomy, it is incumbent on the clinician to become skilled in basic and alternative intubation techniques. The bougie is a basic adjunct to direct laryngoscopy, yet it takes experience to build up a "mental library" of how the clicks of the tracheal cartilaginous rings feel in different patients, and where, relative to the teeth, the resistance occurs with bougie advancement into a small distal airway. To this end, the device should ideally be used in an array of patients, including those anticipated to be "easy", to attain the needed experience. The same goes for use of a fiberoptic stylet as an adjunct to DL. Similarly, experience is needed to attain and maintain competence in an alternative intubation technique, such as the LMA Fastrach or Trachlight. This experience can be attained on lower acuity patients (anticipated difficult patients should be treated with a familiar technique) or on elective surgical patients in the operating room (OR). Having said this, arranging OR time can be "a hassle," and there will be days that one wishes to simply go to work, and complete one's shift without going to the effort of using an unfamiliar technique on low-acuity cases. This is a trap into which the clinician should not fall: competence in the difficult situation can only be attained by gaining experience in easier cases.

Getting Hassled

As outlined above, lower acuity emergency cases may present an opportunity to seek experience with less commonly used alternative techniques. On occasion, some team members may state their discomfort with this scenario. In addition, inconvenience to the care team may be incurred, as carts require restocking, and equipment must be cleaned. However, the ethical issue of "practicing" on real patients is a reality of medical practice, and the requirement for skills acquisition and maintenance must be advanced with firmness and resolve. Obviously, patient safety must remain the priority when considering the use of less familiar tools.

The Bigger Picture: Risk-Benefit Analysis

Airway management is all about risk-benefit analysis, and the clinician should never allow the risk of an intervention to outweigh its benefit. Common examples of situations where this may happen during airway management include the following:

- **The trauma patient with C-spine precautions:** The blunt trauma patient has an increased risk of associated C-spine injury. However, fear of causing a secondary spinal cord injury during tracheal intubation should not interfere with the decision to manage the patient's airway according to the usual indications. The post-motor vehicle crash (post-MVC) patient who has sustained deceleration from high speed, yet does not present with a cord injury after extrication and transport, is generally unlikely to sustain further injury during tracheal intubation—particularly when care is taken with the appropriate application of manual in-line neck stabilization (MILNS).[13] Although MILNS will make attaining a view at laryngoscopy more difficult, it should be applied during the attempt. However, the benefit of allowing just a few millimeters of movement during an intubation attempt (e.g., to visualize the interarytenoid notch, with bougie use thereafter[14]) may well outweigh the risk of encountering a failed airway.
- **The "full-stomach" patient:** The typical patient requiring emergency intubation is not fasted. Their "full-stomach' status will have

dictated interventions such as application of cricoid pressure during RSI. However, cricoid pressure, while standard of care, has never been conclusively proven to improve outcome, while it *has* definitely been shown to cause difficulty with both BMV[15–17] and direct laryngoscopy.[18–20] The risk of continued application of cricoid pressure (i.e., failed airway) in a difficult airway situation may thus outweigh its benefit (i.e., prevention of aspiration). Airway patency and oxygenation are prioritized before "might regurgitate, and might aspirate."

A second example of risk-benefit analysis in the full-stomach patient arises when considering rescue oxygenation options. Certain LMA devices (e.g., the LMA-Classic or Unique) do not necessarily fully protect the airway against aspiration of gastric contents. Knowing this, some may consider their use contraindicated in the full-stomach patient. However, once again, in a failed airway situation, the benefit of successful rescue oxygenation far outweighs the potential risk of tracheal soiling.

Assessment of risk-benefit analysis can only occur if the clinician is maintaining an overview of the "bigger picture"—so-called situation awareness. This requires the absence of fixation on one aspect of the paradigm—often direct laryngoscopy. This is one reason that the **failed intubation** definition of the failed airway (see Chap. 12) has been presented: once three attempts have been made, even if oxygenation with BMV is possible, it is time to stop, "regroup and re-muster," and reassess things.

▶ SUMMARY

Airway management is often the entry point of acute-care management and is a key determinant of a safe patient outcome. At a minimum, success requires a sound knowledge of relevant airway anatomy, physiology, and pharmacology. Complex psychomotor skills must be acquired and maintained for a variety of specialized techniques. In addition, for safe clinical decision-making to occur, cognitive and affective barriers to success must be appreciated and managed. Ultimately, to improve patient outcomes, educational efforts should address each of the psychomotor, cognitive, and affective domains. While promoting success, these programs should also allow supervised failure in a simulated setting, to help maximize the chances of both attaining and maintaining the necessary skills for competent airway management.

REFERENCES

1. Kovacs G. Procedural skills in medicine: linking theory to practice. *J Emerg Med*. 1997;15(3):387–391.
2. Mulcaster JT, Mills J, Hung OR, et al. Laryngoscopic intubation: learning and performance. *Anesthesiology*. 2003;98(1):23–27.
3. Kovacs G, Croskerry P. Clinical decision making: an emergency medicine perspective. *Academic Emerg Med*. 1999;6(9):947–952.
4. Hall RE, Plant JR, Bands CJ, et al. Human patient simulation is effective for teaching paramedic students endotracheal intubation. *Acad Emerg Med*. 2005;12(9):850–855.
5. Levitan RM, Goldman TS, Bryan DA, et al. Training with video imaging improves the initial intubation success rates of paramedic trainees in an operating room setting. *Ann Emerg Med*. 2001;37(1):46–50.
6. Croskerry P. The theory and practice of clinical decision-making. *Canadian Journal of Anesthesia*. 2005;52(suppl_1):R1.
7. Sloman S. The Empirical Case for Two Systems of Reasoning. *Psychological Bulletin*. 1996;119(1):3–22.
8. Croskerry P. Critical thinking and decisionmaking: avoiding the perils of thin-slicing. *Ann Emerg Med*. 2006;48(6):720–722.
9. Gladwell M. *Blink: The power of thinking without thinking*. New York: Brown and Company; 2005.
10. Mamede S, Schmidt HG, Penafort JC, et al. *Reflective practice in medicine*. Fortaleza Brazil Expressao Grafica e Editora Ltda; 2006.
11. DaMasio A. *Descartes' Error: Emotion, Reason and the Human Brain*. Itasca Illinois: Putman; 1994.
12. Yerkes RM, Dodson JD. The relation of strength of stimulus to rapidity of habit-formation. *Journal of Comparative Neurology and Psychology*. 1908;18(5):459–482.
13. Manoach S, Paladino L. Manual in-line stabilization for acute airway management of suspected cervical spine injury: historical review and current questions. *Ann Emerg Med*. 2007.
14. Nolan JP, Wilson ME. Orotracheal intubation in patients with potential cervical spine injuries. An indication for the gum elastic bougie. *Anaesthesia*. 1993;48(7):630–633.
15. Hartsilver EL, Vanner RG. Airway obstruction with cricoid pressure. *Anaesthesia*. 2000;55(3):208–211.
16. Mac GPJH, Ball DR. The effect of cricoid pressure on the cricoid cartilage and vocal cords: an endoscopic study in anaesthetised patients. *Anaesthesia*. 2000;55(3):263–268.
17. Hocking G, Roberts FL, Thew ME. Airway obstruction with cricoid pressure and lateral tilt. *Anaesthesia*. 2001;56(9):825–828.
18. Snider DD, Clarke D, Finucane BT. The "BURP" maneuver worsens the glottic view when applied in combination with cricoid pressure. *Can J Anaesth*. 2005;52(1):100–104.
19. Levitan RM, Kinkle WC, Levin WJ, et al. Laryngeal view during laryngoscopy: a randomized trial comparing cricoid pressure, backward-upward-rightward pressure, and bimanual laryngoscopy. *Ann Emerg Med*. 2006;47(6):548–555.
20. Haslam N, Parker L, Duggan JE. Effect of cricoid pressure on the view at laryngoscopy. *Anaesthesia*. 2005;60(1):41–47.

Index

Page numbers followed by *f* or *t* indicate figures or tables, respectively.